ROLE OF THE FAMILY
IN THE
REHABILITATION OF
THE PHYSICALLY DISABLED

ROLE OF THE FAMILY IN THE REHABILITATION OF THE PHYSICALLY DISABLED

edited by
Paul W. Power, Sc.D.
Director, Rehabilitation Counseling Program
University of Maryland

and

Arthur E. Dell Orto, Ph.D.
Chairman, Department of Rehabilitation Counseling
Boston University

University Park Press
Baltimore

UNIVERSITY PARK PRESS
International Publishers in Science, Medicine, and Education
233 East Redwood Street
Baltimore, Maryland 21202

Copyright © 1980 by University Park Press

Typeset by University Park Press, Typesetting Division.
Manufactured in the United States of America by The Maple Press Company.

Library of Congress Cataloging in Publication Data
Power, Paul W.
Role of the family in the rehabilitation of the physically disabled.
Includes bibliographies and index.
1. Physically handicapped—Rehabilitation—United States—Addresses, essays,
lectures. 2. Physically handicapped—United States—Family relationships—
Addresses, essays, lectures. I. Orto, Arthur E. Dell, joint author. II. Title.
HV3023.A3P68   362.4   79-26356
ISBN 0-8391-1549-0

CONTENTS

PREFACE

This book has evolved from the realization that effective delivery of services to the families of the physically disabled represents a current challenge for health care providers. Advances in medicine, while improving the productive lives of the disabled, have at the same time reformulated the aims of rehabilitation and have created new opportunities for rehabilitation professionals. Traditionally, health care and rehabilitation have been directed primarily to the patient as an individual without considering the utilization of significant others, especially the family, as a potent rehabilitation force.

Fortunately, the trend today is to look at and understand a number of influences that have a bearing on the management of an illness (Barsky, 1976). Efforts directed at the enhancement of the quality of life for the chronically disabled suggest that rehabilitation interventions be undertaken within the context of total human involvement (Feldman, 1974). Special problems, however, are posed to family members who are capable and willing to provide some support, such as realigning their home responsibilities, disrupting social activities, or simply dealing with their own feelings of loss from watching the family member slowly deteriorate.

Human illness and disability occur in the context of a complicated web of interpersonal relationships. A person with a severe disability requires considerable attention from family members. From the perspective of family interrelationships, the family has a vital function as a determinant of behavior in the physically disabled. To answer the challenge that advances in medical science have brought to health professionals, emphasis should be given to those factors that can both ease the burden of the family of the disabled person and utilize the family as a resource for rehabilitation.

One of the primary goals of rehabilitation is helping the disabled individual come to terms with the reality of the disability. This often demands readaptation of the person's life-style in order to achieve meaning and purpose for living. Such a reorganization takes place more readily when the family members can discover resources within their environment that increase the family's and, in turn, the person's ability to cope with the crisis of disability. Although we are aware of the reported fragility of the American family, we believe that the family is in no danger of disappearing and will continue to be a potential rehabilitation resource, even though the traditional family may be modified.

All families, of course, do not have the resources to cope with the demands of chronic disability and may well fragment under its burden. This reality indicates the need for a more comprehensive system of alternatives that permits families to provide what support they can rather than being forced to choose between total responsibility and total rejection of their ill or disabled family member.

Unfortunately, although the literature has provided some helpful insights into how the family can be utilized in the rehabilitation of the physically disabled, the depths of this topic have not been fully explored. This book, building on the information already available, attempts to provide further knowledge to health professionals on how the family can be a resource in rehabilitation by showing how the family can be a determinant in the rehabilitation of the disabled person, how an understanding of the psychological meaning of an illness to the patient and family can be an important tool in helping the patient and family to deal with the implications of a disability, and how relevant helping skills can assist the family to adjust to chronic illness.

The format of this book is a combination of original material, existing literature, and personal statements by the disabled and their families. The original material is presented as a reflection of our thoughts based on our professional experience and interpretations of the work of others. The articles included in the book represent the results of several years of searching for material that provided a comprehensive and timely perspective on the role of the family and disability. The vast amount of literature existing in this area challenged us to select the material that was most relevant to the message and goals of the book.

These dimensions of the book are put into perspective by the personal statements that precede and conclude the major sections. These statements represent a contribution by our clients, friends, and family and create a framework for the other material in the book. We feel they contain issues relevant to the rehabilitation and health care process. The personal statements were prepared by the disabled and their families or, in a few cases, by us. They are presented as a vehicle to balance the largely academic focus of the book and to provide an opportunity for those who have lived and are living the "challenge" to share their experiences with those who help others.

In our presentation we are not working from one established, family-oriented, helping model. We have found that no single theoretical construction can encompass all aspects of what is needed to work with families during their rehabilitation process. The many contributions of social science knowledge relevant to the family require a more comprehensive framework as well as a broad outlook on rehabilitation. What is necessary is an approach that will help the reader to integrate various perspectives with the explosion of material that is available today on general, assorted family issues. From this integration the reader will discover more effective ways to involve the family in treatment care and also learn some answers to the following questions:

1. How does the family influence the adjustment of a disabled family member?
2. What are the role and resources of the family in the rehabilitation process?
3. How can health care providers assist the family of the disabled to function with a disabled family member?

In this book the terms *health professional* and *helper* are used interchangeably to identify those people who, in some way, include in their job responsibilities an involvement with the family. Physicians, nurses, social workers, rehabilitation counselors, psychologists, physical therapists, occupational therapists, audiologists, and recreational therapists are just some of the professionials for whom this book is intended.

Following each of the three sections of the book is a list of recommended readings. These lists are the result of a careful review of the literature on topics relating to the family and disability. They supplement the references and articles after each chapter and provide a more extensive resource to the reader for comprehensive information on the family's role in rehabilitation.

The actualization of this book is a result of the combined efforts of many persons. We would like to thank Jackie, Joe, John and Louise, Linda, Richard and Ilene, Margaret, Sabine, Ted, Charlotte, and Lois, each of whom gave us their personal statements to be included in the book. We would also like to acknowledge the support of our professional colleagues and especially our wives, Barbara Ann and Barbara Ann, who spent many hours reviewing the manuscript, typing, and providing valuable suggestions. Also, special mention is given to Mrs. Barbara Germann, whose typing helped bring the book nearer to its completion.

In particular, we also wish to acknowledge the grateful support of the University of Maryland. The grant award given to the authors helped to defray many of the book's publication costs.

REFERENCES

Barsky, A. Patient heal thyself: Activating the ambulatory medical patient. *Journal of Chronic Diseases,* 1976, *29,* 585–597.

Feldman, D. Chronic disabling illness: A holistic view. *Journal of Chronic Diseases,* 1974, *27,* 287–291.

This book is dedicated to the nine persons and their families who have lived or who are still living with the realities explained in these pages. In sharing their personal statements with us they are showing us that the family is an integral part of the rehabilitation process.

ROLE OF THE FAMILY
IN THE
REHABILITATION OF
THE PHYSICALLY DISABLED

INTRODUCTION

It is the authors' premise that the family is a vital determinant of rehabilitation success. However, the family does not exist as an isolated entity. The family is constantly interacting with the surrounding community, such as educational, political, economic, and health resources, and is deeply affected by changing social patterns and conditions. Families cannot be understood without understanding their sociocultural background. Culture is the means by which a family can adopt and adjust to changes in the environment with some feeling of security and familiarity. Rheinhardt and Quinn (1973) view culture "as all the accumulated ways a group of people solve problems which are reflected in the people's language, dress, food, and a number of their traditions and customs. It also includes material items and the many social institutions that embody and sustain all those elements" (p. 33). Health professionals must consciously design and implement their services by giving much thought to integrating their efforts with the cultural and social milieu in which the family functions.

In this book the term *family* is used to mean classic family forms, newly emerging forms, or the social groups with which the individual is most intimately involved. Robischon and Smith (1977) define the family as an interdependent group system that may consist of the biological or adoptive family and/or influential others. Because of the many existing, nontraditional family structures the meaning of the family must be comprehensive.

The expression *family today* conveys different meanings to different people. Such structures as the open marriage, group and multilateral marriage, the communal family, and the one-parent family are identified as viable styles of family life. Rakel (1977) outlines these family forms in the following way:

Nuclear family Husband and wife and their children
Extended family A family extended to include parents and sometimes other relatives
Alternate family Single-parent families, married adults without children, unmarried adults (heterosexual and homosexual), communes, others

In a disability situation these varied family structures also represent different resources of influence on the patient. Relatives living in the family household or in close proximity can become added sources of support to a disabled person. In contrast, the nuclear family, which may not have relatives living nearby, could feel very much alone when attempting to cope with a handicapped child or adult. An awareness of these family influences promotes a broader perspective for the delivery of health care and rehabilitation services to patients.

One of the basic themes of this book is that the health professional should understand as many influences as possible that can affect the rehabilitation of disabled persons. This understanding is called the holistic approach and is described concisely in Daniel Feldman's article, which follows in the Introduction. He emphasizes that the nature of the environment in which the patient functions is of great importance in planning health care. For improved patient rehabilitation he suggests a new conceptual model, which stresses psychoeconomic function as a critical area to understand when implementing an intervention approach. This holistic approach integrates a knowledge of the person's disabling condition, the emotional responses to the disability, and the patient's living environment. It recaptures the whole person as the focus for rehabilitation efforts.

The personal statements of Jackie and Joe, also included in this Introduction, provide a practical application of this holistic perspective. Jackie's account highlights the need to explore carefully the psychological and social factors that may contribute to a person's recovery or restoration. In her poignant story she shows how a caring physician who is concerned about the whole person is a decided factor in one's response to a life-threatening trauma. During her medical experience Jackie especially wanted to be viewed not simply as someone with a cancerous breast, but as a person with unique needs and feelings. She identifies some of these needs, such as supportive listening, accurate information, and reassurance from friends.

Joe's account is a unique description of personal courage and the emotional impact of a disabling condition. His struggle was a fight against giving up or becoming bitter because of perceived medical neglect. The story suggests to the reader the many ways it could have been different for Joe. It stimulates reflection on how his life might have been more satisfying after the initial diagnosis and surgery.

The personal statements personalize the content of this book and illustrate to the health professional how rehabilitation services could be improved. Dr. Feldman's article provides the underlying philosophy for developing a more effective intervention approach. All of the contributors to this book believe that a person's environment can set the atmosphere and greatly determine the motivation for rehabilitation. This book focuses on a substantial part of that environment—the family.

REFERENCES

Rakel, R. *Principles of family medicine.* Philadelphia: W. B. Saunders Co., 1977.

Rheinhardt, A., & Quinn, M. (Eds.). *Family-centered community nursing.* St. Louis: C. V. Mosby Co., 1973.

Robischon, P., & Smith, J. Family assessment. In A. Rheinhardt & M. Quinn (Eds.), *Current practice in family-centered community nursing,* pp. 85–100. St. Louis: C. V. Mosby Co., 1977.

PERSONAL STATEMENT ......
Jackie

There's just something about a beautiful day in May that makes one want to live forever. The sky, the air, spring at last. It's all the best.

For me it was that kind of day in late May when I was racing around the house getting ready to go out when a conversation on the television caught my ears. Minnie Ripperton, a popular soul singer, was being interviewed on a show and she was sharing her recent personal experience with cancer, breast cancer. She seemed confident and strong and then she knocked me dead. She said, "If a woman has a lump she'll know it. . . and if you're not sure . . . check it out. . . ." And there I was dumbstruck in front of the TV with "check it out" echoing and ringing in my ears.

I wasn't sure of myself or my lumps. I had an important meeting to attend, I had an important presentation at juvenile court, and May was too alive to check anything out today.

Tomorrow arrived as beautiful as before, a Thursday. After I finished at juvenile court downtown I called the school and spoke with the headmaster, who said not to bother to return to school because the school day would be over in 10 minutes. Three cheers for me! I felt as if I were on holiday and headed for Filene's Basement. "Check it out" kept ringing in my ears. I couldn't shop. I went to the pay phone . . . called Harvard Community Health Plan. . . the nurse came on and I began my litany . . . Sorry to bother you. . . I really think it's nothing, but I'm not sure—would you. . . could you . . . check it out? My appointment was at 4:00 pm.

I knew I was in trouble when the nurse examined my left side and her facial expression

tightened as she fired questions—how long. . .
when. . .family history. My blood was turning
to ice. . .less than an hour ago I was minding
my own business enjoying spring. My doctor
came in, examined me, and left the room, obviously concerned. He returned and said
quietly, "This is probably nothing. It appears to
be fibroid adenoma, which is not unusual. Go
downstairs to surgery—I'd like you to meet Dr.
Christian. I want you to know that if I needed a
surgeon, Christian would be my man."

I dress. I leave walking like a robot. I enter
surgery yellow. I am quieted by a lilting British
accent attached to a bright, happy looking
nurse practitioner. Undressed again in those
marvelous "johnnies" I watch the surgeon eyes
and mind click. "You have two lumps and they
have to be removed as soon as possible. I'll send
you across the hall for your preops and then we
can talk. Also I'll set you up for a mammogram
tomorrow at the cancer center."

There it was—surgery—cancer—only a possibility. It wasn't even 5:00. I called my dearest
friend and told of my last 40 minutes and asked
for a ride home. They took my blood, they
x-rayed my chest, they EKG'ed my heart.

Back to surgery—my heart, my head, my
world was racing. Words danced in my head—
"It's probably nothing. . .they have to come
out!"—over and over. My eyes were burning
with tears that wouldn't allow themselves to
come. I was shaking in every corner of my in-
sides. My only question was, "If it's the worst,
could I survive?" "Usually." The doctors and
nurse practitioners were kind. I was picked up
. . .I went home. . .I cried. . .I was scared to
death. I didn't say too much. There wasn't
much to say.

Friday I alerted my employer that I needed
time that afternoon. I explained briefly. I was

fortunate that I worked for a marvelous administrative team. They were and are always in my corner.

Time for the mammogram. The technician was young and vivacious, chattering away at how routine this was for people of my age and how many friends had lumps that were nothing, and away she chirped as the machine was squeezing the life out of me. I quietly thought to myself, "How could this be so normal? It's me and I've never been in so many paper johnnies, staring at so many white ceilings and walls in all my life. What did my age have to do with such a frightening, humiliating experience?" The mammogram was complete, and I was told to wait in my "cubby"—2 square feet of space with a curtain. Happy as a lark the technician asked me if I would step back into the room to see the radiologist. My face must have tightened because she tapped me on the shoulder and said, smiling, "Remember, it's just routine!"

Nice doctor...probing...feeling...looking ...expressionless with the hopes of my life tied to a silent x-ray.

I left, to wait at home for a call from Harvard Health. It came. The mammogram did not confirm anything and I was scheduled for surgery on Wednesday regardless.

My weekend was the most outrageous experience of my life. My family and friends that were aware were so convinced that all was well that I thought I would lose my mind...quietly ...everyone was so busy being convinced... they wouldn't have known that I had gone crazy. Medical friends, everyone was convinced. But in the quiet of my heart I **felt** otherwise. I cried and finally trained people to say "I understand" and then begin their reassurances. To those who glance at these words, keep in mind that this family and these friends were and are caring people who **wanted** to do their best and couldn't. I was a wreck. I felt I knew something dreadful was wrong...only two dear friends responded with the possibility of what could be.

It was a long weekend because of a holiday
—long for many reasons. The doctor called Mon-
day. He was pleasant, he was concerned; he
could see me Tuesday morning. He wanted to do
a biopsy.

Nine am Tuesday. Could this be me? Was I
really in charge of this 5' 1" body? Another office, this time at the hospital, another paper to
fill out.

The doctor's face, his eyes of concern and
care, good conversation, some pair. . . not too
bad by comparison to the mental anguish. It
was 1:00 pm . . . I dressed and waited . . . another
waiting room . . . stale magazines. My friend was
with me; we were just quiet. Time seemed like
days . . . it was only about 20 minutes.

Dr. Christian came back. His long, lanky
stride was sad and deliberate, so I thought. I
went into his office. My heart was dancing on
his desk, or so I was convinced. His words were
straight. The biopsy was and is malignant. . . I
had cancer. In a sense any news is better than
no news, but this . . .

His words were straight and honest. I could
see a radiologist for another opinion instead of
surgery. A hundred options at my frightened
feet. I stopped my world, let out all the stops
and looked this stranger straight in the eye and
stumbled with these words trying to save my
life. Look doc, I don't know you. You don't
know me. I'm not rich, famous, or making
headlines. I want to live with all my heart. Just
tell me. What would you do if I were someone
you really loved—your wife, your mother, anybody—what would you do?

The answer was straight and sincere: "I
would advise a modified radical mastectomy for
someone I love."

For me it was senseless to speak with more
specialists doing experimental work—I know
nothing about the field. I couldn't possibly
make a decent decision.

It's important to mention that simply by
asking "what to do for someone you love" does

not guarantee integrity or expertise. For me, it
did. I was fortunate in having positive medical
experience with the doctor who said he would
have chosen this surgeon also.

Dr. Christian asked me what I wanted to do
and what he could do to help. In the shock of
my confirmed disbelief I said, "Let's go for
surgery tomorrow." I felt that if he always told
me the truth about everything and didn't isolate
me from the people I loved I could survive anything. He said ok, and asked me again what he
could do to help. He wrote down my mother's
name and number and my two friends, my
dearest friends. I asked if he would explain
everything to my friends. He did openly, patiently, and honestly—he promised he would
make sure that they would be with me every
step of the way. The doctor made his word
golden.

First I went to nuclear medicine for my zap
of radioactive material, only to return in 3
hours for my bone scan. Sounds impressive,
doesn't it!

Home for pizza and my toothbrush. I called
the school. Told the headmaster I had cancer
and needed surgery the next day. Over and
over, "It can't be" was his reply. He led the
chorus. The voices of assurance were stilled and
spring had turned to fall—chilled and bleak as
the night before winter.

Dropped by school to put things in order.
My team was supportive and held a stiff upper
lip, but I read the disbelief in their eyes and almost visibly buckled when the secretaries began
to cry. I thought to myself, "How can I be van-
quished on such a beautiful day in June?"

Time passes slowly and so did the bone
scan. Huge machines—bleeping and clicking up
and down. "God I hope it doesn't fall on top of
me." Technician's name was Danny—he lived
on the north shore and liked his job. Three
cheers for my communication skills. When it
was over my two complete skeletons hung on

the screen. "Good God I'm short," I thought to
myself. Mother was there during the scan so the
two of us waited for the results. I kept looking
at myself, wondering how cancer could be living
within me. Wanting to discover it like a mos-
quito and slap it into oblivion.

The doctor came out of the office with a big
smile and thumbs up sign! We all gave each
other a squeeze and for the first time in 6 days
I had received good news.

Off to my hospital ward. The doctor was
right. He had said the ward isn't attractive at
all but you'll have the best medical care in the
world.

What a merry-go-round. Doctors, questions,
nurses. . . I also had a paper due for a course!

A ward. . . sick people. . . everywhere. . .
Here I was on the edge of the bed with my great
white jeans and favorite jersey and my trusty
sneakers. How could this be?

Well it was and is. Night came. It had
rained all the long day. There were friends visiting and flowers arriving already. It was getting
time for my family to leave—my mother and
two dear friends. My stiff upper lip crumbled
and I dissolved into tears and begged **anyone** to
please just take me home and don't let them
hurt me. It lasted about 10 minutes. I shook, I
trembled, I begged heaven and earth to have it
all pass away. It didn't pass away and with
some strong hugs and the deepest and dearest
of love from so many people I changed my
clothes and buckled up, determined to survive.

I refused a sleeping pill, and watched the
TV sign off the air. Finally I gave in and took
the pill. Morning came. Doctors, doctors; nothing to eat or drink. Mum and friends arrived.
Medication to slow me down. (I was still trying
to finish my paper.) Then it was time.

The people I loved surrounded that big
stretcher and I was so sedated that an army
could have marched over me. Their faces tight
but trying to reassure me. . . the anesthetist

promised to wake me up after the operation.
That was one of my biggest fears. The elevator
ride all the way to the doors of the OR and we
said goodbye. . .I was so drugged I was almost
fearless. I couldn't believe I had survived this
long without a straightjacket.

The OR was big and green. . .familiar faces
and then NOTHING. I woke up and thought
they must have canceled it. I didn't realize 6
hours had passed. My eyes opened—there were
Dr. Christian and my mom. I had made it!

Such warmth and support at such a delicate
moment. I returned to the ward. Flowers, cards
were everywhere. . .I was oblivious to how
many. . .I was alive. . .in and out of drowsiness
. . .love and care surrounding my bed.

Pain is not a strong issue in the recovery of
a modified radical. It's not as bad as a lot of
surgery. Your arm feels sore and stiff. I
couldn't believe I was minus part of myself.
Where had "me" gone? What would it be without a breast? Those questions were important.
Most of all, would I—could I—live?

The only person I had known personally
with a mastectomy had died the year before. I
wanted to live so badly. There wasn't anyone to
talk with. The internist visited often. But the
pathology report wasn't in and frankly he
wasn't sure to mourn the loss of my breast or
the loss of my life! I thought those words would
suffocate my mind. How could this be me. . .my
body. . .my life.

Friends. . .warmth everywhere. It was
more than touching. It was a miracle. But there
wasn't anyone around who had walked a mile
in my shoes or even someone that could explain
what maybe dying like this could mean. All
things considered I felt fairly good.

Days passed with no news. Patients on our
ward helped each other. One lady was really
fighting for her life, her husband was all alone,
waiting for news from the OR. To him we were
strangers. He was so frantic he couldn't re-

spond. He was alone. No one visited him with information or support. We watched him pace.
Long after the sun came up our friend came
back. What a feeling to see that bed occupied
with its rightful owner. Each day we saw each
other improve. Mrs. B. and Mr. B. became our
friends in a bond that few words will ever describe. Each of us had seen the "promised
land" and had made it down the mountainside,
hoping we would all live forever.

I went home Tuesday morning feeling
pretty good, after a tough week of being weak
and being allergic to some medication. It felt
strange and a little lonely to leave part of myself
behind. The sun was almost shining. It had
rained for days. I walked up the steps of school
and felt I would beat this thing somehow, especially if I kept going. Warmth and friendship
were grand and Wednesday I was teaching
again. Less than a week and here I was, teaching the kids. Who could believe it!

No pathology report arrived and there was
fear in my heart. My birthday was next week
and I was almost resentful of getting presents I
couldn't use immediately, just in case my number was up.

The phone rang. It was Dr. Christian. He
asked my permission to give me good news—I
told him I wanted the report given face to face.
Three cheers for us! It was negative. My
chances were getting better. Next question:
Would I need chemotherapy and/or radiation?
Parts of the tissue were a nasty form of cancer.

Weeks passed. Stitches were taken out,
school finished, and finally the news: no further treatment. The sun shined that day inside
and out. Maybe Christmas would be in December and not moved back to July.

What's it like going through these experiences as a helper and a helpee? It's a long, hard
time. For me there was not a person who had
my experience available to speak with. There
was not a particular person available that one

could feel comfortable with to even discuss how
to overcome the cosmetic loss, let alone a life
loss.

My medical care was excellent. But I
quickly discovered that a helping listener was
not available for patients anywhere. I often
used my skills training on myself. I just had to
make it. I used every resource I could think of.
Often I would think, "What would I try to say
or do for a person in my shoes?" This mental
exercise helped me try to do the helpful things I
needed physically, emotionally, and intellectually.

Now when I am called, as I have been since
July, to visit and listen to another woman who
faces cancer and the loss of her breast, and
maybe her life, I remember my days and nights.
This, combined with solid helping skills, builds
a bridge for people who are facing a mountain
climb that is awesome.

Specific support people are not available in
a consistent way for many people in need. When
we must ask ourselves, "Where do I send someone I love?" when they need medical help, we
all need pause. Often some of the helping professions are not there. No one should face so many
things in life all alone. Be assured, whatever
your profession or philosophy, that no one
should face a life-threatening experience like
cancer alone.

As a personal thought, women who have
had mastectomies lose their breasts—not their
minds. When help is offered it's good to remember that we are still the same individual. At different times, in different ways, for different reasons we will need a good word, a helpful sentence, an understanding moment, just like the
rest of the human race. Perhaps the problem
lies in the fact that most of the human race
misses these responses too.

My experiences have blessed me with the
opportunity to meet some of the most wonderful
medical people in the world, some of the most

courageous people in the world. It's also reminded me that too many people have no place
to send the people they love, and there's no
place for those who are loved to get the best
when they need and deserve it most.

CHRONIC DISABLING ILLNESS
A Holistic View

Daniel J. Feldman[1]

Recent advances in the knowledge of the fundamental processes of disease have been formidable. The influence of this knowledge on the thinking of the health professions has been profound. It is likely that many diseases now considered irreversible and incurable will, in the future, be preventable and curable but how long this will take cannot be predicted. Under these circumstances, concern with components of illness other than the disease process per se may be the only 'clinical' management possible. Sociocultural and behavioral factors have considerable input both on the ultimate expression of the illness and the patient's response to it. Research into the nature and influence of these components has not been done with the same intensity so apparent in the biological aspects. Admittedly, much more needs to be done, but their importance should not be depreciated. They are significant in the formation of that complex entity—sick man.

The holistic view of illness postulates that it is a composite phenomenon, contributed to and shaped by a number of influences which may or may not bear a direct causal relationship to each other. It follows that management of illness requires understanding of as many of these influences as possible. This is particularly important for those patients with chronic disabling illness; they are not only involved with the 'medical' problems of their illness, but with a great spectrum of social, economic and behavioral complications as well. Chronic illness can only be partially managed by treating the patient as an isolated entity, no matter how sympathetic such treatment may be. The nature of the environment in which the patient functions is of great importance as is the patient's behavioral response, which contributes significantly to the meaning of the illness. It follows that chronic disabling conditions must be examined within the context of total human involvement.

The intrusion of a significant illness, especially of a chronic and disabling nature, is a major life crisis posing a formidable challenge to what was previously a workable adaptation to life. The crisis generated thereby is 'ongoing' in that there is little possibility of a complete return to the pre-

Reprinted with permission from *Journal of Chronic Disease 27*, pp. 287-291, © 1974, Pergamon Press, Ltd.

[1]From the Department of Psychiatry and Human Behavior and Department of Physical Medicine and Rehabilitation, University of Calfornia at Irvine, College of Medicine, Irvine, CA 92664.

morbid state. Certain general mechanisms of coping seem to operate in this circumstance. They appear early, and are undoubtedly necessary for immediate emotional survival.

Hamburg and Adams (1969) have pointed out that the threat of, and therefore the response to chronic disabling illness, is heavily influenced by a succession of past environments and experiences. They state, somewhat surprisingly, that despite the plausible expectancy of uniformly disastrous emotional sequellae, clinical experiences indicate a substantial proportion of severely involved people make impressive 'psychological' recoveries.

Turning to the specific mechanisms of early coping, a general denial of the frightening implications for the future seems to be the first response. Undoubtedly, this is necessary to avoid being completely overwhelmed by the catastrophe. As denial is relinquished, and reality fearfully approached, periods of depression are regularly encountered. Mourning the loss of the pre-morbid self and its potential is to be expected. Absence of such mourning is unusual and disturbing. In its way, mourning facilitates the structuring of a future-oriented existence, which may not be possible until what has been lost has been grieved for.

The possibility of continued membership in highly valued groups increases the ability to cope with the crisis of serious illness. This in some way may imply the possibility of continuance of the pre-morbid way of life, even on an abbreviated basis. Together with the mourning process, it facilitates the construction of a new self-concept, new self-meaning, and a new 'mode of being'. Valued groups include family, close friends and, in the instance of prolonged hospitalization, fellow patients. It is possible that such continued group relationships make easier the identification of a future role, within the limitation imposed by the illness. These early coping responses to the crisis of serious illness are necessary for emotional survival, and make possible progress to the only viable resolution of the situation—a transition from 'sick' to 'different'.

When these ways of coping are continued beyond their usefulness, however, they become techniques of resistance rather than aids to survival and progress. There are various reasons for continuing these beyond their usefulness. Early recognition of the maladaptive aspects is of the greatest importance if physical survival is to lead to the redevelopment of self-meaning and a new way of being.

Avery Weisman observes, *'The meaning of being disabled includes an awesome recognition that organs and body parts are no longer conspicuous compliant instruments that carry out their owner's intentions. Instead, the affected parts become alien and alienated objects with a distinct existence ...indeed an autonomy of their own...Because he (the involved individual) is unable to bring about significant change in his familiar world, his sense of being able to cause and control is transformed into an antithetical sense of being acted upon by impersonal forces, interpersonal displacements and intrapersonal anguish. . . The sick person becomes an object to be manipulated by forces beyond comprehension and control.'*

A responsibility of any treatment plan for chronic illness must be to bring about change in the involved individual which will avoid or reverse the feelings and behavior that Weisman so vividly describes. Such a change implies the surrender of the sick role, with its passive object-like state, for another identity—one which allows maximum independence and freedom of choice, in which 'being responsible' again becomes possible. This transition must take place within the context of external reality if it is to be genuinely effective.

The transition from 'sick' to 'different' requires relinquishing the sick role. It should be kept in mind that illness is the only condition that permits the giving up on responsibility by an adult, and condones his dependency in a work-oriented culture. The cultural exemption of the sick was based on the 'temporary' nature of the illness. The process was expected to end in recovery or death within a relatively short period of time. Further, the exemption implied that every effort to recover would be made.

There are, however, powerful incentives to continue in the sick role, particularly with those illnesses in which one does not 'get well' in the ordinary sense. The secondary gains of illness may offer a temporary opportunity for the satisfaction of the patient's unconscious needs. When such needs are sufficiently demanding, it takes considerable effort and understanding to counter their regressive influence. The possibility of secondary gain must always be borne in mind, and not only as it applies to the patient.

It can be reasonably assumed that the reaction and response to the trauma of serious illness is influenced by the pre-morbid personality, life style, and level of psychosocial competence. Successful readaptation is immeasurably enhanced by a sensitive awareness of these factors by those responsible for treatment. One should bear in mind that the patient is vulnerable to the pressures of unconscious needs formed long before the specific event of the illness.

It becomes obvious that a complete life history is important if the full impact of chronic illness is to be fully appreciated. Erik Erikson noted that the more advanced an individual's psychosocial development, the more successfully he has integrated previous conflicts, the more capable he is of meeting present crises and coping with new adaptational demands. The behavioral and emotional response to significant chronic illness is influenced by factors involving a person's entire previous life experience and will, in large measure, reflect his pre-morbid style of dealing with crisis and conflict.

Regardless of previous life experience, to be the victim of catastrophic illness poses an awesome reality. The stricken one must accept that life is irrevocably different, and because of that difference, a new meaning and way of life must be found. This is clearly an existential decision. The alternatives are to remain 'sick', with no realistic hope of cure in the usual sense of the word, or to relinquish life itself. Either choice is equivalent to 'non-being'. To discover a new meaning in life in the face of the dissolution of the old meaning, to accept the difference imposed by the illness, and to still maintain one's dignity and worth is the essence of the transition from sick to different. When one has accomplished this, there is no longer a need for illness as a primary life style.

When it does occur, the transition from sick to different is obvious. Why it occurs relatively easily in some people, while in others it manifests itself only after long suffering, or not at all, is not completely clear. Premorbid self-concept and life style appear to be important factors. When one observes the response to chronic illness over a period of time, much of what happens seems to be related to how a person 'sees' himself. People seem to behave in ways appropriate to a 'held' self-concept whether that self-concept is realistic or not. The response to illness may be related to the degree that it prevents one from behaving congruently with a 'held' self-concept. When illness does not significantly interfere with the capacity to sustain that concept, giving up sickness and moving to differentness proceeds more easily and smoothly. When there is a marked discrepancy between the pre-morbid life style, influenced strongly by the 'held' self-concept and the options available within the restrictions of the illness, giving up being sick may become a threatening and challenging decision. Until the satisfactions of being different outweigh those of being sick, the transition will not occur. The individual must desire such satisfactions more than the safety he derives from the sick role.

By using an oversimplified system of classification, one can divide people into basically motor and cerebrally oriented groups. The first includes those who see themselves essentially as physical beings, for whom strength, stamina, athletic skills and motor excellence in general have great meaning. The latter encompasses those primarily involved with cognitive, intellectual and creative activities. Such people generally seem more likely to make a successful transition.

The question of dependency warrants critical consideration. Dependency generally has a negative connotation. To be dependent implies weakness, while to be independent is a sign of maturity and responsibility. For virtually all of the chronically ill, total independence is nearly impossible. The constant emphasis of 'independence' in our culture, therefore, can act as a subtle barrier to those who are attempting to give up sick behavior. In actuality, independence is a relative term. As our social structure becomes more complicated, we become progressively more interdependent. Perhaps it is more relevant to speak of positive and negative dependency. Positive dependency recognizes and accepts a need for help in order to achieve maximum functional potential. It represents a realistic and pragmatic acceptance of the limitations imposed by illness and disability. Negative dependency, on the other hand, exhibits behavior whose purpose, essentially, is regressive. Its main function is avoidance of responsibility and maturity. It is a major secondary gain of illness.

The degree of dependency (and therefore the need for help) is a function of the severity of the disability and the demands of the environment. The important thing is that, as opposed to avoidance, the goal of positive dependency is greater involvement. By relying upon and utilizing others appropriately, the capacity to cope and achieve is increased. The use of positive dependency takes a special skill. To utilize others positively requires honest acceptance of one's differentness and the special needs and conditions it imposes. It requires further recognition of the fact that many, if not most, 'normal' people are uncomfortable with the disabled; and the equanimity to be neither angered nor embarrassed by their discomfort. Far from being regressive, positive dependency is perhaps the most significant quality of the readapted disabled individual.

Readaptation (the French use this term in preference to rehabilitation) is coming to terms existentially with the reality of chronic illness as a state of being, discarding both false hope and destructive hopelessness, restructuring the environment in which one must now function. Most importantly, readaptation demands the reorganization and acceptance of the self so that there is a meaning and purpose to living that transcends the limitations imposed by the illness.

The time may have come to consider a new conceptual model within which to understand and treat the chronically ill and disabled. Such a model would stress psychosocioeconomic function as the critical area in dealing with the problem. It would emphasize readaptation and maximal social function as the major tasks faced by such patients. Obviously, such a new model would utilize diagnostic, therapeutic and restorative procedures and benefits, but it would channel and direct these currently fragmented (and frequently isolated) components of medical care toward a realistic and socially meaningful goal. In its way, it would be an affirmation of Rudolph Virchow's frequently forgotten aphorism, 'Medicine is a social science in its bone and marrow'.

While the components of comprehensive care may exist in many areas, a coordinated service is not easily found. This is in large measure due to the fragmentation inherent in the present system as well as the incapacity of organizations, as presently constituted, to assume overall responsibility for the problem of chronic illness. Thus, it may be that the present model of a health care system tends to encourage and maintain the sick role, and thus discourage the transition from sick to different.

To conceive and establish a different system requires a significant change of thinking as to the nature of the problem of chronic illness, and consequently the methods necessary for its management. If chronic illness is, in large measure, a problem of behavior and function, the traditional disease-oriented medical model may not be the best one within which to operate.

The primary concern of a new model would be with the behavioral and social impact of chronic illness: its aim, the minimization or elimination of these impacts as far as possible. It would assume responsibility for seeing that individuals received necessary diagnostic, therapeutic and rehabilitation care, but always within the *goal-oriented* approach of maximum psychosocial function and maximum quality of life. Its operation, by the very nature of its task, must involve every aspect of the community in which it functions. The human aspect of the illness, which is of primary concern to the patient, and the meaning of the illness as a personal event to the patient, would be dealt with and assessed more realistically. The 'wholeness' of this model's approach confirms the value of the patient as a human being in the fullest sense. If these objectives are to be met and the concepts disseminated, it is important that the staff consist of people who share the model's values and objectives.

The whole purpose of such a model is meaningful and continuous involvement with the patient as a person. This involvement must include realistic and sophisticated recognition of all of the problems that the illness has raised for a particular individual, and the knowledge to deal with as many of them as possible. Such a conceptual model makes possible broad humanistic involvement with those enmeshed in chronic disabling illness, opening new vistas for truly comprehensive care.

REFERENCES

Engel, G. L. A life setting conducive to illness: The giving in-giving up complex. *Annals of Internal Medicine*, 1968, *69*, 293–300.

Feldman, D. J. Medical rehabilitation—The clinical management of disability. *Journal of Chronic Disease*, 1963, *16*, 1313–1316.

Feldman, D. J. The impact of long term illness on human work as a sociobehavioral phenomenon. *Proceedings: Research conference of applied work physiology*. New York: New York University Medical Center, Department of Rehabilitation Medicine, 1968.

Feldman, D. J. *Coping and behavioral response to physical disability—Their importance in the rehabilitation process.* London: British Council for the Rehabilitation of the Disabled, 1969.

Field, M. *Patients are people* (3rd ed.). New York: Columbia University Press, 1967.

Goffman, E. *Stigma: Notes on the management of spoiled identity.* Englewood Cliffs, N.J.: Prentice-Hall, 1968.

Greaves, M. *Work and disability*. London: British Council for the Rehabilitation of the Disabled, 1969.

Hamburg, D. A., & Adams, J. E. A perspective on coping behavior. *Archives of General Psychiatry,* 1969, *17.*

Kimball, M. D. Conceptual developments in psychosomatic medicine: 1939–1969. *Annals of Internal Medicine,* 1970, *73,* 307–316.

Schoenberg et al. (Eds.). *Loss and grief: Psychological management in medical practice.* New York: Columbia University Press, 1970.

PERSONAL STATEMENT ......
Joe

Life can be unfair. This is a conclusion one could
reach having studied the following presentation of the
life of Joe.

As a 47-year-old man, Joe had reached the point
in his life when his children were married and grand-
children were born. His job was secure and it was the
time to reap the harvest of a toil of a lifetime. There
should be the opportunity for fishing, building, and
the realm of creative tasks for which there had not
been time. The "should be's" did not equate with the
realities of what would fall on Joe and his family over
the next several years. The following is a statement
reflective of Joe's struggle as told to and observed by
the author.

Friday, December 6, 1968, was a day like
all days. It began with work and ended with the
relief of another day gone and a weekend to
look forward to. An unexpected snowstorm resulted in my having to shovel out the driveway
to prepare for going shopping the next day. I
had completed about half of the job when I felt
a pain in my leg and I decided that I should go
inside. I told my wife Helen that I must have
pulled a muscle because the pain got worse. I
realized that something was wrong when I fell
over and could not get up. She called an ambulance and I wound up in the hospital. I had a
terrible time adjusting to being in the hospital
because I am primarily an independent person
and I was not used to being sick. Having been a
paratrooper in World War II, I had experienced
danger, but never injury. So this was all new to
me. What had begun as a pain had now turned
into a major event. I was told I had a blood clot
and that I would have to have my right leg am-
putated below the knee. To me, this was traumatic information. I who was active, worked

hard, would now be without a leg? I never was
so afraid in all my life. But I knew I did not
have much of a choice—it was this or die from
gangrene.

I talked this over with my wife Helen, who
had just had a mastectomy, and we agreed that
things would get better. I felt badly about my
situation since Helen had not fully recovered
from her operation and now I was placing more
strain upon her. My operation was more emotionally than physically painful. It seemed no
one attended to me or my needs. Someone came
in, taped my leg, and said this is where they
will cut tomorrow. During the operation I was
awake and could hear the saw cutting through
the bone. No one responded to me. They only
cared about their operation.

After it was over, I was determined to beat
the odds. I worked hard during my rehabilitation, was fitted for a prosthesis, and was back
at work and driving my standard shift car. I
had made it, done the impossible. Life was wonderful. All until I realized that my stump was
not healing. I went to the doctor who operated
on me and he did not give me a satisfying answer. As a mechanic by profession, I felt something was wrong and that I wanted it fixed. As
a veteran I felt my best bet was to go to the Veterans Administration Hospital.

It was at this point when my world began to
fall apart. The doctor who examined said, "Who
took off your leg, a shoemaker?" This was
scary and I knew I was in trouble. She was an
excellent doctor and attempted to improve the
stump. However, it was too late and more had
to come off. At this time I was alone. No one understood. No one was there in the hospital to
explain and encourage me.

On a weekend pass home and with the help
of a few drinks, I cut my wrists in an attempt
to end the pain, frustration, and uncertainty.
My cat saved my life. His meowing woke up my
wife and she called the ambulance. Because I

was on blood thinners for my blood clot, the cuts were almost fatal.

At this point I was taken to the VA Hospital, where I felt secure and hopeful. Unfortunately, the odds were not in my favor. Complications set in and I was informed that my other leg had to come off. This was the point of total desperation. With one leg I could manage. With two gone, how could I survive? Amazingly I decided that I had suffered too much to give up at this point. I devised a system in my head that would give me complete mobility in the house. It was sort of a monorail on the ceiling powered by electrical motors. Having designed and built many things, I knew it would work. It was very disappointing when family members did not encourage this idea. I asked them to buy certain items and drew up specifications but they did not respond. It would have been a worthwhile project for me to keep my mind busy.

The most difficult thing for me to bear was the pain I saw in my family's eyes, when they visited me. Here I was, two legs gone, plagued with gangrene, still fighting for life, and only a few people could encourage me. It was at this point I knew I was a dying man. How I wished I could live again the past year, to enjoy a drink, to sit in the sunshine. I felt that I was deprived and missed many of the important moments. I had a lot to say to my family but I could not. I did not want to burden them with my pain, fear, and regrets. The best I could do was pretend to be optimistic while dying in a strange bed, wanting to be home.

On December 22, 1970, at the age of 49, Joe died.

SECTION I

BASIC CONSIDERATIONS FOR UNDERSTANDING THE FAMILY AND DISABILITY

The materials in Section I were selected to help the reader understand the dynamics that have an impact on the family today and appreciate those individual, illness-related factors that can determine the family's reaction to disability. The authors' text, the articles, and the personal statements also identify the many influences impinging upon the patient's rehabilitation. The disabled person's adjustment and current social and family forces are interrelated, and the many contributions in this section accentuate the vital connections between the patient's emotional response to disability, the family, and effective rehabilitation approaches.

Understanding the operative forces from the community can assist the health professional to develop an awareness of why the family members emotionally react as they do to the severe illness or disability of a family member. How an individual copes with a disability will further affect how the family deals with the implications of the condition in their everyday life. In turn, the coping style of the family can influence the disabled person's own response to rehabilitation demands.

Chapter 1 deals with the current status of the family, and Chapters 2 and 3 explore the varied emotional effects that disability or chronic illness can have on either the adult or child. The last two chapters of this section present different theories on how the family may react to adult or child disability. All of these chapters are establishing a base of understanding for the reader, from which can be developed an effective helping approach for families with a disabled or chronically ill member. A knowledge of the different family reactions to disability can generate added understanding of these forces within the patient's environment that can influence rehabilitation efforts. A helping approach should be designed with such an awareness.

The personal statements of Maria and Karen give actual examples of many of the emotional reactive theories explained in the chapters. Maria's account was written by her father and identifies the many family traumas accompanying the birth of a handicapped child. Feelings of helplessness and frustration pervade the family scene, to be replaced later by the needed strength and energy to cope with the endless demands of treatment care. Yet even these diminish as the years progress. Maria's father explains how the other children react to family pressures, but also describes how these children are an effective resource for rehabilitation care. At the end of the account he gives some suggestions for health professionals on how to improve their responsiveness to parents in a disability situation.

The story of Karen concerns the hope and disappointments in raising a child with cerebral palsy. It focuses on the time at birth, and recalls the many feelings a mother can have when the event becomes traumatic. In writing the story the mother also wanted to relate her own uncertainty for the child. She lives with guarded hope—a lingering suspicion for the child's future and a confidence in her ability to provide necessary care. This acknowledgment is not only a reflection of her love but identifies a continued, positive source of influence on the child's life adjustment and daily coping.

PERSONAL STATEMENT . . . . . .
Maria

Maria was lucky enough to be born at home to
Louise and I, who recognized the presence of
spina bifida and were able to get her to the
Crouse-Irving Memorial Hospital, which specialized in the care of such infants.

The chronology of Maria's first 8 years was
punctuated by crises severe enough to test both
her physical and emotional stability as well as
those of her family.

November 5, 1969   An uneventful pregnancy and excellent delivery ended with the
shock of a birth defect of a very serious nature
that was not known in either family tree. We
rushed Maria to the hospital instead of remaining together as a family unit to savor the joy of
the first-born child. The first test was of
Louise's strong Roman Catholic faith and the
self-doubts that assailed us both: What did I do?
What could we have done? Explain it to us
please! How were we to respond to the resident
doctor (a pregnant female, no less) who told
Louise that "it serves you right" for having
Maria born at home with no doctor in attendance?

November 19, 1969   Maria's first operation. A shunt valve to control the developing hy-
drocephalus was inserted, but her head was
shaved and misshapen, her eyes crossed. She
was no longer the same pretty baby of 2 short
weeks ago.

December 3, 1969   The second operation,
to close the meningomyelocele, proves to be almost fatal and our mixed feelings of wanting
her to die, to save us the lifelong upbringing,
and needing her home to love, tear at us. She is

27

a pathetic sight in the incubator; insulated from us, out of reach, little body heaving for each gasp of air, really fighting to stay alive, naked and helpless.

December 24, 1969   We get Maria home for Christmas, a great joy. At 7 weeks she is regressed, needing love and attention, but now she is ours. Maria develops quickly into the normal baby routine of food, sleep, and activity. I exercise her legs looking for movement, Louise prays for a miracle, we enjoy our first-born, but continue to seek the answer to "Why?"

Our general pattern of life is not very different from other families while she is a babe-in-arms. We work hard at exercising both her physical and intellectual capabilities; testing, working, and extending her range.

Louise becomes pregnant and we decide to have a hospital delivery, which goes well, and Tommy is born on May 8, 1971. All the fears of a second congenital malformation, those spoken and unspoken misgivings, are fortunately allayed.

Preschool for disabled children helps to lighten some of the demands we have placed upon ourselves, but we question the degree of effort made to push Maria's skills and develop her competencies.

Our own feelings of strength and the energy to keep working begin to wane as the years progress. Other parents we meet seem to have survived the zoo-like clinics with rows of babies and lines of interns, specialists, nurses, and others, not to mention the prohibitive hospital costs of operations, prostheses, braces, wheelchairs, and the seemingly incessant travel to clinics, meetings, and search for funds to pay for some of the larger expenses. From this peer group we obtain a reinforcement and reaffirmation of our role.

As Maria grows she begins to make demands and develop her own sensitivity to some of the insults inflicted upon her by simpering

people and calloused professionals. Treated as
an inanimate object, spoken about rather than
with, her disability the focus of most attention,
she learns to turn people off, ignore demands,
and emotionally resist any attempts to cajole
her cooperation.

Louise and I reacted as defensive parents,
angry at the insensitivity, and consequently received write-ups from staff professionals such
as "highly emotional," "disturbed and angry,"
"we suggest immediate counseling. . ." Our demands were rarely addressed as either reasonable or legitimate, let alone legally ours to
make. We have learned to question, doubt,
threaten, and insist—not an easy thing to do
when you are defensive and weary knowing
that the system has its own inertia and that the
medical model needs it passive patient.

September, 1975   Public school at last appears to be at hand: 5 years, 10 months of age
with 3 years of preschool, Maria was a veteran
of numerous psychologists, tests, and evaluations. The principal of the local school has a
thousand reasons why Maria, the teachers, and
the other pupils would find her presence in **his**
school untenable: we go elsewhere to main-
stream her. But it is all in vain, the testing had
not detected the learning disability (though we
had warned the core evaluation team of our
misgivings at a first grade entrance for her) and
she gets put back to a kindergarten class after 4
weeks in first grade. The following year she enters first grade at a private school for the physically disabled because the public school says
that she still will not be able to cope with their
first grade curriculum.

Again the failure is ours as parents; it was
we who fought for a regular school with an
aide. We hoped that Maria would be a regular
school child, who just happened to be in a
wheelchair, in a regular grade in a public
school. Thus she could develop intellectually
and socially in a realistic setting with the nondisabled population.

It is almost impossible to convey the base-line level of family existence without it appearing to be a series of obstacles, crises, and running battles with architectural barriers, emotional confrontations, or physical restrictions. A fully accessible public school that has ramps that are impossible for a 5- or 6- (even older) year-old child to negotiate, and a trip to the ballet is potentially a battle with fire regulations for a wheelchair person who cannot see the stage from a regular seat. Or trying to see the Children's Museum with all its stairs and different levels—very attractive but impossible and inaccessible. Each time we meet new service people (teachers, therapists, doctors) we try to ensure that Maria is fully consulted and informed and that she actively participates in her program. It comes as a surprise to some people that we objected to Maria being unceremoniously stripped and poked to observe her reactions. Living in the northeast, winter stops her individualized mobility, older houses with stairs prevent impromptu visits, camping and hiking have to be more carefully routed and planned, public transportation is almost impossible to negotiate.

Despite the chronic nature of the physical restrictions, Maria grows and matures as other children do. Her insights into the motivations of lay and professional people continue to surprise us. Inappropriate behavior and attitudes of others is recognized and later questioned. Maria's ability to verbalize her disappointments, needs, and emotions tells us that she is becoming her own person, that she is attempting to understand herself and others and so to control her own destiny.

April, 1978   We face another crisis: two operations (at minimum) 2 weeks apart to fuse and straighten her spine, 4 to 5 weeks in hospital and then 6 months in a body cast. There are bright spots: our insurance will probably cover most of the costs, the surgeon is good, and

Maria likes his quiet and reassuring manner.
She has been doing a lot of talking about it, her
fears, anger, apprehensions, and the necessity
for the operations. We had been told to have a
partial fusion when she was 4 years old, but
Louise objected, found a doctor that would
brace her until she got older, grew more, and
better able to deal with the trauma involved. So
we did buy 4 additional years and Louise has
accepted the lack of a miracle, which makes the
need for the operations inevitable. Maria is a lot
more mature and better able to verbalize all the
things she was not able to when she was only 4.
With the added advantage of talking things out
is the ability to be consoled and even convinced
that in fact it will be a good thing not to have to
wear her brace, which is uncomfortable, gives
sores, and gets hot in summer. Our decision 4
years ago has turned out the way we had hoped,
and as such makes the coming ordeal easier to
accept. We are finally vindicated.

Looking back at our 8 years as Maria's parents we can appreciate the unique strengths
that each of us has: Louise has a strong faith
and carries the primary burden of everyday
care and health visits; I try to serve as the supportive member since I am less emotionally involved, with a more pragmatic approach to
Maria's development as well as keeping in touch
with Louise's physical and emotional needs. Because we have very different attitudes and techniques in dealing with Maria and health professionals we have had to learn to talk out differences, which often allows the involved partner
to do it his or her way with the other serving as
a support and back-up.

Caring for a disabled child is a physically
and emotionally draining exercise for all concerned. Daily routines must be developed that
allow the child and parents some flexibility and
a break from constant contact and interdepen-
dence. Emotionally the child has to develop independence and toughness to make demands as

well as go it alone. The parents have to balance
support with demands: Are we asking too little,
enough, or too much? Should we push or hold?
It is an ongoing reassessment procedure.

How have the other children reacted to
these family pressures? Essentially by resenting
the extra attention and physical involvement
that Maria receives. This we have attempted to
address in three ways: in their infancy the children (the four who have followed her) have been
given all the attention they ask for, with breast-
feeding, handling, and play on demand. As they
develop speech and understanding skills they
are given responsibilities, and demands are
made of them as family members. What is good
for one should be good for the whole family and
mutual support becomes a central theme: opening a door for Maria will result in faster action
for all of us. Finally, if the resentment becomes
anger, we sit and talk it out either individually
or in a family conference to show how there is a
balance of love and attention in degree if not in
kind: does a wheelchair equal a bicycle? Is it
worth going to the hospital to get attention and
presents? How do we all feel about Maria going
to camp for 2 weeks?

The talking out of parent anger/frustration
is, we feel, a technique that many health professionals fail to address when confronted with
parents and patients. An 8-year-old is less likely
to verbalize fear and anger as such; Maria becomes resistant, passive, or weepy. We have
found that the nonverbal language of professionals implies censure, derision, or shock at attitudes, behaviors, or procedures we parents
use with Maria. We can still remember those
few that sat down and responded to us. Nonjudgmental attitudes must be combined with
gentle, caring, verbal responses to parents who
need support and constructive advice, not self-
righteous censure with a condescending approach.

It is difficult for a parent who has been
waiting for an hour, after a delayed appoint-

ment, to be calm, cool, and collected with the receptionist, nurse, therapist, intern, and doctor
when no one addresses the parent as a fellow
team member, let alone primary care person
and essential life support for the patient. In our
8 years we feel that there has been a real improvement in the quality and sensitivity of the
health care that we as a family have received,
but the occasional "downer" takes the family
months to recoup.

During our ongoing crisis we have learned
in part to cope with the traumatic as well as the
practical problems that face us. The spinal fusion operation is one of the most traumatic for
it signals the end of one hopeful era and the
beginning of another reality. While the results
of the operation are scary, Louise is fearful of
the operation itself. After all, it is major and
can be life threatening. This issue has been one
that we differ on. While we both recognize the
possibility of Maria's dying, Louise sees it as a
blessing if it would spare Maria from a life of
pain and sorrow. I, on the other hand, believe
that we can cope with anything and that we can
help Maria live a fulfilling life. One explanation
of our differing of opinions is that Louise is the
person who is responsible for the day-to-day
caring of Maria. While I do certain tasks, such
as the catheterization in the morning, I have my
job and other activities to which I can "escape."
However, I do recognize Louise's needs and I attempt to support her and she supports me so we
work as a team. This aspect of mutual support
has been critical for our emotional survival
because we understand one another and do not
blame ourselves as a unit or as individuals for
what happened to Maria.

When Maria was born, Louise almost gave
up religion and went through a phase of not
needing God. Now religion is a major support
for Louise. Religion has been the constant factor
that has provided a perspective on our situation
and some direction for our managing our
unique situation. While I am not as religious as

Louise, I see the value of it and can benefit from it in my own way.

I was more angry at the situation. I could not understand why the child had to be so afflicted and why it had to happen to us. I personally feel I am beyond this point and that I can relate to Maria as a caring father who is able to go beyond his needs and respond to the needs of Maria and the family.

As parents of a child with a disability we have had a unique opportunity to interact with the medical community in a variety of ways. Reflecting upon these experiences has both its positive and negative dimensions. On the positive side, there have been many people who have attempted to respond to our unique needs and situation by providing excellent medical care. On the negative side, many of the rules and philosophies of hospital care have not attended to the needs of Maria. For example, during most hospitalizations, she was not permitted to have visits from her siblings. This was and is a point of contention for us since we do not believe in such a philosophy and will respond accordingly.

As far as suggestions for health professionals related to improving their responsiveness to parents and children in our situation we can suggest:

1. Spend time at the initial period of crisis
2. Involve the total family
3. Expose them to alternatives and resources
4. Share your personal feelings: If you feel bad, tell us
5. Treat the child as a person, not as a disability

CHAPTER 1

UNDERSTANDING THE FAMILY

Paul W. Power and Arthur E. Dell Orto

This chapter is divided into four sections: 1) reflections on the modern family, 2) roles in modern marriage, 3) life stages in marriage, and 4) cultural considerations in health and illness. These aspects of the family and society give an overview of what is happening to modern family life and especially describe the changes that are still taking place in the different roles of family members. A family is helped in the context of its values, beliefs, and cultural heritage. Family life stages and cultural considerations will give readers added perspectives to explore when implementing their rehabilitation approaches.

REFLECTIONS ON THE MODERN FAMILY

Today there is widespread belief that the family is in a state of decline. Peters (1974) believes that "the American Family is today experiencing conflict as a result of rapidly changing and diversifying cultural and value orientations" (p. 33). It has been indicated that this is the "age of the fragile family and the family in transition" (Nordheimer, 1977, p. 4). This is supported by a good deal of statistical evidence: rising divorce rates, declining fertility rates, rising numbers of women leaving the home for paid work, and the disappearance of the extended family (Bane, 1976).

Nordheimer (1977) reports statistics showing dynamic trends of basic change within the family:

a. The divorce rate has doubled in the last 18 years.
b. Two out of every five children born in this decade will live in single-parent homes for at least part of their youth.
c. The number of households headed by women has increased by more than a third in this decade, and has more than doubled in one generation.

d. More than half of all mothers with school age children now work outside the home, as do more than a third of mothers with children under
the age of 3 years.

e. Day care of irregular quality is replacing the parental role in many
working families. There has been extraordinary growth in the classification that sociologists call "latch key children"—children unsuper-
vised for portions of the day, usually in a period between the end of
school and a working parent's return home.

All of these changes that supposedly have contributed to the decline of
the family have important implications for the family and disability. Because there are more opportunities available to enter the work world,
women have the renewed chance to help maintain the family unit when the
crippling disability of the husband-breadwinner has minimized possibilities
for economic support. Yet the disappearance of the extended family means,
for example, that when disability strikes many families are very much alone
in bearing this emotional and physical burden. Rehabilitation for such families usually becomes especially difficult. If a family member incurs a disability in a family that is living close to a poverty level, their ability to cope is
diminished. If home is just a place where family members sleep and wait
to be fed, and where communication tends to be minimal, then the family's
ability to deal with a disability will be lowered.

Although most of the literature has strongly indicated that the family is
in serious trouble, Bane (1976) turns the coin and states "that the time has
not yet come to write obituaries for the American family or to divide up its
estate" (p. xiv). Her research indicates that discontinuation in parental care
is not greater than it was in the past, and that changes in fertility rates may
lead to an environment that is more beneficial for children. In carefully examining census statistics and general social surveys, Bane affirms that
children of the 1970s face a predominantly adult world because they make
up a smaller proportion of society, and the trend toward more mothers in
the paid labor force has probably not affected parent-child bonds mate-
rially. She also reports that census figures show that the majority of marriages do not end in divorce, and the vast majority of divorced people re-
marry. Consequently, we are a long way from a society in which marriage is
rejected or replaced by a series of "short-term liaisons" (p. 31). Marriage
and family are still an exceedingly important part of American life, although Bane believes that men and women will do more similar work and
will approach each other more equally as partners.

Sussman (1974) believes that the popular theory of "the isolated nuclear family" is based mainly on fiction, and suggests that kin ties, particularly intergenerational ones, have far more significance than we have been
led to believe in the life processes of the urban family. The family is closely
integrated within a network of mutual assistance and activity, which can be

described as an "interdependent kin family system." Bane (1976) supports this statement by explaining that "recent sociological studies have shown that Americans maintain close ties with many of their relatives and that the American nuclear family is not as isolated from kin as was once thought" (p. 37). Neighborhoods, communities, and kin networks are probably most important to the lives of families.

There are, consequently, two contrasting views on the status of the current American family. One presents an optimistic picture, the other a pessimistic one. The latter suggests many difficulties for rehabilitation workers, because seldom can a fragmented family become a resource for the patient in rehabilitation efforts. The former offers hope for the rehabilitation worker, because if research does indicate the potential availability of parental substitutes and minimizes the relative degree of social isolation of family members, then the family is in a much better position, not only to cope with physical disability, but actually to play a part in its rehabilitation. Within this supportive environment, disability may not produce as many negative consequences.

ROLES IN MODERN MARRIAGE

One of the striking changes in the American family during the past 20 years has been in the roles of the family members. Role is defined as a learned behavior. The role a person learns to play in relation to others not only determines behavior toward others but also influences the way that person behaves toward himself. The roles of family members are assigned by the family and its cultural history (Peters, 1974).

Overs and Healy (1973) believe "that increasingly the family has come to be seen as an integrated system of reciprocal roles" (p. 87). Thus the family as a unit functions adequately or inadequately according to the degree of role perception and the interaction among the role performances of the various members. Marital success or adjustment can be defined by the degree of congruence between the husband's and wife's perceptions of their perspective roles (Overs & Healy, 1973).

Parsons and Bales's (1955) theory has stimulated more research than any other role theory, but it is important to realize that the roles that they define are in a process of change. They identify two main roles in marriage, the instrumental and the expressive. The instrumental role belongs to the husband. His task is getting things done, namely, earning money, paying bills, and maintaining the outside relationships with the economic and school systems. The wife has the expressive role; she is primarily concerned with maintaining satisfactory relationships within the family and with the expression of feelings that are a part of intimate relationships. However, these functions are not exclusive. The wife may shop for groceries and call the school about her children, and the husband may settle quarrels among the children and tell his wife that he loves her. Swenson (1973) believes that this theory suggests which person assumes primary responsibility for which area. The husband is primarily concerned with instrumental functions and secondarily with expressive function, whereas for the wife the situation is reversed.

Today roles in marriage are becoming increasingly less rigid and defined. In a modern, nuclear marriage the husband and wife are colleagues, and there is a blurring of the edges of primary responsibility. Women are granted or have assumed increasing authority when they become responsible for the welfare and socialization of the children. Now there is more sharing of tasks, with the "companiate marriage" being seen as the hallmark of contemporary family life.

In role theory there are four concepts that are basic in understanding disability and the family. They are role complementarity, role change, role conflict, and role reversal. Each of these concepts can be identified in the family who experienced the trauma of a young family member with leukemia:

> Jennifer, age 15, was hospitalized with the diagnosis of leukemia. The illness went into remission following medication and hospital treatment care. Upon returning home, the family became aware that new, continued demands were to be made upon them, i.e., frequent clinic visits and coping with their own anxiety and grief over the illness situation. The mother was particularly affected, feeling guilty that perhaps she was neglectful in the care of her child before disease onset. She became temporarily depressed, and during this time withdrew from many of her social contacts, and asked her daughter, age 14, and son, age 17, to assume many of the household chores. The husband also began to perform many more household duties, and accompanied his wife, whenever possible, to the clinic for treatment. Eventually her guilt feelings were alleviated, and through the assumption of added responsibilities in the home the family members found new strengths within one another to cope with the trauma.

Because there was a fluidity of roles among the family members—each family member could either adapt to or assume new responsibilities—the family was able to adjust to the daughter's illness. This equilibrium could not have been achieved without what is called a "complementarity of roles." Roles in the family did not exist in isolation but were patterned to mesh with those of other family members. The mother first expressed a need to share her role responsibilities with another, to transfer for awhile many of her tasks to another family member.

The husband and father, in addition to his role as breadwinner for the family, enlarged his role within the home by cooking for the children while the wife had to be with their daughter at the hospital. This can be referred to as a temporary role change. This change can cause role relationships within this family to become delicate. For example, as a mother changed her methods of disciplining her child or made a decision about the daughter's health care, conflicts could arise in her relationship with her husband, or she could become confused and inadequate in her role as wife, or the complementarity of roles could break down. In either instance, role conflict is generated and role complementarity is not restored until the family members become aware of the demands of the illness situation and are willing to make the effort to modify their accustomed family behavior.

One way to resolve role conflict is through role reversal. This involves looking at what is happening in the family from the other person's point of view. It requires a good understanding of what really is occurring within the family because of the disability situation. Role reversal can begin with such a statement as, "I see what you mean...."

The changes in family life reflect a high complementarity of roles. When family members have to retreat from their customary roles, however, the family can become vulnerable. If the husband has been performing many household tasks and has taken much responsibility for the care of the children, or if the wife has been working or feels confident to enter the work market, then the limitations on family life caused by a disability can be minimized. Family role complementarity enables the family members to re-pattern their lives in such a way that family needs can still be met in an efficient manner.

FAMILY LIFE STAGES

When a disability occurs in a family, it occurs at a definite stage in the family's life cycle. The reaction of family members to a disabled husband and father can be quite different in the earlier stages of a marriage and family life than when the couple and family have been living together for many years. For example, the factors of role expectations, intimacy, and dependency, which are strong determinants of how a family copes with disease or disability, will vary during different stages of family life. A disability can disrupt the balance of these factors, and the extent of the disruption depends upon the life stage of the family.

The severe cardiac patient illustrates the intermeshing of these factors and the disability. For example, when a husband has a heart attack and has been married for many years, the family's emotional system might find it very difficult to meet the patient's needs for self-esteem and competency. The patient-husband may have left all household chores and child-rearing decisions to his wife, and now, because of physical restrictions, has no other readily available role within the family. His self-esteem may be closely tied in with his ability to provide, so that the loss of this role is perceived as a loss of worth. In contrast, in addition to her role as homemaker, the wife may have to explore opportunities for a part-time job to augment the dwindling family income. The lack of a definite role for the husband and the possible added role for the wife may create conflict and disharmony for the couple. True, such conflict may occur whether the couple is newly married or has just celebrated a 25th wedding anniversary, but because the functions in the home have been so well established the health professional has a more difficult helping task. The health professional must shape a model of intervention from this particular, patterned home environment and utilize the family members in a distinctive way in order to assist in the care of the husband.

Within each stage certain family tasks emerge. These family tasks reflect the assumption that developmental tasks of individual family members have an overriding influence on or affect the nature of family life at a given time. Adequate task handling at early stages also strengthens the family's ability to handle subsequent stages effectively. Disability and illness, therefore, can be better understood within the family when each of the family stages is explored, because each stage has its own demands, responsibilities, problems, roles, and challenges. The way the family comes to terms with the disability-related crisis may vary according to the respective family stage.

Two of the most frequently used systems for understanding family life stages are those containing eight life stages as described by Havighurst (1953) and Duvall (1971). Cavan (1974) has merged these two systems, and Rhodes (1977) has identified stages in the life cycle of the family in the tradition of Erik Erikson's life cycle of the individual. Much of the material on the following pages is an adaptation, interpretation, and clarification of the beliefs of these four researchers. The names of each stage are provided by Cavan (1974), although they are based primarily on the research of Duvall (1971). They give the reader a body of knowledge that the authors of this volume apply to rehabilitation work with families.

Beginning Families (Married Couples without Children)

The beginning families stage is characterized by the spouses building their relationship, assuming responsibility for each other in the relationship, and negotiating differences and conflicts with one another. The partners are attempting to find mutually satisfying ways to nurture and support each other. During this time the couple often dwells on themes of mutual understanding, caring, shared interests, and enjoyment of each other's company (Duvall, 1971). In the marriage almost exclusive attention is given to personality characteristics and emotional responsibility. Usually minimal reference is made to marital roles (Rakel, 1977), although the husband is attempting to establish himself in an occupation and the wife is learning to manage a household (Cavan, 1974).

A disability in one of the partners occurring during this time often represents a disappointment for one of the spouses, and can engender much conflict. The spouses are attempting to achieve intimacy and to discover the joys within each other. A severe disability can represent a serious obstacle to developing intimacy and can inhibit the beginning of workable marital roles. Disability can also aggravate the difficulty generally present during this time when each partner attempts to resolve the unrealistic expectations of the other (Duvall, 1971).

Child-Bearing Families (Oldest Child Birth to 30 Months)

At the child-bearing time of their marriage the spouses' ability to succor and to be available and responsive to the needs of very young children is being tapped. Their response depends on the presence of both their inner resources and a caring environment established by them (Rakel, 1977). The couple that has achieved intimacy during the first stage of married life is in a position to make the necessary adaptations to a new family member who is both helpless and demanding (Rhodes, 1977). With the arrival of children, of course, there may be a period of some disillusionment as the husband, especially, realizes that there are new demands for the wife's attention. The better integrated the marriage partners, the less could be the disillusionment.

The occurrence of disability usually complicates the adjustment to the child. Needed treatment care, the perhaps negative emotional reaction of the adult to the disability, the early readjustment to customary marital tasks all serve as a challenge to the couple, and the disability itself may represent a difficult hurdle for the spouses to overcome in adjusting to each other as parents. A newly disabled husband, experiencing his own loss and depression, may resent the attention given by the wife to the children. However, with many couples, one of whom is newly disabled, the new presence of a child can become a source of joy and a resource for coping with the limitations imposed by a disability.

Families with Preschool Children (Oldest Child 30 Months to 6 Years)

Most of the abilities needed by parents with small children are certainly carried over to the preschool stage. The succorance, nurturance, and availability must continue as children develop.

However, the mother may become totally involved in maintaining her home and caring for her children (Cavan, 1974). Outside opportunities may be necessary for personal replenishment. The husband and wife should spend time together in order to prevent the possibility of losing their marriage in family life.

If the presence of a severe disability in one of the spouses limits this opportunity, special problems can develop between the husband and wife. A disabled child may demand all-absorbing attention from the mother, and the husband may feel excluded. Frustration, anger, and tension will occur frequently.

Families with School Children (Oldest Child 6 to 13 Years)

Rhodes (1977) believes that during the school age period families must shift the primary attention of their energies from family concerns to individual interests. She claims that the major struggle for the partner, released from the early dependence of children, is to prepare for an identity that is not defined by that partner's roles and responsibilities within the family. The danger in this stage is when a family limits opportunities for development outside of itself. If the children feel free enough to enter into peer networks and community institutions, then parents might feel capable of developing resources for personal satisfaction outside of the home (Rhodes, 1977). If the parents are accustomed to seeking replenishment outside of the home, then the beginnings of this new identity will be facilitated. The same is true with disability. If the family members have utilized community resources apart from the family, then this particular family stage will intermesh harmoniously with previous stages of the marriage. The caring responsibilities associated with disability may not become as much of a burden when appropriate outlets have been established.

Families with Teenagers (Oldest Child 13 to 20 Years)

Such factors as role models, a consistency of family life, the giving of parents, and who is the dominant person in the home assume continued importance for the family (Duvall, 1971). At the teenager stage separation themes surface within the family, themes that may be difficult for family members to tolerate if a disabled parent has become very dependent on the children (Rhodes, 1977). The resolution of a major crisis for family members rests with their ability to develop companionship inside and outside the family. These bonds will ease the pain of loss stemming from the children who are leaving home for college or for their own living arrangements.

During this stage a new kind of parent-child relationship should be established, based on a recognition of the child's growing independence. If disability strikes a parent during this family period, and if this parent has not adapted constructively to the disability, then such a recognition will generally not be achieved. Too much attention may be focused on the disabled parent, or the latter may become very demanding. The children may feel isolated and eventually leave home abruptly (Power, 1977). Tension and fear may characterize the marital relationship.

Families as Launching Centers
(First Child Gone to Last Child Leaving Home)

Seeing their children leave home may be hardest for women who feel that their home-related competencies are no longer needed or valued. This phase of family life is usually experienced as particularly difficult for the mother and wife since there is also a renewed demand on the family's ability to foster and support individuation (Rhodes, 1977). The viability of the marital relationship is a strong determinant of how the family negotiates this stage.

When disability has caused severe dependency and aroused conflicts or resentments among the marital partners and family members, individuation for the children may be thwarted. The attention may be focused almost exclusively on the ill family member. The children may be asked to assume a large role in treatment responsibilities, or may be often ignored because of caring for the disabled person. The older children may feel guilty in leaving home to begin their own life. Disappointment may pervade the family scene, and the parents may not help their children make the transition from the home to a more independent life.

Families in the Middle Years (Empty Nest to Retirement)

The middle years can be particularly difficult for a couple, one member of which is disabled. It is a time for a renegotiation of the adult-adult relationship. Rediscovery is all important, because usually in the later years of marriage there is a general drop in marital satisfaction and adjustment, which can be conceived as a process of disenchantment (Rhodes, 1977). The cessation of parent functions seems to leave a vacuum and often demands major reorientation of purposes and goals. The presence of disability may only aggravate a loss of intimacy, especially if the disability severely affects the couple's sexual life or the amount of time given to shared activities. Yet with a renewed interest in the personalities of their spouses, the husband and wife could become a source of support for each other, leading to increased satisfaction in the post-parental and retirement time of their life (Duvall, 1971).

Aging Families (Retirement to Death of Both Spouses)

The retirement stage entails most of the changes related to the aging process. Rakel (1977) states that most people in this stage who maintain a wide diversity of interests remain psychologically healthy and are satisfied with their stage of life. Although at this stage in their relationship roles may have to be redefined, based on the exchange of services, it can be a time of renewed satisfaction if the spouses have coped well with the stresses of their family and have the resources to deal with the loneliness and depression that may accompany growing old. Kin networks and community ties are necessary resources for coping with the aging process. These resources may generate alternate satisfactions and values that permit individuals to maintain a sense of personal usefulness and contentment with life (Rakel, 1977).

Physical infirmities and related health problems are expected to occur to the spouses. If the couple has recaptured a needed intimacy, and utilizes these kin networks and community ties, then the blows associated with the aging process can be softened. Physical and emotional closeness among family members is an important source for adaptation in stress and illness.

CULTURAL CONSIDERATIONS IN HEALTH AND ILLNESS

Individuals cannot be understood apart from a knowledge of their sociocultural background. Every society is composed of groups who have different interests, beliefs, values, and attitudes. These form the basis of learned patterns of behaviors that are basically acquired through the family (Reinhardt & Quinn, 1973). Such patterns are likely to influence how individuals respond to others, as well as how they respond to health care. Leininger (1970) has stressed that "patients have a right to have their socio-cultural backgrounds understood in the same way they expect their physical and psychological needs to be recognized and understood" (p. 45).

The family, in their response to the illness or disability of a family member, will be influenced by cultural attitudes and values. An awareness of these norms further aids the health professional to understand the distinctive reactions that family members will have to the disability of the family member. For example, presuming that among varied ethnic groups disabled persons will show differences in their response to medical care, so the family will generally show corresponding differences in their utilization of resources to aid them to cope with the experience of disability.

Although the family is continually being shaped by all the social forces surrounding it, because of time demands imposed by treatment care it is difficult for the health professional to understand all these forces. Many practitioners can find useful the identification of those aspects of family life that can be particularly affected by cultural influences. Such an understanding can assist the worker to plan rehabilitation interventions. Leslie (1976) has suggested the following characteristics of family life, and to this list the authors have added the factors of roles and illness behavior:

1. *The family's value system*   This includes the family's social norms or rules according to which family life is structured.
2. *Geographical mobility*   Among many American families the home may not be a particular structure on a given block in a certain town, but is more a set of relationships, goals, and needs among its members. Approximately one family in every five in the United States moves each year (Leslie, 1976).
3. *Socialization*   This includes the family's financial resources, their utilization of community resources, their openness to changing social opportunities, and their financial means to afford social outlets.
4. *Parent-child interaction*   For certain ethnic families this interaction is bound up intimately with the nature of the interaction between the par-

ents; for other ethnic groups parental interaction as an influence upon the children is not that important. In many families women are expected to devote themselves to their children, and the daughters are raised to continue that pattern.

5. *The kin network*   This includes relationships among in-laws, visiting relatives, and mutual aid between related conjugal families. It is important for many ethnic families living in urban areas to have their home located fairly close to relatives, and close relationships among the families are a major source of solidarity.

6. *The family's achievement, religious, and work orientations*   For many ethnic families a strong commitment to work is apparent at both ends of the economic scale. Also, many ethnic families, as well as certain socioeconomic levels, may have more pronounced higher educational aspirations. The church has also been a conspicuous extrafamilial organization among many ethnic groups, and for those families is a steady source of solace and of moral standards.

7. *Roles of husband and wife*   Among many families with a strong, predominant ethnic background the duties of husband and wife are clearly demarcated, and the same is true of families belonging to certain socioeconomic classes. Yet other families who have not preserved these traditions have found that a mutuality of tasks is preferable, and often in such families the working wife and mother is looked upon as a family asset.

8. *Illness behavior*   Defined by Mechanic (1962) as "the ways in which given systems may be differentially perceived, evaluated and acted upon by different kinds of persons" (p. 189), ethnicity can be an important determinant of illness behavior. The utilization of medical care, cooperation with a treatment agent, and the availability of family support needed to direct many people toward needed medical care could depend on cultural norms, practices, and beliefs.

CONCLUSION

Understanding what is happening to the family today and being aware both of the changing roles in modern marriage and cultural considerations in health and illness will aid the professional to utilize helping skills in a relevant manner. Realizing that a marital relationship will develop through life stages, with each cycle bringing its own crisis, provides a framework for more feasible intervention. If the health professional is alert to the way these crises have been handled, a perspective is gained on how a present trauma can be managed effectively.

Added to this perspective is a need for an understanding of the impact of disability on the child, adult, and family, as well as a knowledge of the varied forms of family classification. These topics are discussed in the next two articles and developed more extensively in the succeeding chapters of this section.

Lawrence Fisher's article provides an extensive review of the literature on family classifications. The classification schemes are based on broad, encompassing dimensions. He shows the diversity of approaches when attempting to understand the family. His explanation of Voiland's classification has especially important prognostic implications for health professionals. For example, understanding the makeup of the inadequate family can suggest appropriate intervention approaches. In times of chronic illness this family particularly needs external supports, and the prognosis is good for family intactness and their help in treatment care when the external support is provided. Generally, however, Fisher's article strongly suggests that the "type" of family is an influence in itself on the disabled family member and, in turn, on rehabilitation efforts.

Clara Livsey's article is a comprehensive treatment of the impact of illness on family dynamics. She discusses extensively the importance of family role intactness and the development of coping patterns. As an introduction to the material that is elaborated upon in this section, it is an excellent beginning. Her review of the literature highlights family coping and adjustment patterns, and the reader will find unique and valuable her suggestions for clinical applications.

REFERENCES

Bane, M. J. *Here to stay*. New York: Basic Books, 1976.

Cavan, R. S. Family life cycle, United States. In R. S. Cavan (Ed.), *Marriage and family in the modern world—Readings,* pp. 91–104. New York: Thomas Y. Crowell Co., 1974.

Duvall, E. M. *Family development* (4th ed.). Philadelphia: J. B. Lippincott Co., 1971.

Havighurst, R. J. *Human development and education.* New York: Longmans, Green & Co., 1953.

Leininger, M. M. *Nursing and anthropology: Two worlds to blend,* pp. 45–47. New York: John Wiley & Sons, 1970.

Leslie, G. R. *The family in social context.* New York: Oxford University Press, 1976.

Mechanic, D. The concept of illness behavior. *Journal of Chronic Diseases,* 1962, *15,* 189–194.

Nordheimer, J. The family in transition. *The New York Times,* November 27, 1977, pp. 1, 4, 275.

Overs, R., & Healy, J. Stroke patients: Their spouses, families and the community. In A. B. Cobb (Ed.), *Medical and psychological aspects of disability,* pp. 87–117. Springfield, Ill.: Charles C Thomas Publisher, 1973.

Parsons, T., & Bales, T. R. *Family: Socialization and interaction process.* New York: The Free Press, 1955.

Peters, L. The family and family therapy. In J. E. Hall & B. R. Weaver (Eds.), *Nursing of families in crisis,* pp. 33–42. Philadelphia: J. B. Lippincott Co., 1974.

Power, P. Chronic illness and the family. *International Journal of Family Counseling,* 1977, *5*(1), 70–78.

Rakel, R. *Principles of family medicine.* Philadelphia: W. B. Saunders Co., 1977.

Reinhardt, A., & Quinn, M. *Family-centered community nursing.* St. Louis: C. V. Mosby Co., 1973.

Rhodes, S. A developmental approach to the life cycle of the family. *Social Casework,* 1977, May, 301–312.

Sussman, M. The isolated nuclear family: Fact or fiction? In M. Sussman (Ed.), *Sourcebook in marriage and the family,* pp. 25–29. Boston: Houghton Mifflin Co., 1974.

Swenson, C. *Introduction to interpersonal relations.* Glenview, Ill.: Scott, Foresman & Co., 1973.

ON THE CLASSIFICATION OF FAMILIES

Lawrence Fisher[1]

From the beginning of family therapy as a relatively distinct clinical approach, many have expressed the need for a useful and meaningful family typology. Several typologies have emerged over the course of the 20 years between the mid-50s and the mid-70s, and as the title indicates this article is a progress report, a review of these existing classification schemas.

Two strategic points need to be made at the outset. First, we shall focus on family classification as opposed to family diagnosis. The term *diagnosis* implies, to some extent, a distinction between sickness and health, or between normalcy and pathology. Such distinctions are particularly blurred in the field of family and couple therapy, and the single most discriminating characteristic between health and disease is often whether or not a family or couple has sought professional assistance. Clearly, what is needed is a system(s) of family classification and not an addition to the perennial controversy over what constitutes pathology. Second, it is apparent that families have been classified and pigeonholed on the basis of a plethora of variables, and the resulting literature spreads across a broad range of scientific questions and academic disciplines. Clearly, any single review could not be all-inclusive. With this in mind, this review will focus on those writings that are specifically geared toward creating a classification schema as opposed to those that do so indirectly or with an ancillary focus.

SYSTEMS OF CLASSIFICATION

Strauss (1973) has proposed a useful grouping of approaches to the diagnosis of individual patients that may be helpful as we review the rather complex field of family classification. The "topological diagnostic model" creates discrete categories of disorder, which implies some degree of mutual exclusiveness of causation as well as intervention techniques. The "dimensional model" does not categorize but instead attempts to locate individuals at some point within multidimensional space. Last, is the "mixed model" in which broad categories of disorder are identified and dimensions are specified within each. It may be helpful to keep these models in mind as each schema is reviewed. These models may provide a general frame of reference for reviewing systems of family classification.

Reprinted from *Archives of General Psychiatry 34,* pp. 424–433, ©1977, American Medical Association, with permission.

[1]From the Department of Psychiatry, University of Rochester School of Medicine and Dentistry, Rochester, NY.

Describing and comparing a large number of schemas of family classification requires some degree of organization and classification of the schemas themselves. Hill and Hansen (1960) have proposed a five-point outline of conceptual approaches to the family that includes the interactional, structural, situational, institutional, and developmental frameworks. Using this as a starting point, five major groups or approaches to classification have been selected based on a review of the existing literature. 1) "Style of Adaptation" incorporates the family's approach to the world, its pattern of handling stress, and its characteristic tendencies for dealing with crisis. It may involve broad family reactions or it may, on the other hand, relate to behaviors of individual members within the family context. 2) "Developmental Stage" characterizes some approach to denote a family developmental level. Some aspects of the developmental levels of individuals in the family can be used or alternatively, a broad, more abstract family base level may be established. 3) "Presenting Problem or Diagnosis of the Identified Patient" characterizes a popular approach to family classification and it has a relatively long history. Typically, the diagnosis or a particular aspect of the individual who brings the family to treatment becomes a criterion for grouping families. 4) "Family Theme or Dimension" is somewhat of a catch-all group. Schemas in this section differentiate families on the basis of some relatively objective dimension such as type of family power allocation, or specific kinds of family structure. 5) "Type of Marital Relationship" is the last of the five approaches to family classification. Since the marital relationship clearly sets the tone of the family's function, a decision has been made by the author to include types of marriages as one approach to the overall problem of family classification.

This five-point organization emerges as one possible logical structure in that each point applies to a major premise underlying the development of the respective schemas. The primary aim of these categories is to facilitate presentation, and while such an organization makes conceptual sense, other equally logical organizational structures could have been proposed.

Style of Adaptation

Three schemas are included in this first category, and all three relate to a classification of families based on an approach to the world or to a style of dealing with stress, either internal or external to the family.

Gehrke and Kirschenbaum (1967) proposed the repressive, delinquent, and suicidal family types. They suggest that children display symptoms when the family communicates a message that the survival of the unit is in some way dependent on them. "Survival myths" are an illusion that each member must maintain a given role to ensure family integrity and balance. 1) The repressive family contains the myth that the expression of feelings brings with it the threat of loss of love and possible abandonment, especially if other family members have opposing feelings. Affect is experienced in the children as tension, and they tend to manifest internalized aggressive symptoms. Conflict is never expressed and everyone must feel the same way about everything. 2) The survival myth in the delinquent family is that one parent cannot survive the sexual-aggressive impulses of the spouse, if expressed openly. The identified patient acts out these impulses to relieve the resulting tension, enabling the spouse to displace impulses and protect the weaker parent. 3) In the suicidal family, the myth states that unless the family remains whole, no member can survive. If one member leaves, destruction of all will occur. Role boundaries are blurred in these families and all conflict is eliminated with disqualified interaction and communication.

Richter (1974) described two general kinds of family disturbances: family symptom neurosis and family character neurosis. In the former, a family member drains off family tension by becoming "sick," and following such an event a remarkable calm often settles over the family. The scapegoat allows one part of the family to impose its unresolved problem on others, but if the scapegoat becomes "well," the "healthy" person falls victim. The second of Richter's two main categories is the family character neurosis, which occurs when the family as a group creates and maintains distorted perceptions and ideas in an effort to reduce family tension. The family becomes uniform in its adherence to an ideology or point of view such that the illness becomes egosyntonic with the family. No scapegoat emerges as such, although symptoms may appear in one member when family denial and distortion becomes too great. There are three subtypes of family character neurosis: 1) The anxiety-neurotic family builds a protective world that keeps out anything that is potentially anxiety-arousing. 2) The paranoid family builds a fortress. Instead of denying anxiety-arousing stimulation, it reconstructs the world and redirects intolerable stress outward toward other groups or individuals. 3) In the hysterical family, a central figure is selected who then assigns artificial roles to each family member in order to escape major family depression. The central figure is a stage manager, and the roles are part of a prescribed play for audiences outside the family.

Reiss (1971a, b, c) contrasts two types of disturbed families, based on a shared "view or explanation of its environment and the patterns or principles that govern its people and events." These family contructs relate to perceptual and cognitive abilities in individual family members and are also apparent in determining how members interact with each other in response to environmental situations: 1) The environment-sensitive family sees the world as enticing, predictable, manageable, and understandable. 2) Consensus-sensitive families see the world as unorganized and threatening. There are no laws or rules for explaining environmental events, and life is seen as outside of one's control.

These three authors, then, typify family classification based on style of adaptation. Richter's distinction between a family symptom neurosis and a family character neurosis may provide the format under which these three schemas may be subsumed. Gehrke and Kirschenbaum's repressive and suicidal families appear to be general family styles and could be categorized under Richter's family character neurosis heading. The delinquent family utilizes a clearly identified patient or scapegoat and sounds more appropriate within the family symptom neurosis group. In addition, Reiss's consensus-sensitive family designation could be placed within the character neurosis group as well.

Developmental Family Stage

Interest in developmental family stage emerged out of family sociology and it has only been recently that developmental concepts have been actively incorporated into clinically oriented family work. Glick and his colleagues (1955; Glick & Parke, 1965) have used population census data to study a number of social and economic variables as they relate to the development of the family over time. Glick has demonstrated that family stages are more useful than age of spouses in understanding and predicting a large number of family parameters. A main emphasis in the field has been a search for appropriate, reliable, and relevant family stage criteria.

A report of the National Conference on Family Life (Duvall & Hill, 1948) established seven stages, and Duvall (1967) revised these seven some 20 years later by broadening the developmental perspective to include Ericson's notion of developmental task. These seven stages appear to be the foundation on which much research has been generated: 1) beginning families; 2) child-bearing families (oldest child 30 months); 3) families with preschool children; 4) families with schoolchildren (oldest 6 to 13 years); 5) families with teenagers; 6) families as launching centers (first child gone to last child gone); 7) empty nest to retirement; and 8) retirement to death of one spouse.

Both Hill (1964) and Rodgers (1973) assert the need for clarification of the variations that exist in the broad middle range of family life. One approach (Rodgers, 1962) has been to include the age of the youngest child in the family and another has been to insert a new stage between Duvall's stages 5 and 6 (Hill, 1964).

Solomon (1973) has proposed one of the few clinically oriented life stage breakdowns that also includes a developmental task principle. Like Grunebaum and Bryant (1966), Solomon refers to each stage as posing a life crisis situation that must be resolved if adaptive growth is to continue. Stage 1—marriage—involves two tasks: ending each spouse's primary gratification with their own parents and redirecting these energies into the marriage. Stage 2—birth of first child and child bearing. This stage requires the solidification of the marriage as well as the establishment of parental roles. A frequent difficulty in this stage is the sacrificing of marital roles for parental roles. Stage 3—individuation of family members. This is the broad mid-range of family life in which the task becomes the continual modification of roles and the evolving individuation of each member over time. Stage 4—actual departure of the child. The primary task of this stage is the reworking of parent roles so as to establish a position as parents of adult children. Stage 5—integration of loss. This stage involves the acceptance of social, economic, and physical changes that occur in old age. Solomon has attempted the first steps of an application of family developmental theory to clinical process through his emphasis on the types of pathology that emerge when developmental tasks are not appropriately completed.

Grunebaum and Bryant (1966) have made a similar contribution by suggesting an epigenetic model. Their view is that a breakdown occurs within a family when it is unable to meet the developmental crisis posed by a particular stage within the family life cycle.

The use of a developmental stage format for the classification of families suggests at least two fundamental views vis-à-vis the nature of family pathology. The first, as evidenced by Haley's (1971) writings as well as by Duvall and other family sociologists, is that family pathology is derived from a combination of life stage events plus external circumstances. The second view is derived from more clinically oriented work; it suggests that pathology emerges as a function of the construction of the family system itself, and that the developmental stage simply colors its expression or defines the nature of its symptoms.

These two views emphasize somewhat different directions for clinical intervention. The first stresses environmental manipulation as well as involvement with specific family members. The second stresses more of a systems conceptualization of family pathology that leads to an intervention program involving all family members and dealing with the structure of the family unit. While this is clearly not a black-and-white distinction, it does serve to show that one's view of family development and its relationship to other aspects of family life will directly relate to therapeutic strategy.

A review of the severe developmental classifications presented above indicates some similarity, with differences being more in emphasis than in actual content. How useful these particular stages are in clinical work is yet to be demonstrated. While most family clinicians incorporate some developmental notions in their approach to families, there has as yet been no demonstration of how existing family stage formats empirically relate to family pathology.

Initial Problem or Diagnosis of the Identified Patient

As implied by the title, this section will focus on those family classification systems that distinguish among families on the basis of the individual diagnosis, initial problem, or some other aspect of the identified patient.

Serrano et al. (1962) presented a four-point schema based on the function the identified patient serves in keeping the family stabilized: 1) Infantile maladjustment reaction in adolescence. The schizophrenic teenagers in this group serve the function of providing a needy parent with a full-time occupation. The parents tend to hide their lifelong friction, but there are frequent outbursts, usually over tangential matters. The ill child becomes the eventual outlet for the mother, who identifies him as the "sick one," and this process saves other siblings from a similar fate. 2) Childish maladjustment reaction in adolescence. These are arrogant, aggressive, negative, and impulsive adolescents, with a penchant for irresponsible behavior leading to guilt and shame in the parents and other adults. Fathers in these families tend to see their sons as intruders, and by functioning somewhat passively such fathers are reluctant to assert leadership or authority. The adolescents tend to act out this problem by confronting their father's attitudes and by becoming unlikeable to others. Treatment often includes bringing the father back into the family. 3) Juvenile maladjustment reaction in adolescence. These are anxious and tense adolescents with many somatic complaints and poor school performance. Their fathers are authoritarian and aggressive as a cover for their own feelings of inferiority. The children are seen as rivals, and any challenge or expression of assertiveness on the child's part is met by overreaction; hence the children internalize their hostilities to prevent guilt and reduce the challenge to their father. 4) Preadolescent maladjustment reaction in adolescence. These older adolescents have a relatively acute onset of rebellious and antisocial behavior. The negative behavior tends to reflect an overidentification with the peer group at a time when other youngsters are becoming more individualized. Parents tend to be socially oriented and they are also passive-aggressive critics. The four types described by Serrano et al. tend to emerge with no general set or model underlying the schema. Hence, these patterns tend to "hold together" on a pragmatic clinical level rather than on a conceptual or theoretical level.

Goldstein et al. (1968) presented a more unified classification system, or at least directed effort at creating a classification system based on family concepts. The referred adolescents and their families were grouped into the following types based on the behavior of the adolescents themselves: 1) Aggressive antisocial. These are externalizing youngsters who have difficulty restraining impulses, have some degree of inner tension, and tend to act out conflicts. 2) Active family conflict. These are youngsters with inner tension and somatic complaints but who primarily are disrespectful of parents, are belligerent, defensive, and antagonistic as well. The negative behavior is focused inside the family almost exclusively. 3) Passive-negative. These adolescents do poorly in school, are sullen and somewhat depressed, and are not disruptive but express indirected, passive hostility and defiance. 4) Withdrawn-socially isolated. These are fearful teenagers who show marked signs of anxiety and tension, who are withdrawn and isolated socially, and who are highly dependent on one or both parents. This four-way grouping is based on two underlying bipolar dimensions: locus of conflict, that is, focus inside the home or outside as well; and overt versus covert activity as expressed in pathology, that is, aggressive acting out as opposed to a passive-negative stance. The authors demonstrated that direct and intrusive forms of social influence by parents are associated with aggressive-antisocial adolescents, whereas rational techniques of control are associated with active family conflict.

The Serrano and Goldstein typologies are descriptions of adolescent behavior rather than styles of family functioning. The adolescents described by these two authors can be combined into two generic clusters. Cluster 1 includes Serrano's juvenile maladjustment reaction and Goldstein's passive-negative groups. Adolescents in this cluster are described as passive and depressed; they display somatic complaints. They tend to come from constricted families where indirect methods of emotional expression are common; and in at least several cases, the fathers are somewhat dominant and controlling as a cover for their own feelings of inferiority. Cluster 2 includes Serrano's childish maladjustment reaction and Goldstein's aggressive-antisocial groups. These adolescents are depicted as acting out and irresponsible, and they tend to get into trouble at home, at school, and often with the police. They can be hostile, aggressive, and at times destructive. From description at least, clusters 1 and 2 may reflect the well-known internalizer and externalizer dimensions of personality, respectively. Internalizers direct anxiety back to the self, and, as would be expected, they come from families where acknowledgment of a variety of issues on an overt level is prohibited. Externalizers act out impulses directly and tend to come from families where parental control is reduced or where the family has lost its direction due to overt conflict, usually within the marital dyad. Additional support for this dichotomy comes from the more empirical schemas of Jenkins (1968) and Waring and Ricks (1965).

Beavers et al. (1975) classified adolescent pathology into four groups: healthy, neurotic, behavior disorder, and psychotic. Their clinical and rating scale data indicated differences between midrange families, that is, families with neurotic and behavioral disorder children, and the extreme groups, that is healthy and psychotic, as well as differences between the midrange families themselves. In the midrange families 1) separation and individuation is successful; 2) ambivalence, anger, and sexuality are viewed with disdain; 3) an abstract code or morality is adhered to, often personified in a particular person—the grandparent, religious leader; 4) a rigid rule system is adopted that often leads to scapegoating; and 5) the rigidity resulting from the tight rule system often leads to power struggles between the parents. Neurotic and behavior disorder families were distinguished in the following ways: 1) Both family types adhere to rigid and authoritarian rules. In the neurotic group, the parents form a coalition to maintain enforcement of family roles in such a way that one spouse is dominant and the other subservient. In the behavior disorder group the need for adherence to a highly structured family system is the same, but there is no parental coalition to maintain it. 2) The neurotic family uses repression to rid itself of unacceptable feelings and thoughts as prescribed by the moral code. Hence, these impulses are unconscious and are not seen as part of the self. In the behavior disorder family, denial and projection are used, but frequently such defenses are ineffective and open rule breaking occurs. Hence, the impulses are identified as part of the self and efforts are placed on their control by internal and external means. 3) Last, neurotic families have few crises and their efforts at maintaining status and power are successful. Behavior disorder families display frequent crises and these often serve to maintain equilibrium by pointing to an increased need to control and restrict impulses.

Riskin and Faunce (1970) utilized severity and number of family problems to classify their family sample into five groups. Group A are multi-problem families where several neurotic and psychotic level difficulties ranging from severe psychosis to underachievement in school were present. These families disagree more than they agree; there is a potential for explosiveness; and the tone of the families is one of unfriendliness, chaos, and competition. Group B are "constricted" families with two or three labeled difficulties. Problems are on a neurotic as opposed to a psychotic level, but more than one family member is affected. They are "compulsively clear" and concise, although they cannot stick to a topic for any length of time. The mood is one of depression, and spontaneity is severely reduced. Group C has acting out or underachieving child-labeled problems. Children appear quiet, sullen, and argumentative. Deeply rooted struggles are covert, clarity of communication is low, and often one member is scapegoated. Group D contains families with significant but undiagnosed problems. They are quite diffuse and do not stand out on their own. Group E contains well-functioning, normal families who are clear, rational, affectively expressive, spontaneous, tolerant of differences, humorous, and so on. The significance of this study is not only its establishment of measures for the assessment of family interaction, but its classification system based on what may be termed the degree of pathology as defined by initial problems.

Family Theme or Dimension

The classification schemas presented so far are based on broad, encompassing dimensions that incorporate major thrusts in thinking about families. The schemas presented in this section are very much of a potpourri. They tend to tap major themes that emerge in clinical interviews or to divide families on the basis of a variety of theoretical concepts.

Ackerman (1956, 1958) presented one of the first typologically based classification systems. He collected extensive clinical data on 50 referred families and on that basis developed seven family types: 1) The externally isolated family is isolated and displays a failure of emotional integration into the community, instead tending to redirect energies internally. 2) The externally integrated family, in contrast, displays overactive participation in the community, perhaps due to a failure in internal unity and gratification. 3) The internally unintegrated family is characterized by a split between the parents and an alliance between at least one parent and one child. There is usually a good deal of hostility that maintains the split, and the resulting isolation keeps the inappropriate pairing in operation. 4) The unintended family is characterized by a mutually protective alliance between the parents. Of importance is the satisfaction of parental needs, often at the expense of the children. 4) In the immature family, the immaturity of the marital couple creates a breakdown in the boundaries separating parents and grandparents. Each spouse tries to parentify the other and both remain dependent on their own parents. 6) The deviant family displays marked rebellion against the standards of the community and they adopt somewhat deviant goals and values. 7) The disintegrated or regressed family is marked by open conflict, hostility, and lack of integration such that a potential for breakup of the family is great. Ackerman's system for classifying families is difficult to comment on from a conceptual point of view because each of the seven types appears to tap a somewhat different family dimension. The externally isolated family and the externally integrated family deal with boundary or directional issues, the internally unintegrated family and the disintegrated or regressed family pertain to family organization and structure, and the remaining groups deal with level of parental maturity, egocentrism, and conflict. Although these seven may be a meaningful division of family types, the lack of a useful way to conceptualize and structure them reduces their applicability in theory or model building. Ackerman's main contribution in these early schema was to present relatively clear and concise family types before a clinically based system or structural vocabulary was even developed.

Fallding (1961) interviewed 38 urban Australian families to establish types of adaptive or normal families using the dimension of internal versus external focus. The adaptation family is characterized by each member claiming a broad area of personal life outside of the family. In the identification family parents at times overfocus their personal interests and energies on the family itself, and a premium is placed on contributing to a positive family atmosphere. The false-identification family falls between these two, and one or both parents have difficulty deciding what role extrafamily activities should play in family life.

Voiland's (1961, 1962) work is significant insofar as it is the only extensive empirical study aimed exclusively at establishing a system of disordered family types that includes prognostic indicators. The schema is based on the nature of psychosocial dysfunction in the family using highly specific assessment criteria. An individual, socially based dynamic focus, as opposed to an interactional focus, is maintained and pathology is defined as a breakdown of social functioning as manifested by a failure in fulfilling the requirements demanded by either society or the family.

Four family types were identified: 1) The perfectionistic family is characterized by their high expectations to conform to social rules and mores, and to avoid mistakes at all costs. Prognosis is favorable, especially since the adults assume responsibility and value intervention. 2) The inadequate family is immature and relies on the presence and support of others to maintain internal stability. They anticipate poorly and are unable to be self-reliant in times of even mild distress. Specific problems tend to emerge in financial management, child rearing, and especially in issues to do with pregnancy and family planning. Prognosis is good and treatment often focuses on training in parental roles and in bolstering certain parts of family structure. 3) The egocentric family seeks the goal of personal status and prestige. Family members become important to each other only insofar as they serve as need gratifiers; they become objects, not people. Friction and hostility dominate and intimacy is lacking, for each acts as a means to an end for the other. Contact with an agency usually is sought by a spouse as a hostile, retaliatory act to the other, or a child will act out the conflict outside the home. Because of the primitiveness of the need gratification pattern, prognosis is guarded. 4) The unsocial family has difficulties establishing adult relationships and impulses are often acted on directly, leading to psychosis or delinquency. These are chaotic families where responsibility is shunted from one to another, major decisions occur impulsively, work records are poor, and home management is weak. Prognosis is described by Voiland as fair as long as contact is continued. Treatment is often on a crisis basis, with maintenance and support provided as needed to ward off the destructive and chaotic aspects of the family.

Markowitz and Kadis (1964) classified families on the basis of "centerness" or the person on whom the family revolves. In father-centered families, the father attains major importance and his gratification becomes primary. Similarly, in mother-centered families, the mother assumes the magical quality of the all-giving female and the maintenance of her position in the family is crucial. In child-centered families, the child and his or her welfare seems to hold the family together and gives it status in either the community, with the extended family, or alternatively by the child's definition of motherhood or fatherhood in the parents, which is highly valued.

Last, family-centered families place an overemphasis on family cohesion, and individual needs are often sacrificed for the sake of the larger unit.

Wertheim (1973) made predictions about the response to family treatment on the basis of three dimensions: morphostasis, morphogenesis, and family system. Morphostasis refers to those aspects of family life that produce stability and solidarity, whereas morphogenesis relates to those aspects that permit growth and change within the family system. These concepts are introduced in an effort to broaden systems theory to include growth and change as inherent in family life. Consensual morphostasis refers to a consensually validated distribution of power. Forced morphostasis relates to an enforced power system, not consensually validated. Spontaneous morphogenesis is defined as the family's expected adaptive change in the face of life events; induced morphogenesis refers to a capacity for change when such change is an induced intervention, as in treatment.

The family systems dimension is divided into three types: 1) open family systems are articulated families with a network of subsystems connected by permeable boundaries; 2) closed families systems are rigid settings where rules are dogma and boundaries are not open; and 3) externally open systems operate freely within the environment but communication is minimal within the system. Its opposite, the internally open system, is also described. These three concepts, then, lead to a description of eight theoretical family types. At present, however, there are no clinical or empirical data to support Wertheim's typology, and hence the eight-point typology will not be presented here. The classification system does propose, however, a theoretical model for the prediction of differential response to family treatment in terms of accessibility, duration of treatment, and probable outcome. It deserves concentrated clinical testing, and even if the specifics are not fully supported it should provide the impetus for the development of more elaborate schemas.

Ford and Rarrick (1974) described "family rules" that reflect the overriding life style of the family and the manner in which they approach the world. Five family rules or styles are described: 1) Children come first. These are somewhat chaotic child-focused families in which both parents have careers, although the wife often sacrifices hers for the children. Children are seen as attempts toward intimacy between the spouses, but this is not successful since only the children can receive the desired emotional closeness. Parental gratification can only be received by becoming childlike and burdening the other spouse. 2) Two against the world. This situation develops when two people view the world with fear and they collude together to join hands in mutual defense. 3) Share and share alike. This reflects the family where a true partnership never develops, but instead, the spouses take turns being parent and child. 4) Every man for himself. This occurs in families where the spouses are joined not for emotional reasons but to achieve a goal or complete a task. Lack of trust is common, and individuals use others for what they can get. 5) Until death do us part. This occurs in families where dissolution of the family is sensed, yet that kind of parting is seen only as a consequence of death. So, everyone loves hopefully but pessimistically and the anger and frustration lead to bitterness. Children tend to continue this pattern and homicide and suicide are common. Because the above rules are unstated, their formulation can be directly related to therapeutic techniques, and Ford and Rarrick suggest that therapy should focus on the constant, explicit restatement of the diffuse, inappropriate rule. Hence, in this case, family classification becomes directly related to treatment technique.

Minuchin (1974) described a bipolar dimension on which to classify families: disengaged versus enmeshed. Enmeshed families turn in on themselves and the boundaries around members of subsystems of the family become blurred. Disengaged families have rigid boundaries, where contact across subsystems and between people is reduced. These terms can apply as a descriptor of entire families or parts of families, and the status of boundary integrity can vary developmentally as well as over the course of treatment.

Some interesting similarities emerge among those schemas reviewed in this section. First, both Voiland and Ackerman refer to uncontrolled, almost chaotic families entitled unsocial and disintegrated, respectively. Second, Minuchin's emphasis on the establishment of appropriate boundaries with sufficient permeability and stability is reflected clearly in Ackerman's isolated, integrated, and unintegrated families.

Third, Voiland's egocentric and Ackerman's unintended families both reflect the focus on parental need gratification, often at the expense of the children; whereas their respective inadequate and immature families seem to reflect the constant need for external support in the maintenance of family equilibrium. Fourth, is the similarity among Ackerman's externally isolated, Ford and Rarrick's "two against the world," and Markowitz and Kadis's family-centered families—all of which reflect internally focused families which see the outside world as a threat to their very existence as a unit and which tie family members together in a rigid, unhealthy knot. Last, Markowitz and Kadis's child-centered and Ford and Rarrick's "children come first" families describe situations in which the children assume unusual importance and prominence in the maintenance of family life. So while each of these authors appears to describe families on the basis of somewhat different dimensions, concepts, or points of view, the descriptions of family types are quite similar in many respects.

Types of Marital Relationships

Although types of marital relatedness have been mentioned in the classification schemas described above, the emphasis was in most cases family-oriented as opposed to couple-focused. Those systems reviewed in this section will focus on attempts at classifying marriages alone, without necessary reference to broader family issues. The classification systems included in this section fall into three rough groupings: 1) those based on the dynamics of the individual spouses; 2) those relating to types or patterns of conflict and associated power within the marriage; and 3) those focusing on broad types of "normal" marital relationships.

Individual Dynamics   A small group of authors have described particular patterns of marriage based on the individual dynamics of each spouse. Mittlemann (1944, 1956) described five complementary marital styles based on this individual dynamic model: 1) A spouse is aggressive and dominating to the point of humiliating the partner, whereas the other spouse is passive and submissive. 2) Emotional detachment in one spouse (usually the wife) leads to a craving for support in the other. 3) Intense competition for domination exists between the spouses, yet each is frightened at the prospect of losing the other. 4) Extreme helplessness in one spouse occurs in conjunction with extreme considerateness in the other. The weak partner requires an omnipotent mate, which, when not realized, leads to more depression and neediness. 5) Alternating sequences of helplessness and assertiveness occur in each spouse. As can be seen in this brief summary of five marital types, Mittlemann appears to focus on issues on dominance and need satisfaction.

Pittman and Flomenhauft (1970) described the "dollhouse marriage" in which inadequacy in a spouse is required for the maintenance and stability of the marriage. Attempts at altering this somewhat one-sided relationship may lead to destruction of the marriage, raising the point that structural changes in marital therapy are not always exclusive goals.

Conflict and Power   Conflict and its resolution is often related to marital stress and, hence, marital therapy. With this in mind, two authors have classified couples on the basis of type of conflict or style of handling conflict.

Gehrke and Moxon (1962) described five marital patterns based on the content of the conflict: 1) Masculine-feminine roles. In this marriage, the spouses tend to reverse sex roles, the wife being relatively more masculine and the husband relatively more feminine. Conflict results from the resulting somewhat ambivalent stance each spouse takes. 2) Sadomasochistic conflict. Here, the male's hostile and negative feelings toward women are expressed through the marriage. Since the wife has a poor view of herself to begin with, she submits to the abuse. In the 3) detached, demanding conflict, both spouses are immature and require parenting from the other without demanding anything in return. In the 4) oral dependent conflict, both partners require rather primitive need gratification, and both are dependent, somewhat helpless people. Last is the 5) neurotic illness conflict, in which the wife displays pervasive and diffuse somatic complaints and appears helpless while the husband dotes in an attempt to fill her every need. He does so out of his own feelings of inadequacy.

Raush et al. (1974) evoked conflict in newlywed couples and they described two types of couples. In discordant couples, conflict becomes a battle of wills where, depending on the content of the conflict, one or the other spouse will assume a coercive attacking stance. Disruption and escalation result. Harmonious couples have less heated exchanges, where in one subtype conflict is easily settled, and in another the couple tends to avoid the conflict altogether. It should be noted that none of these couples were referred by a clinic and therefore they may not demonstrate more extreme forms of marital distress.

Power has been an important dimension on which couples have been classified. Because it is abstract, power is most often assessed by the observation of conflict and its eventual resolution as well as by patterns of decision making. Hence, power as a dimension for the classification of families and couples needs to be seen as a higher-order variable, conceptualized one step from observable data.

Lederer and Jackson (1968) described three types of power relationships: In the symmetrical relationship, differences between spouse roles are reduced and each has equal power in all areas. The complementary relationship is characterized by the more traditional dominant/nondominant marital pattern. Last, in the parallel relationship, the couple sets up a rather elaborate set of roles that vary between symmetrical and complementary relationships, depending on the context of the decision making.

Zelditch (1964) described eight types of power allocation in families and couples. He suggests that such a classification must take into account Parsons and Bales (1955) concept of multiple power structures. His view is that it is rather simplistic to believe that all power is exercised according to one hierarchy regardless of content. Different aspects of family functioning call for different power structures and alliances, a view similar to Minuchin's (1974).

If indeed more than one power structure is in operation, then Zelditch suggests that either decisions are made jointly by the couple or they are made separately by one spouse alone. These marriages are referred to as colleagueship and autonomic, respectively. If, on the other hand, a single power structure is in operation, decisions can be also made jointly or by one partner alone. In the former case, this leads to husband-dominant, equal partnership, or wife-dominant marriages. In the latter case where one partner makes the decision, the results are patriarchal, interchangeable roles, and matriarchal marriages.

Jackson (1959) described four kinds of marital relationships based on power and dominance: 1) A stable-satisfactory relationship occurs when a couple explicitly and overtly reaches agreement about who is in control of specific areas of family life. 2) An unstable-satisfactory relationship is usually temporary and occurs during periods of change when the couple is in the process of working out a definition of the relationship. 3) An unstable-unsatisfactory relationship contains virtually no completed transactions, and although both parties desire some sense of definition, each maneuvers to control the other and denies the action at the same time. Psychosomatic and hysterical symptoms often result. 4) The stable-unsatisfactory relationship is withdrawn, cold, and distant in an attempt to preclude any issue that might make its instability overt. A united, pseudomutual front is often presented in an effort to avoid potential conflict.

Normal Couples   Cuber and Harroff (1965) undertook an extensive study of nonreferred couples in an effort to determine if social and financial success is related to marital success. Using a detailed open-ended interview technique, the authors established five types of marital relatedness: 1) Conflict habituated. This most frequent type is characterized by well-controlled but rather pervasive conflict that is kept under the surface but emerges in the privacy of the home. Physical violence rarely occurs and caring is only delivered around periods of crisis. 2) Devitalized. These are couples who share a great deal of sexual and emotional intimacy in the early years of the marriage but who lose their closeness in middle life. Interests are centered outside the family and the marital relationship is restless but devoid of open conflict. 3) Passive-congenial. This group is characterized by apathy and restlessness but, unlike the devitalized couples, the passive-congenial couples never had the emotional closeness to begin with. The marriage was formed intentionally for a variety of reasons but there was never any deep caring. 4) Vital. There is in these couples a psychological bond and relatedness that ties their lives together. Disagreements are settled quickly and conflict is avoided. 5) Total. This is somewhat of an idealized group who share almost all aspects of life in a deep and vital way. It should be kept in mind that these are couples who do not experience sufficient stress in their relationship to consider therapy, separation, or divorce. If one can generalize from Cuber and Harroff's sample, it would appear that the vast majority of successful middle-class people have constricted, conflict-ridden, or zestless marriages. This is a sobering realization in terms of understanding baselines of marital life in American Society.

Ryder (1970) established 21 patterns or types of marriages using a large sample of nonreferred newlywed couples. Five conceptual dimensions were established on the basis of a factor analysis of extensive interview and paper-and-pencil schedules: husband's potency or affectiveness; husband's degree of impulse control; degree of wife's dependency; wife's attitude toward sex; and wife's orientation toward the marriage. Twenty-one marital patterns were identified and, because of space limitations, the reader is referred to Ryder's original article for a complete description. Ryder's approach is useful from a methodological point of view in that empirically demonstrable dimensions were converted into scalable, nonreferred marital groups.

A DESCRIPTIVE COMPARISON OF FAMILY SUBTYPES

It is apparent that no single family nosology is presently available that will serve to pragmatically unify the various purposes that need to be served. Regardless of how a family schema has been classified, however, and regardless of what dimensions have been used, certain similarities among the descriptions of family types emerge. From a review of all the schemas presented above, six clusters of family types seem to fall together. They were created by comparing the subtypes of each family schema with each other and grouping together those subtypes that, by my understanding of the original authors' description, displayed a reasonable degree of similarity. Figure 1 lists each family cluster, the original author, and the specific family subtype involved.

It should be kept in mind that no concept or model underlies these six clusters; they tend to fall together only on a simple, descriptive basis. Each family cluster contains an entire range of psychopathology, although because most of these were derived from samples of referred families, each implies a maladaptive tendency or direction. The descriptions of each cluster are overviews of the several subtypes included. Although each subtype may not fit the overall description totally, sufficient similarities were present to warrant inclusion.

Constricted Family Types

These families are characterized by an excessive restriction of a major aspect of family emotional life, such as the expression of anger, negative affect, or ambivalence. Affect is then internalized into anxiety, depression, and somatic complaints. The passive, depressed, internalized child or young adult is often the presenting patient. There may be a concerted effort to protect a "weak" or "ill" family member or family relationship, and adults with particular problems of low self-esteem or past emotional difficulty are often present. Outcome of family treatment is primarily dependent on the degree of constriction. Following some of Wertheim's (1973) views on highly constricted families, family intervention is often viewed by the family with antagonism and resistance such that individual or couple approaches may be more beneficial in the long run. In families with mild to moderate degrees of constriction, a family approach often has favorable results. Such families tolerate the move toward openness and respond to more direct forms of communication and feeling expression.

Family Clusters

1. Constricted Family Types
  1. Gehrke & Kirschenbaum—Repressive
  2. Goldstein et al—Passive-negative
  3. Serrano et al—Juvenile maladjustment reaction
  4. Voiland—Perfectionistic

2. Internalized Family Types
  1. Ackerman—Externally isolated
  2. Fallding—Identification
  3. Ford & Rarrick—Two against the world
  4. Gehrke & Kirschenbaum—Suicidal
  5. Jackson—Stable-unsatisfactory
  6. Markowitz & Kadis—Family-centered
  7. Minuchin—Enmeshed
  8. Reiss—Consensus-sensitive
  9. Richter—Family character neurosis

3. Object-focused Family Types
  1. Child-Focused:
    a. Ford & Rarrick—Children come first
    b. Markowitz & Kadis—Child-centered
  2. Externally Focused
    a. Ackerman—Externally integrated
    b. Cuber & Harroff—Devitalized
    c. Fallding—Adaptation
  3. Self-focused
    a. Ackerman—Unintended
    b. Ford & Rarrick—Every man for himself
    c. Voiland—Egocentric

4. Impulsive Family Types
  1. Gehrke & Kirschenbaum—Delinquent
  2. Goldstein et al—Aggressive-antisocial
  3. Serrano et al—Childish maladjustment reaction

5. Childlike Family Types
  1. Ackerman—Immature
  2. Gehrke & Moxon—Detached, demanding & oral
    dependent
  3. Voiland—Inadequate

6. Chaotic Family Types
  1. Ackerman—Disintegrated
  2. Voiland—Unsocial
  3. Riskin & Faunce—Group A

Figure 1. Family clusters.

Internalized Family Types

Such families are inwardly focused and tend to view the world with fear, pessimism, hostility, and threat. A constant state of vigilance maintains the boundary between the internal and external world in a rather stable state of defense. The family has a well-defined role structure with strongly held values and powerful sanctions for misbehavior. Although members may stray from the fold, the threat of possible family disintegration and fears of chaos pull them back before complete separation occurs. Family loyalty runs high and there is often a pseudomutual relationship between the parents. Internalized families view the family therapist cautiously and hesitantly as an outsider and an intruder into the fortress of the family. Prognosis is variable depending on the thickness of the fortress walls and the therapist's patience and perseverance in tolerating small gains over long periods of time.

Object-Focused Families

These families are characterized by an overemphasis or excessive reliance on the children, the outside community, or the self. 1) In the child-focused subgroup, the children serve in some way as a link between the spouses, maintaining their relationship as a guilt reaction to unacceptable desires for parenting from the other spouse. Often there is competition between the spouses for the children's affection and life is guided by decisions made ostensibly "because of the children." 2) In the externally focused subgroup, family members turn outside of the family for areas of interest and sources of support. Hypothetically, what is lacking inside is sought outside. 3) Members of the self-focused subgroup stay together to fulfill personal needs, and the emphasis is clearly tipped in favor of self as opposed to family issues. Family cohesiveness and emotional closeness are low, and people are used for personal purposes, often resulting in explosions of anger and hostility when personal needs go unmet.

The child and externally focused subgroups indicate an inappropriate reliance on other sources for need satisfaction. The emphasis on children or external sources may point to a family system unable to effectively fulfill the needs of its members. The self-focused group may point to a different dynamic insofar as the personal ability to delay gratification and to gain for the self by giving to others is lacking. All three groups point to an overemphasis in one area of gratification, whether it be due to deficiencies in other areas or to certain individual personality dynamics.

The prognosis for object-focused families in family therapy is generally good. The child and externally focused subgroups display a sufficient degree of internal structure and integration for favorable outcome. Motivation for treatment is primarily dependent on the willingness of the marital pair to renegotiate the marital relationship in terms of commitment and allegiance. One runs the risk of possible separation and divorce in such families, because as the therapist points out the excessive reliance on external sources or on the children the couple may begin to realize that there is little left of an emotional relationship between them. The prognosis for the self-focused subgroup is more variable, for such individuals may not be able to tolerate sharing the therapists or they may need to first work through a variety of personal issues in individual treatment.

Impulsive Family Types

The majority of these families are characterized by a troublesome adolescent or young adult who displaces his or her parental-based anger onto the community and acts on feelings in a socially undesirable way. Alternatively, many of these adolescents act out the parental conflict or they become the "expressor" for an angry but constricted adult. In any case, the identified patient is brought to treatment by the police, school officials, or exasperated parents who feel helpless to exert functional controls. Family therapy would appear to be a preferred approach to this kind of problem. The acting out against parents or the adolescent's role as a voice for marital or other difficulties implicates other family members and requires their major participation in treatment. Prognosis, however, is probably more dependent on the characteristics of the family than on the presence of acting out behavior alone.

Childlike Family Types

These are often young families or families where the adults have never thoroughly separated from their family of origin. They are needy, dependent people who rely on their own parents, the community, or other sources for emotional support, decision making, and parenting of their own children. Some are simply immature and frightened, although capable; others are inadequate in ability and aptitude. The presence of major and perhaps destructive emotional ties between first and second generations opens a number of possibilities for family treatment, including single- or multiple-generation sessions. Where the issue is one of inadequacy and not immaturity, however, such couples may need continued "parentlike" assistance from the therapist in the form of long-term supportive work; chances for major improvement leading toward totally independent functioning are slim.

Chaotic Family Test

This somewhat rarer group is composed of poorly structured and decompensating families where chronic psychosis and delinquency are often rampant. There are few rules for anything, reliability of family members is quite low, and family members are constantly leaving and reentering the family. These families are often of low social class where undependability keeps adults unemployed and living standards variable. The lack of integration and the marked instability of these families make treatment outcome extremely variable. This is often due to a lack of commitment to the family unit.

CONCLUSIONS

Progress in family classification has developed by collecting large amounts of varied data on relatively large samples of families. Then, by a process of theoretical, clinical, or statistical inference, a hypothesis or two has emerged about how families tend to "fall together." At present, however, insufficient data and experience are available to consider the establishment of a typological classification system as defined by Strauss (1973), one that proposes clearly distinct family types that are mutually exclusive and that assume distinct causes. Although many clinicians have displayed some degree of similarity in their definitions of given family types, we are still at a descriptive level and not sufficiently sophisticated to propose discrete family entities. An alternative, however, is a more thorough adherence to Strauss's dimensional or multidimensional model, which would classify families on the basis of previously specified, well-defined dimensions; and then a determination of the relationships of that classification to a limited number of dependent measures (see Riskin and Faunce, 1970).

The development of a single, prominent classification schema, however, may be more restrictive than helpful. I speak here to the nagging uncertainties and inappropriatenesses of traditional unitary diagnosis to many settings and circumstances. As an addition to the proposal for adopting a dimensional model, we may need to focus on developing several mini-classification schemas rather than aiming for a single classification system. Given kinds of research and clinical endeavors require the inclusion of different family variables, and perhaps no single system should be sought. Our aim may be to focus on narrower, more problem-oriented systems that will display more limited application but that will be based on more solid ground.

The present review, however, demonstrates that family classification on given predefined dimensions can be helpful in both clinical and research efforts. It also points out the fact that certain similarities in types of systems and kinds of families and couples is emerging and that these efforts call for continued study. Coupled with the increasing problems of insurance, record keeping, and governmental needs, research in this area must continue on an accelerated basis.

REFERENCES

Ackerman, M. W. *The psychodynamics of family life.* New York: Basic Books, 1958.
Ackerman, M. W. *American Journal of Orthopsychiatry,* 1956, *26,* 68–78.
Beavers, W. R., Lewis, J., Gossett, J. T., et al. *Family systems and individual functioning: Mid-range families.* Read before the American Psychiatric Association meeting, Anaheim, California, May, 1975.
Cuber, J. F., & Harroff, P. B. *The significant Americans: A study of sexual behavior among the affluent.* New York: Appleton-Century-Crofts, 1965.
Duvall, E. R. *Family development.* Philadelphia: J. B. Lippincott Co., 1967.
Duvall, E. R., & Hill, R. *Report of the committee on the dynamics of interaction.* Prepared for the National Conference on Family Life, Washington, D.C.
Fallding, H. The family and the idea of a cardinal role. *Human Relations,* 1961, *14,* 329–350.
Ford, F. R., & Rarrick, J. Family rules: Family life styles. *American Journal of Psychiatry,* 1974, *44,* 61–69.

Gehrke, S., & Kirschenbaum, M. Survival patterns in family conjoint therapy. *Family Process*, 1967, *6*, 67–80.

Gehrke, S., and Moxon, J. Diagnostic classification and treatment techniques in marriage counseling. *Family Process*, 1962, *1*, 253–264.

Glick, P. C. The life cycle of the family. *Marriage and Family Living*, 1955, *18*, 3–9.

Glick, P. C., & Parke, R. New approaches in studying the life cycle of the family. *Demography*, 1965, *2*, 187–202.

Goldstein, M. J., Judd, L. L., Rodnick, E. H., et al. A method for studying social influence and coping patterns within families of disturbed adolescents. *Journal of Nervous and Mental Disease*, 1968, *147*, 233–251.

Grunebaum, H. V., & Bryant, C. M. The theory and practice of the family diagnostic: Theoretical aspects and resident education. *Psychiatric Research Report*, 1966, *20*, 150–162.

Haley, J. A review of the family therapy field. In J. Haley (Ed.), *Changing families: A family therapy reader*. New York: Grune & Stratton, 1971.

Hill, R. Methodological issues in family development research. *Family Process*, 1964, *3*, 186–205.

Hill, R., & Hansen, D. A. The identification of conceptual frameworks utilized in family study. *Marriage and Family Living*, 1960, *22*, 299–312.

Jackson, D. D. Family interaction, family homeostasis, and some implications for conjoint family psychotherapy. In J. H. Masserman (ed.), *Individual and family dynamics*. New York: Grune & Stratton, 1959.

Jenkins, R. L. The varieties of children's behavioral problems in family dynamics. *American Journal of Psychiatry*, 1968, *124*, 1440–1445.

Lederer, W., & Jackson, D. D. *The mirages of marriage*. New York: W. W. Norton & Co., 1968.

Markowitz, M., & Kadis, A. L. Parental interaction as a determinant in social growth of the individual in the family. *International Journal of Social Psychiatry*, 1964, *10*, congress issue.

Minuchin, S. *Families and family therapy*. Cambridge: Harvard University Press, 1974.

Mittelmann, B. Complementary neurotic reactions in intimate relationships. *Psychoanalytic Quarterly*, 1944, *13*, 479–491.

Mittlemann, B. Analysis of reciprocal neurotic patterns in family relationships. In V. W. Eisenstein (Ed.), *Neurotic interaction in marriage*. New York: Basic Books, 1956.

Parsons, T., & Bales, R. F. *Family, socialization, and interaction process*. Glencoe, Ill.: The Free Press, 1955.

Pittman, F. S., & Flomenhauft, K. Treating the doll house marriage. *Family Process*, 1970, *9*, 143–155.

Raush, H. L., Barry, W. A., Hertel, R. K., et al. *Communication, conflict and marriage*. San Francisco: Jossey-Bass, 1974.

Reiss, D. Varieties of consensual experience. I. A Theory for relating family interaction to individual thinking. *Family Process*, 1971a, *10*, 1–28.

Reiss, D. Varieties of consensual experience. II. Dimensions of a family's experience of its environment. *Family Process*, 1971b, *10*, 28–35.

Reiss, D. Intimacy and problem-solving: An automated procedure for testing a theory of consensual experience in families. *Archives of General Psychiatry*, 1971c, *25*, 442–455.

Richter, H. E. *The family as patient*. New York: Farrar Straus Giroux, 1974.

Riskin, J., & Faunce, E. E. 1970. Family interaction scales. I. Theoretical framework and method. *Archives of General Psychiatry,* 1970, *22,* 504–537.

Rodgers, R. H. *Improvements in the construction and analysis of family life cycle categories.* Unpublished thesis. Western Michigan University, Kalamazoo, 1962.

Rodgers, R. H. *Family interaction and transaction: The developmental approach.* Englewood Cliffs, N.J.: Prentice-Hall, 1973.

Ryder, R. G. A topography of early marriage. *Family Process,* 1970, *9,* 385–402.

Serrano, A. C., McDonald, E. C., Goolishian, H. A., et al. Adolescent maladjustment and family dynamics. *American Journal of Psychiatry,* 1962, *118,* 897–910.

Solomon, M. A. A developmental, conceptual premise for family therapy. *Family Process,* 1973, *12,* 179–196.

Strauss, J. S. Diagnostic models and the nature of psychiatric disorder. *Archives of General Psychiatry,* 1973, *29,* 445–449.

Voiland, A. L. *Family casework diagnosis.* New York: Columbia University Press, 1962.

Voiland, A. L., & Buell, B. A classification of disordered family types. *Social Work,* 1961, *6,* 3–11.

Waring, M., & Ricks, D. Family patterns of children who became schizophrenics. *Journal of Nervous and Mental Disease,* 1965, *140,* 351–364.

Wertheim, E. S. Family unit therapy and the science and typology of family systems. *Family Process,* 1973, *12,* 361–376.

Zelditch, M. Family, marriage and kinship. In R. E. L. Faris (Ed.), *Handbook of modern sociology.* Chicago: Rand-McNally, 1964.

Rodney Shapiro, Ph.D., John Strauss, M.D., and Mary Anna Ham provided helpful comments and critical review.

PHYSICAL ILLNESS
AND FAMILY DYNAMICS

Clara G. Livsey[1]

INTRODUCTION

Serious physical illness in an individual creates a family crisis. This paper discusses the importance of recognizing intrafamilial factors when illness occurs, the processes of disruption and restoration of equilibrium that follow it as well as the importance of the coping mechanisms that are a part of both these phases. Pertinent literature is reviewed and clinical examples are presented. Suggestions are made for management, for necessary changes in the training of psychiatric and non-psychiatric medical personnel, and for areas of future investigation.

Traditionally the physician has regarded the individual patient and his symptoms as the unit for observation and treatment (Lipowski, 1969). 'A paradoxical situation has resulted in that the physician treats the individual while being overwhelmingly aware that the psychological factors and stresses in operation are tied up intimately with the important relationships of his patients' (Livsey, 1969). The drive of individuals to relate intimately is crucial to human nature. Since the family is a universal institution where basic relationships exist, investigators should explore the *intrafamilial environment* to better understand symptoms that may result from or be exacerbated by disturbed family relationships.

In the field of psychiatry family investigations have become an area of special interest in the last two decades. Dissatisfied with an individual, intrapsychic point of view, some investigators began to look at the family. They have evolved different theoretical frameworks to do so: some see the family as a *system;* some see it in terms of *communication networks;* others still view it in terms of *role* theory.

It is beyond the scope of this chapter to discuss family theory in general; for a review, see Meissner (1964). The clinical applications of the thinking of investigators in the family field are flourishing. To consider the family when one member is sick makes so much sense that clinicians are increasingly less preoccupied with the validity of this approach. In this respect, the advent of 'family psychiatry' has brought the awareness of the

Reprinted from *Advances in Psychosomatic Medicine 8*, pp. 237–251, ©1972, S. Karger AG, with permission.

[1]Associate-Chief, Department of Psychiatry, Sinai Hospital of Baltimore, Inc.; Assistant Professor of Psychiatry and Consultant, John F. Kennedy Institute for Handicapped Children, Johns Hopkins University School of Medicine.

complexity of this area of investigation. As Haley (1969) puts it, 'Compared with traditional research on individuals or artificial groups, family research was a new kind of venture. No one had ever described and measured the habitual behavior of a group of intimates who had a history together and a future association. Sampling families instead of individuals raised unique problems, and developing ways to measure how people deal with each other had to be explored.'

LIFE STRESS AND FAMILY EQUILIBRIUM

The way a family functions as such is significant. In some families there seems to be a drive toward individual development and differentiation. Bowen (1966) has related such drive to the integrity of self in the parental couple. There is sufficient evidence, especially from experienced clinicians who treat families, that those that are in serious trouble are frequently those where the primary couple in the nuclear family transmit the kinds of messages that cripple growth. In those troubled families the capacity to adapt to change and to life stresses is deficient, and only fixed, restricted methods of communication are available. All this is conducive to an unstable equilibrium, one that is frail, unhealthy. Breakdowns occur when such equilibrium is disturbed, as when one individual becomes sick or sicker. It is particularly when the family equilibrium is unsteady that illness may be viewed differently from an 'individual' than from a 'family' point of view. To illustrate: Mr. A. had a coronary at the age of 56. He was a top executive in an important business concern. His working hours seemed to be endless although one would never have guessed it by his calm, benevolent appearance. He was highly respected in his place of work and had considerable social prestige. He was very considerate of his subordinates, covering his distant attitude with a veneer of warmth. He was married and the father of a daughter and a son in their early twenties. His wife was very devoted and had always been a great support to his self-made-man image. They both befriended people from his place of work and constantly entertained, especially those who were still low on the executive ladder. Prior to his coronary, there had been some problems that greatly upset Mr. A. As a business merger occurred, it was discovered that a couple of middle-management people had been very negligent in their duties. Though he had been aware of their laxity, Mr. A. had tried to ignore it. His tendency had been to surround himself with people who admired and supported him, but in this case the two people had proved to be incompetent. When Mr. A. finally fired them, they put up a fight and partly succeeded in degrading him.

   The above description reflects the patient's view of the situation. Let us now look at what transpired in the description of the *family system* of which Mr. A. was a part: The life style of the A.'s was a stereotype of a 'perfect family.' The family myth was that Mr. A. was not only a VIP, but a super

VIP. This had been so even in his family of origin. Both Mr. and Mrs. A. were patronizing toward other people. Although Mr. A. was an intelligent man, he was no genius; however, he had to keep up the pretense that he was, as did his wife. As the complexities of the business grew, there was no room for complaining or becoming overtly anxious or depressed. Nor was there room for learning new ways of coping. Both husband and wife were intensely interdependent although spontaneous communication between them was distorted. Mrs. A. was at all times ready to do anything that would further his success. Part of the couple's system of communication consisted of confused messages. For instance, while constantly presenting her husband as a VIP, Mrs. A. made frequent insinuating comments and, in fact, indoctrinated her daughter with the idea that women are supposed to keep their mouths shut and let men 'shine.' She let it be known that she played the fool so as not to harm her husband.

The implications of this clinical vignette are that: 1) the husband had to maintain at any cost his image as an independent and self-sufficient, strong man; 2) as a consequence of item 1, he could not afford to communicate to his wife his distress related to disturbed relations at work; 3) his serious illness made it impossible for him to maintain his usual role within the family, whose precarious balance became destroyed as a result; 4) the rigid roles and skewed communication within A.'s family both increased his premorbid stress and, possibly, facilitated his coronary and made it most difficult for him and his family to cope with his illness.

DISTURBED FAMILY RELATIONSHIPS AS PSYCHOLOGICAL STRESS

Stress in human relationships is believed to precipitate and/or intensify somatic illness. For instance, the mother-child relationship, especially a pathological one, has been hypothesized to predispose to physical illness and to certain undesirable forms of illness behavior. Sperling's (1967) work should be mentioned because it deals specifically with the psychosomatic aspects: 'The method of concomitant psychoanalytic treatment of psychosomatically sick children and their mothers reveals the essential role of a specific mother-child relationship in the etiology and dynamics of a psychosomatic illness. In this psychosomatic relationship, which originates during the pregenital phase and which remains active throughout life (although it may not become manifest until precipitated by a traumatic life situation), the child is rewarded by his mother for being sick—that is, for remaining helpless and dependent—and is rejected when he is healthy—that is, when he evidences overt aggression and strivings for independence. In other words, there is a premium for being sick and a punishment for being healthy.'

Other works dealing with the relationship of family-related stress and physical illness will be discussed here as they pertain to this paper. It is only in recent years that there have been any publications dealing with physical illness in relation to the family interaction.

Schmale (1958) studied a series of 42 patients admitted to Strong Memorial Hospital for different ailments and found that before the onset of their illness most of them had experienced an object loss in reality or in fantasy. Such sense of threatened loss is most often experienced with regard to another family member. There is thus some evidence that certain types of stress within the family may co-determine the time of onset of physical illness.

The author is engaged in a study of the pre-morbid life situation of a series of men under 55 years of age who suffered coronary heart attacks. The importance of interviewing other members of the family has proved to be great. Sometimes little was said by the patient that would give an inkling of a chronic, very distressing life situation or of stressful events prior to the coronary. Important facts were added that were not received from the patients. To illustrate: Mr. L., a jolly, ingratiating man, reported that prior to his heart attack he had been very tense because of a promotion. From a position as an inspector in the plant, he had become a foreman, with over 40 men under his supervision. Mr. L. recognized that approval from others was very important to him and that, conversely, lack of it upset him. He saw it as his overriding responsibility trying to please these 40 men and make them happy. Mr. L. was self-conscious about his lack of education, and some of the men were more educated than he. When his wife was interviewed, she seemed to welcome the opportunity to talk about a matter that greatly worried her: the *father-daughter relationship*. She felt that her husband has always given an inordinate amount of attention to their only daughter. Mrs. L. talked about her distress upon learning a few years back that the girl was pregnant out of wedlock. She also mentioned that prior to his coronary her husband was very upset when his stepfather died of a heart attack. She was aware that he was worried when he received the promotion, but somehow his distress about this matter did not seem to touch her. She felt that her husband tried to hide his own worries from her because he found it very difficult to see her anxious. The following is a verbatim abstract of the interview with the daughter: '...My father is everything to me...I just adore him...He is the most wonderful person in the world...He worries about everything and everybody...He really cares about people...His first attack came after I got married. I guess you know what happened...I did not go to college and it hurt him a lot. He never had an education. In February of 1966, I was hospitalized. It was because of my nervous condition, but my doctor just put me in a regular hospital for a complete rest. Two days after I came back from the hospital, he went in with a coronary. . .'

This case illustrates the importance of interviewing other members of a patient's family to obtain a fuller picture of the social setting in which his illness occurred. Further, we note aspects of the family situation which were clearly stressful to this particular patient and may have helped precipitate his heart attack.

Engel (1955) described the family constellation of patients with ulcerative colitis. He saw the patients as having an intense relationship with the mother or a mother surrogate, at times reaching symbiotic proportions. 'In many instances only a very shadowy, stereotyped picture of father was obtained and that chiefly on direct inquiry.'

Jackson and Yalom (1966) studied a small sample of families in each of which one of the children had ulcerative colitis. They saw the families in conjoint interviews. They found striking similarities among them. All the families appeared to be severely *socially restricted* and at the same time restricted each other's behavior. The study compared these families to those of schizophrenics labelled by Wynne et al. (1958) as 'pseudomutuality families'.

McCord, McCord, & Verdon (1960) used the data from a comprehensive study over a number of years to relate conditions in the home with the incidence among children of obesity, acne and gastrointestinal disorders. They divided the children between intropunitive, those who express distress by punishing themselves and who have psychosomatic problems as a result; and extropunitive, those who punish the environment with their delinquent behavior. Such a classification presupposes a sweeping generalization that cannot be accepted in the light of our present knowledge. For one thing, some people use their symptoms, or willful neglect of their illness, to punish and control significant people in their families. They usually punish themselves at the same time. Notable among these are diabetic patients and those with skin disorders, as well as those who are overweight. In some of the children McCord reported an apparent causal relationship between tension and conflict in the family and the children's symptoms. They also saw a relationship between such symptoms and families where the parents themselves had a strong tendency to adopt the sick role.

Sheldon and Hooper investigated the relationship between health and adjustment in early marriage. They found a questionable relationship between variations of health and adjustment, especially in women. Hall-Smith and Ryle (1969) used psychometric tests to study marital patterns in relation to illness. They conclude that current interpersonal relationships are of significance in many psychosomatic and psychiatric disorders. They feel that the use of interpersonal tests is promising and should be further explored.

Friedman et al. (1960) studied the family adjustment to children with familial dysautonomia. They describe the complexity of the total picture, where a child's neurological disorder may be complicated by a personality disturbance because family relationships have become conflicted as a result of his disorder.

It is important to think of the family from an ecological perspective. Hinkle (1966) points out that 'more than half of all the episodes of illness that occur among adults of similar age seem to be experienced by fewer than one quarter of that number'. In his study of a group of Hungarian refugees in whom he found a propensity for illness, he noted that the tendency was not related to environmental stress. His analysis revealed that people who had experienced frequent illness in Hungary were the same people who had experienced frequent illness in the States. Although his paper is concerned with ecological observations, there is no reference to the intrafamilial environment of the refugees. Those interested in a family point of view would regard such data as of paramount importance. It is important to go beyond individuals and to investigate family patterns which often reveal interactions that have a significant bearing on illness. In what family settings do dysfunctions manifested in physical illness occur? Is illness in some cases part of an intricate communication system? If so, how does the individual utilize his body as a means to respond to or deliver messages?

Some investigators have attempted to answer these questions. Meissner (1966) suggests that somatic illness often occurs in families that are tense and in conflict. He sees these factors as being in operation without attempting to explain how they operate. Meissner proposes that 'disruption or disequilibrium within the family system' is related to the development of symptoms. In the opinion of this author such a disruption may be a potent source of psychological stress, which acts as an intervening variable between environmental events and illness in the individual.

THE IMPACT OF ILLNESS ON FAMILY DYNAMICS

Jackson (1966), who years ago presented his ideas on family homeostasis, points out that somatic disorders often play an unexpected role in maintaining emotional balance within the family. 'The outbreak of such disorders, conversely, can be utilized by the physician as a barometer of family emotional difficulties.' In another paper he describes the difficulties that such an approach presents to the physician who is trained to think of the individual's symptoms as isolated occurrences.

Dysinger and Bowen (1959) reported on the handling of health matters by a group of families, each with a schizophrenic son or daughter, who were under observation and lived for a period of time in a ward at NIMH. In these families where the involvement among parents and child was intense, the handling of health matters was not based on realistic factors but was highly colored by feelings. The distinction between feelings and facts was blurred. Implied in Dysinger's observations are different coping mechanisms that these families used with the schizophrenic and with the well siblings respectively: 'The family functioning was much more realistic and adequate in the few experiences with major acute physical illness (in the well siblings) that occurred during the period of study.'

The occurrence of illness in an individual can be viewed from the point of view of *how such illness affects the family,* what changes take place to cope with its occurrence, and how the family influences the development, maintenance, deterioration or improvement of the patient's condition. In ordinary families when an individual becomes sick to the degree that he cannot function in his habitual manner, a sequence of changes evolves and a series of mechanisms develops to adjust to the care needs of the sick and cope with the changes that are necessary to do so (Ellenberger et al., 1964). Serious illness in a member of a family is a crisis and, as such, produces *disruption and disorganization* of the previous equilibrium. Many elements enter the picture. Some changes are situational, such as financial hardship; some are subjective. There may be lack of precise knowledge of the diagnosis and prognosis, or denial when the facts are known. Covert anger may be present and guilt may be a prominent feature in various members (including the patient) who may see the illness as punishment. There may be misunderstandings and misinterpretations that further complicate the picture. A family member who wishes the sick individual dead may act in an exaggeratedly overprotective fashion. The situation is influenced by who is sick, what the prognosis is, what care needs are necessary and for how long, whether the illness contains elements that can become life threatening, whether prolonged hospitalization is required, or whether certain death is the outcome.

If the father is ill and does not function as the head of the family, a general feeling of insecurity may prevail. Financial problems may arise, depending upon his form of employment or business. By his constant presence in the home, he unwittingly disturbs the daily household routine. His demands for his wife's attention may cause resentment in her and the children. In turn, his change or role may cause him sufficient anxiety to prompt him to resume his usual activities before he has the capacity to do so. The opposite may occur if he assumes a passive role, with serious consequences for the family survival. Regardless of the changes that our society is undergoing, including those in the role of women, when a man's instrumental role in the family is undermined, the family deteriorates.

When the mother-wife becomes seriously ill, a great deal of anxiety may result. At times the anxiety may be mixed with anger, if dependency needs of the various family members remain frustrated as a result of mother's prolonged illness.

Two papers will be discussed at this point that deal with the occurrence of illness in one spouse. Katz (1969) studied a group of wives of diabetic men who presented problems in management. Although the women were the subjects of the study, the paper illuminates areas of marital functioning. Relationship was found between the wives' conflicts, for instance around their own dependency needs, and the needs arising from the husband's illness. At times, 'dietary needs were incorporated into the neurotic conflict in the marriage'. The study also discusses impotence, present in a large percentage of diabetics, in the light of the wives' sexual problems and the marital interaction. It was as though the marriage, rather than the sick individual, had to deal with the diabetes. Of particular interest are the observations about the relationship between the wives and the husband's doctor, which underscore the necessity to train medical men to evaluate the impact of a patient's illness on the members of his family.

Fink et al. (1968) examined the relationships of physical disability and need and marriage satisfaction in couples where the wife was disabled. The authors found that the physical disability of the wife was not a useful predictor of need or marriage satisfaction. The authors point out that 'the woman's reaction...and her effectiveness in the role of homemaker seemed to bear little necessary relation to the relative seriousness of her case. Indeed, some of the physically most limited homemakers seemed to have the best-organized and smoothly operating households.'

The importance of role intactness needs stressing. A wife may be physically disabled, even bedridden, and yet not necessarily relinquish her functions as the home manager and the provider of mothering. It is only when the effects of physical illness become complicated by conflicts within the family, that the sick member relinquishes all his premorbid family roles. Thus, a disabled or chronically ill woman may become the child; a man in the same situation may assume the role of the homemaker, mother or child. As it is a fact that many people with chronic illness or disabilities do not relinquish their roles, the occurrence of deviant behavior should be investigated routinely.

When a child is seriously ill or disabled, the same considerations apply as when a parent is the affected one. The parental couple is the central relationship in the family and conveyor of messages that influence how the child develops. A sick child may become the focus of the parents' own interaction when the marital relationship is troubled. The child complies by becoming an active participant rather than a passive observer. It is well known that a young chronically ill patient may induce dangerous complications of his illness as a weapon and a means of control of his parents as well as to comply with the implicit messages he may be getting from them. To illustrate: Nine-year-old Lisa was referred by her pediatrician. The child had been diagnosed as a diabetic two years prior to the consultation. Problems in her management were marked. She refused to test her urine or give herself insulin injections and dragged her feet about eating at appropriate times. Lisa, a frail-looking, intelligent girl, was the older of two children. There was marked sibling rivalry between her and her seven-year-old brother. The parents expressed a great deal of concern about the child's diabetes; in fact, both they and the in-laws discussed the problem constantly. Both parents praised the child abundantly: how beautiful, how intelligent she was. They also talked about another problem: the child insisted on sleeping with them since she was extremely frightened to sleep in her own bedroom. Refusal to yield to these demands made her hysterical to such a point that the parents feared for her health. When questions were asked to evaluate the marital relationship, Mrs. T. stated that she was very unhappy about her marriage and felt trapped in it. On the contrary, Mr. T. was quite satisfied and felt that there were only money problems, that although he worked overtime he could not provide luxuries for his wife. They had married when he was almost 40 and she was 24 and had a typical 'doll-house marriage.' Mrs. T., an only daughter, had indeed been her family's 'doll' and continued a very close relationship with her parents, especially her father. She considered her parents' marriage 'perfect' and presented her life up to the point of marriage as a paradise. Mr. T. shared her admiration for her parents. Clearly, he saw himself as their ally, forever protecting his wife; Mrs. T. described Mr. T's family as 'sick' and 'sickening.' A brother was still living with the parents, and the only sister was a schizophrenic who had a lobotomy. It seemed that at times Mrs. T. was terrified at the prospect of suffering the same fate should she continue living with her husband. However, her attempts at separation from him in the past had resulted in physical illness, such as acute thyroid crisis. She blamed all her problems on him. He, in turn, was unable to see her as anything but an emotional cripple and seemed to have married her for that reason. After she initiated a discussion of their separation, it became apparent that they could not go through with it. In fact, he could not leave even overnight because he had to give Lisa her insulin shot; mother was afraid to do so.

In this case the ill child responded to her parents' marital conflict by disturbed illness behavior. Further, through her illness she successfully manipulated and held them together. Without this background information her behavior could neither be understood nor corrected.

Rutter (1966) carried out a study of the relation between psychiatric disorders in children and illness in or death of their parents. His aim was to test the hypothesis that there would be a significantly high rate of parental illness of all kinds among children with psychiatric disorders. He compared populations of the Maudsley Hospital Children's Department with children attending the Dental and Pediatric Departments of King's College Hospital and another out-patient clinic. The study shows a clear distinction between the children whose parents had psychiatric illness and physical illness respectively. Rutter found higher incidence of chronic and/or recurrent physical illness in the parents of psychiatrically ill, i.e. Maudsley children.

Parsons and Fox (1960), in their classic paper, have discussed physical illness in the framework of the modern American family. They point out that illness is a heavy load for the small, rather isolated, nuclear family and that this leads to the tendency toward delegating care for the sick to outside institutions: 'In other words, what we are suggesting here is that the optimal balance between supportive-permissive and disciplinary facets of treating illness is peculiarly difficult to maintain in the kind of situation presented by the American family. Medico-technical advances notwithstanding, therefore, therapy is more easily effected in a professional milieu, where there is not the same order of intensive emotional involvement characteristic of family relationships.'

ILLNESS IN THE FAMILY AND THE COPING PATTERNS

Discussion of the effects of physical illness in a family member on the family as a whole raises the crucial issue of what *coping mechanisms* the family and the individual use (Ellenberger et al., 1964). It is a common observation that the nature of the coping patterns adopted by them may profoundly influence the course of the sick member's illness as well as the stability of the family.

Lipowski (1970) distinguishes 'coping styles,' i.e. the individual's enduring attitudes that are put in operation when he is ill; and 'coping strategies,' which reflect the current situational factors. He describes a number of meanings of illness of which one, 'illness as a challenge,' evokes an adaptive, rational response, while the others are colored to a varying extent by irrationality and distortions. It may prove rewarding to apply these concepts to the study of intrafamilial relationships. It may be postulated that a patient's coping strategies are both influenced by and affect his family relationships. One may also speak of coping by the family as a unit.

Earlier in this paper the initial period of disruption of the family equilibrium was discussed. Coping refers to the mechanisms by which the family adapts itself to and deals with the changes resulting from the illness of one of its members. A physically incapacitated husband-father, even if unable to leave his home, may be retrained and able to resume the role of breadwinner. A housewife may, by hiring adequate help, again continue to manage her home; a diabetic child may learn how to take care of himself while being appropriately provided with diet and other kinds of care by the parents. When illness results in a chronic brain syndrome that seriously affects an individual's capacity for judgment, a patient may have to be institutionalized. The ability of a family to function successfully may be affected by conflicts that impair coping and disturb the sick member. This is particularly so in the case of children. The sick or disabled child whom his parents use for displacement of their own conflicts may develop an impaired self-image and body-image. He may grow up with defective sense of autonomy of his self and body. Such relative lack of differentiation may result from the child's being used as a tool and target for attempted solution of the family's problems.

Olsen (1970) stresses adaptive and successful coping and lists the following characteristics of families that make a good adjustment to serious illness: a clear separation of generations; flexibility within and between roles; direct and consistent communication; and, above all, 'tolerance for individuation.'

CLINICAL APPLICATIONS: EVALUATION AND MANAGEMENT

To evaluate the family when a member is sick, it is essential to keep in mind the conceptual framework of the *family as a whole* and not think only of interactions between two or more members. 'A constant observer of the family—or of any other persistent group process—has a somewhat contrary impression that much of what occurs in the way of behavior is not under the control of any one person or even a set of persons, but is rather the upshot of complicated processes beyond the ken of anyone involved. Something in the group process itself takes over as a steering mechanism and brings about results which no one anticipates or wants, whether consciously or unconsciously' (Spiegel, 1960).

One may argue the last sentence, yet Spiegel's (1960) *transactional approach* rings true to any 'constant observer of the family,' and the concept has important consequences for research and medical management. To understand how a family reacts when an individual is ill, one must also be aware of the interactions between the family and the system of care. It is sometimes difficult to decide whether family members are reacting to patterns which existed before the onset of illness and are very difficult to change, or whether what we see at a given moment is partly the result of unavailable or inadequate medical management.

Evaluation of a family where a child has a chronic disease or physical defect may serve us as a model for this discussion (Ellenberger et al., 1964). Cerebral palsy is a good model to use because it presents the whole spectrum from near normalcy to very severe physical and mental disability. Appropriate management from the very beginning may prevent the recurrence of some family-related problems. Focusing on small areas of functioning that contribute little to the total goal of teaching the child how to be self-reliant in his own individual way is common and insufficient. Overlooking possible ambivalent feelings of the parents toward the child and their consequent guilt results in a skewed evaluation. At times the financial burden is so great that it must be given its due weight. Appropriate management in these and similar situations may mean the difference between adjustment and a constructive life or a tragedy that may involve not only the patient but other members of the family as well. There is a tendency among both the parents and the health professionals to deny the disturbing emotional components of the whole situation. Even parents who do not deny such factors are often not encouraged to discuss their feelings about their problems. Leaving out the psychosocial aspects from the evaluation of a family of a physically ill child precludes optimum management. There are some points to keep in mind in helping such families. The parents should be encouraged from the very beginning toward a realistic appraisal of the situation in order to plan realistically. Such planning should concentrate not only on the patient, but on the rest of the family members as well. The approach should be clear and well-structured from the start, even if all the facts are not at hand. As the medical facts are explained, it is important to evaluate what feelings and fantasies the parents have in relation to the child's problem. In the opinion of this author, a psychosocial family evaluation should be part of the total medical evaluation. This author advises psychiatric assessment whenever either a chronic or serious problem affects a member of the family. The family evaluation may take various forms dictated by the needs and limitations of its members. In some cases *conjoint family* or *marital sessions* should take place, while in others they may be contraindicated.

As for treatment, it is neither necessary nor feasible for every family to receive psychiatric help on a regular basis, but it is important to provide opportunity for a periodic consultation. A major form of support involves repeated *clarification* of the problems that may arise. The therapist should function for some as a constant reminder of reality. Sometimes this calls for separation of the sick member which may be necessary because the disability, physically and/or mentally, may be too severe to be handled at home. In other cases there may be, for instance, a clear picture of a child's being infantilized or used by parental conflict, or the child may be having secondary gains by acting out through his illness, perpetuating an unhealthy pattern even if the parents are ready for change. Family evaluation may lead to the recommendation of other forms of therapy of which the most useful, in the opinion of this author, is group therapy, either alone or, preferably, in conjunction with family or marital therapy. In some cases, for example in patients with myocardial infarction, it is wise to refrain from conjoint sessions, especially before the nature of the family interaction has been assessed. Adsett and Bruhn (1968) have discussed group therapy for such patients and their wives in separate groups. Although their results are unimpressive, the concept is a valid one.

SUMMARY

To conclude, in spite of the obvious reasons why we should know more about the family to better understand illness, many physicians consider patients as isolated units. This truncated approach vitiates in many cases the proper management and optimum recovery from or adjustment to illness. The study of the family is providing data which is beginning to filter into medical practice. Evaluation of the family situation of every physically ill and/or disabled patient should become a routine part of medical management. This function may be carried out by social workers but the information elicited is of little value unless the doctor in charge is aware of it and incorporates it into his overall treatment plan.

Longitudinal studies of families where chronic and/or serious illness occurs are sorely needed. They call for a systematic and uniform system of data-obtaining. What we need to know is how to help families cope with physical illness in their midst so as to ensure an optimum recovery of the sick individual and safeguard the integrity of his family.

Changes are needed in the training of psychiatrists and physicians in general. It is important to teach them from the very beginning, that is, in medical school, how to evaluate families. A physician occupies a position of leadership in the delivery of care, in medical teaching and research. He has to have the proper training to understand not only that he cannot escape being a *family* physician, but also how to be one effectively.

REFERENCES

Adsett, A., & Bruhn, J. G. Short term group psychotherapy for post-myocardial infarction patients and their wives. *Canadian Medical Association Journal,* 1968, *99,* 577–584.

Bowen, M. The use of family therapy in clinical practice. *Comprehensive Psychiatry,* 1966, *7,* 345–374.

Dysinger, R. H., & Bowen, M. Problems for medical practice presented by families with a schizophrenic member. *American Journal of Psychiatry,* 1959, *116,* 514–517.

Ellenberger, H., et al. Phases types de l'adaptation familiale à la maladie physique prolongée d'un enfant. *Canadian Psychiatry Association,* 1964, *9,* 322–330.

Engel, G. L. Studies of ulcerative colitis. *American Journal of Medicine,* 1955, *19,* 232–256.

Fink, S., et al. Physical disability and problems in marriage. *Journal of Marriage and the Family,* 1968, *30,* 64–73.

Friedman, A. L., et al. *Family adjustment to the brain-damaged child: A modern introduction to the family,* pp. 555–562. Glencoe, Ill.: The Free Press, 1960.

Haley, J. An editor's farewell. *Family Process,* 1969, *8,* 149.

Hall-Smith, P., & Ryle, A. Marital patterns, hospitality and personal illness. *British Journal of Psychiatry,* 1969, *115,* 1197–1198.

Hinkle, L. E. Ecological observations of the relationship of physical illness, mental illness and the social environment. *Psychosomatics,* 1966, *23,* 290–296.

Jackson, D. D. Family practice. A comprehensive medical approach. *Comprehensive Psychiatry,* 1966, *7,* 338–344.

Jackson, D. D., & Yalom, I. Family research in the problem of ulcerative colitis. *Archives of General Psychiatry,* 1966, *15,* 410–418.

Katz, A. M. Wives of diabetic men. *Bulletin of the Menninger Clinic,* 1969, *33,* 279–294.

Lipowski, Z. J. Psychosocial aspects of disease. *Annals of Internal Medicine,* 1969, *71,* 1197–1206.

Lipowski, Z. J. Physical illness, the individual and the coping processes. *Psychiatric Medicine,* 1970, *1,* 91–101.

Livsey, C. Family therapy. Role of the practicing physician. In Lisansky and Shochet (Eds.), *Modern treatment* (Vol. 6), pp. 806–820. 1969.

McCord, W., McCord, J., & Verdon, P. Familial correlates of psychosomatic symptoms in male children. *Journal of Health and Human Behavior,* 1960, *1,* 192–199.

Meissner, W. W. Thinking about the family—Psychiatric aspects. *Family Process,* 1964, *3,* 1–33.

Meissner, W. W. Family dynamics and psychosomatic processes. *Family Process,* 1966, *5,* 142–161.

Olsen, H. The impact of serious illness on the family system. *Medicine,* 1970, *47,* 169–174.

Parsons, T., & Fox, R. C. Illness, therapy and the modern urban American family. *Modern introduction to the family,* pp. 347–360. Glencoe, Ill.: The Free Press, 1960.

Rutter, M. *Children of sick parents.* An environmental study. London: Oxford University Press, 1966.

Schmale, A. H. Relationship of separation and depression to disease. *Psychosomatic Medicine,* 1958, *20,* 259–277.

Sheldon, A., & Hooper, D. An inquiry into health and ill health and adjustment in early marriage. *Journal of Psychosomatic Research, 13,* 95–101.

Sperling, M. Transference neurosis in patients with psychosomatic disorders. *Psychoanalytic Quarterly,* 1967, *36,* 344.

Spiegel, J. P. The resolution of role conflict within the family. In Bell and Vogel (Eds.), *A Modern introduction to the family,* p. 362. Glencoe, Ill.: The Free Press, 1960.

Wynne, L., et al. Pseudomutuality in the family relations of schizophrenics. *Psychiatry,* 1958, *21,* 205–220.

CHAPTER 2

IMPACT OF DISABILITY/ ILLNESS ON THE ADULT

Paul W. Power and Arthur E. Dell Orto

Often the real deterrents to rehabilitation are those created by the person's emotional concerns. A crippling, disabling disease can be at least as damaging to the personality as to the body. The task of effectively rehabilitating disabled persons is impossible without understanding the impelling psychosocial problems related to chronic illness and disability. The emotional reaction of patients to an illness will usually strongly affect those who share their living environment. If a disabled person is continually angry about his physical limitations, for example, he will frequently project that anger onto others, creating an atmosphere of tension and anxiety. The lingering presence of these emotions in the home can inhibit the family from assisting its disabled family member to achieve productive goals. Optimum treatment of disabled people requires not only sound scientific, medical management, but also an awareness of the consequences of the illness on the lives of their families.

Consequently, there is usually much interaction between the feelings exhibited by the patient and the emotions shown by the family. A determination by the health professional of how the person's emotional reaction influences others about him is important in assessing how the family members can be utilized for the patient's rehabilitation. If the family members are upset, for example, because the disabled family member is demanding more attention and has become overly dependent, then they often will be hesitant to help this person work through personal feelings of loss. Health professionals should know the reactions and typical coping strategies of disabled persons. From this recognition they can prepare or advise family members of events or emotions that are most likely to occur.

Physical disability encompasses a variety of disorders and includes "any impairment of bodily function over a period of time" (Abram, 1972, p. 559). Disabilities arouse certain responses in the afflicted persons, and this chapter outlines many of these emotional reactions. It also contains discussions of varied determinants of the emotional responses. Dr. Kiely's article, which follows in this chapter, explains the coping strategies that patients may use in dealing with a severe disability or chronic illness. All of this material provides the reader with a beginning understanding of the psychology of physical disability.

DETERMINANTS OF PSYCHOLOGICAL REACTION TO DISABILITY

The way a person will emotionally react to a disability or trauma depends upon many factors:

1. *The personality makeup of the individual before disability or disease onset*   If a person is accustomed to being dependent on others for most daily needs, and has always been reluctant to show initiative or independent behavior, then that person usually will react to the threat of disability by becoming even more dependent than before disability onset. Much of this behavior will be unwarranted. If a man views himself exclusively as a vigorous, sexually active, and physically strong individual, a crippling disability will cause in him heightened feelings of depression and even despair. He apparently perceives his basic identity as devastated, and adjustment will usually be very difficult to achieve.
2. *Illness-related factors*   These include the type and location of symptoms, namely, whether they are disfiguring, disabling, painful, or in a body region that carries special importance, like the heart or reproductive organs. Different organs and functions may have a psychological significance that has little to do with biological factors related to survival (Moos, 1977). For example, severe burns to the face or a crippling injury to the leg of an athlete may have greater psychological impact on these persons than severe hypertension directly threatening their life.
3. *The individual's reaction to previous crises*   If the patient has confronted traumas in his personal or family life before the present one, then often there are coping mechanisms that have already been used that will carry over to this new trauma. If it is a completely new experience, however, confusion and anxiety could endure for a longer, more unwarranted period of time.
4. *The person's satisfaction with work*   If a job, a leisure activity, or a household occupation conveys much personal fulfillment, these outlets will provide a sense of satisfaction that will help minimize the emotional effects of the disability. Yet many persons, continually dissatisfied with their work, may find in their illness or disability an excuse not to return to work, or will find that the benefits of being taken care of far outweigh their desire for independence. The disability gives such persons a new, more acceptable identity.

5. *Presence or absence of therapeutic intervention*   This includes the attitude of health professionals, because they can significantly affect the behavioral adaptation to a disability (Moos, 1977). Also, appropriate early intervention could help someone to focus more on the residual assets than the limiting handicaps of a disability, and this perspective could help to minimize a lingering depression, as well as facilitate an aggressive attitude of coping.

6. *Familial and societal reactions to the impairment*   A disabled individual often faces societal inconsistency, social injustice, and a negative attitude from the family. Architectural barriers, stereotypical ideas about disability, hiring prejudices, and negative expectations from family members concerning performance in the home all represent a challenge to the disabled individual and can foster feelings of inadequacy and insecurity.

7. *Religion and philosophy of life*   For varied reasons a person may feel that chronic illness is a punishment for past sins or believe that the acceptance of pain associated with disability may relieve guilt feelings. Turning to God may alleviate feelings of anguish caused by disability-related limitations, or may encourage hope. This hope may facilitate a more optimistic attitude.

8. *The life (developmental) stage of the person*   Research is becoming more available that indicates that adults go through many life stages as they grow older (Sheehy, 1974; Levinson, 1978). The timing of an illness in the life cycle is particularly important. An adolescent diagnosed with juvenile diabetes has concerns different from those of an elderly patient incapacitated by arthritis. Previous experience with illness may be a resource from which the older person can draw for coping. Many younger people have a difficult time coping with an illness because it represents an additional stress to the already existing demands of attempting to achieve maturity.

EMOTIONAL REACTION TO DISABILITY

There are many ways that a disabled person can emotionally react to a disability/illness situation. In studying the behaviors of the patient in chronic illness or faced with the reality of dying, five authors (Shontz, 1965, 1973; Fink, 1967; Kubler-Ross, 1969; Weisman, 1972; Pearson, 1973) describe a pattern of reactions leading to a stage that comprises some form of adaptation, either through denial or acceptance. Dr. Bray's article, included in Chapter 6, also explains a reactive theory to one particular disability, namely, spinal cord injury. In their formulations the authors explain that the patient's reactions form a path on which the patient progressively walks toward some form of illness resolution. It is important to stress, however,

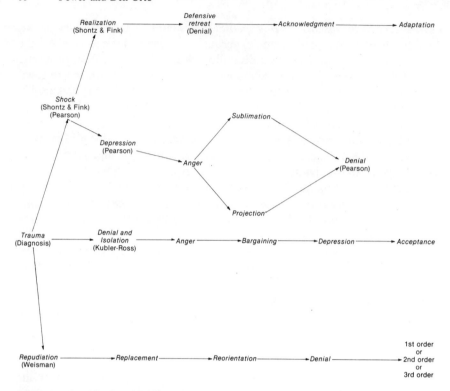

Figure 1.   Combined stages of reactions to chronic illness and dying.

that usually no one particular patient will follow precisely the progressive steps outlined by the various authors. Depending upon pre-disease/illness onset characteristics, patients will show a variety of behaviors that may follow a different sequence than any reported progression leading to emotional adjustment. Yet one of the contributions of the authors is to suggest workable concepts, terms that can be utilized to identify the particular reactive stage of the patient (see Figure 1).

Since the different theories are highlighted in the literature more from the perspective of the authors themselves, rather than by the concepts they employed to explain their findings, the authors provide the framework for the following discussion of varied adaptional resolutions.

Shontz and Fink

After working together for several years with chronically physically ill patients, as well as conducting research on the psychological aspects of physical disability, Shontz and Fink (1961) put their observations together into a formal scheme. They explain that their ideas are guesses, but, if assumed to be correct, have certain implications. Viewing a crisis "as an event in which the individual's normal coping abilities are inadequate to meet the demands of the situation" (Fink, 1967, p. 592), the theory postulates five sequential phases: shock, realization, defensive retreat, acknowledgment, and adaptation. Shontz (1965) and Shontz and Fink (1961) believe that in "shock" the individual perceives a threat to existing structures and reality as overwhelming. There are feelings of panic, anxiety, and helplessness, with an inability to plan or to understand the situation. "Realization" implies a feeling that existing structures have collapsed, and reality continues to be seen as overwhelming. Panic and an inability to plan continue. During "defensive retreat" there is an attempt to maintain old structures, wishful thinking, denial of reality, indifference, and a resistance to change. In "acknowledgment" the disabled individual slowly faces reality as the facts impose themselves, but this is accompanied by depression, bitterness, mourning, high anxiety, a defensive breakdown, and a reorganization in terms of altered perceptions of reality. During the stage of adaptation or change the individual gains a new sense of worth, a gradual increase of satisfying experiences, and achieves a reorganization of present resources and abilities.

Pearson

Pearson (1973), between 1954 and 1962, contacted 13 individuals, 8 female and 5 male, ages 18 to 28, who were the progeny of parents with Huntington's disease. He followed these individuals and their children for 10 years. From a subjective evaluation of his experience over the past 18 years with Huntington's disease patients, Pearson reported that, although there seems to be no consistent pattern or pre-morbid personality traits in victims of Huntington's disease or in their unaffected siblings, there does appear to be a highly consistent pattern in the mental mechanisms or dynamisms that "underlie the waxing and waning of anxiety among the potential victims of the disease" (p. 708). He found that most individuals eventually coped with the continued threat of the illness by denial. They believed they would not contract the disease, and this assumption helped the children to manage their own anxiety. The stages of reaction are presented in Figure 2.

Kubler-Ross

In interviewing over 200 dying patients between 1965 and 1968 in a Chicago hospital, Kubler-Ross (1969) formulated her theory of the stages of dying. Although her published study failed to provide a breakdown of the different types of dying patients, because of occasional references made by her it appears that the majority of the ill persons were terminal cancer patients. Her theory is represented in Figure 3.

Weisman

In Weisman's (1972) study, interviews were conducted with over 350 patients during the period 1962-1965. They were referred from various sources and were in different stages of illness that reportedly could lead to

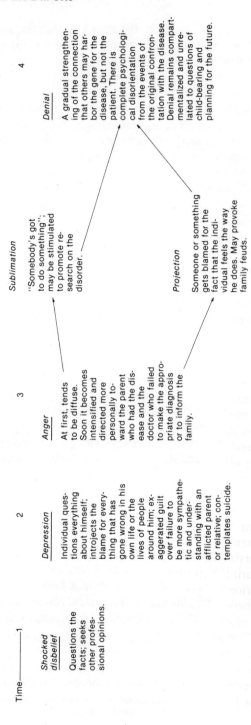

Figure 2.   Reactions to stages of Huntington's disease by Pearson.

Time ——————1

Shocked disbelief

Questions the facts; seeks other professional opinions.

2

Depression

Individual questions everything about himself; introjects the blame for everything that has gone wrong in his own life or the lives of people around him; exaggerated guilt over failure to be more sympathetic and understanding with an afflicted parent or relative; contemplates suicide.

3

Anger

At first, tends to be diffuse. Soon it becomes intensified and directed more personally toward the parent who had the disease and the doctor who failed to make the appropriate diagnosis or to inform the family.

Sublimation

"Somebody's got to do something"; may be stimulated to promote research on the disorder.

Projection

Someone or something gets blamed for the fact that the individual feels the way he does. May provoke family feuds.

4

Denial

A gradual strengthening of the connection that others may harbor the gene for the disease, but not the patient. There is complete psychological disorientation from the events of the original confrontation with the disease. Denial remains compartmentalized and unrelated to questions of child-bearing and planning for the future.

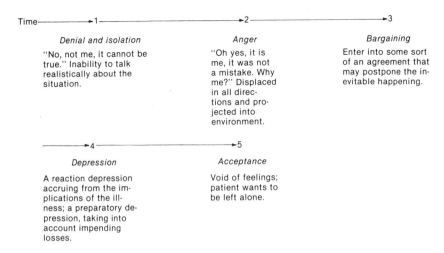

Figure 3.   Reaction stages to dying by Kubler-Ross.

death. In general the bulk of his case material consisted of: a) cancer patients, b) elderly people suffering from different illnesses and degrees of senescence, c) myocardial infarction patients, many of whom were on the danger list when first interviewed, d) pre- and postoperative patients who were thought to be potentially terminal by the staff, the patient, or both, and e) psychiatric patients who were conspicuously preoccupied with death. Children, adolescents, depressed patients who were in no danger of dying, patients who were admitted because of a suicide attempt, and terminal patients who were too moribund, too heavily sedated, or too inarticulate to cooperate in an interview were excluded from his study. Although Weisman only included those who were gravely ill, the concepts that he identifies in the reactive stages can be used to describe persons who are not as seriously disabled. As Pearson (1973) has suggested, many disabled or chronically ill persons, as well as those living in the patient's environment, use denial as an adaptive mechanism. Weisman's explanation of denial is particularly interesting and is represented in Figure 4.

From an understanding of these theories it is evident that the concern of most patients during the early reactive phase is with the impending need for massive evaluation and reorganization of their life, a sober realization that life is not and never again will be the same as before the onset of the illness. It is a period of depression, anxiety, and aggression. Various defense methods are used to control these reactions, with denial the one dominant thread in the fabric of psychological defenses.

Abram (1972) and Blacher (1970) discuss the use of denial; Blacher believes that it is perhaps the most common mechanism utilized in adjustment to chronic illness. In using denial patients keep out of their awareness

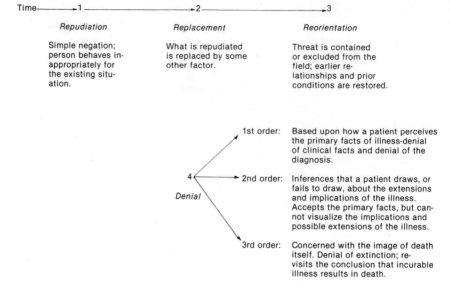

Figure 4.   Reaction stages to dying by Weisman.

the danger that the illness poses to their bodily, psychological, and social functioning. Anxiety is handled by not allowing it to reach consciousness, and patients avoid the conflict by not intellectually or emotionally recognizing that it exists. In working with 25 hemodialysis patients over a 4-year period, and exploring particularly the stages of adaptation to maintenance hemodialysis, Reichsman and Levy (1972) found that the primary and most commonly used mechanism of defense just before the period of long-term adaptation was that of denial. They believed they had not seen denial used as massively as it was by this group of patients. Cummings (1970) maintains that, although denial serves as a protective device to reduce the unsettling impact of chronic renal failure, at the same time it can lead the patient to withdraw from involvement in the demands of being a dialysis patient.

CONCLUSION

With an understanding of both the complexity of the impact of disability on the person and different coping strategies, the health professional is able to become aware of possible causal factors of the family's own reaction to the disability. Family members can reinforce both negative and positive responses to a disabling condition. From this knowledge, effective intervention can then be designed that may help the disabled person to live more adaptively with the physical condition.

The following articles in this chapter describe many emotional responses that one may have to an illness or disability. Dr. Kiely focuses more on the coping process associated with serious illness and explains the strategies that can be employed to deal with illness. He identifies the range of coping behaviors available to a disabled person, as well as reports what may influence the coping pattern. It is a comprehensive article and contains a wealth of information for the health professional. Dr. Weinstein's article emphasizes the concept of the disability process, and especially concentrates on work disability. He talks about reactive stages to disability trauma, and believes that the final adaptive stage is the result of a complex process. In explaining this process he develops concepts that are important to understand when helping the patient and family. Both articles elaborate on the material presented here and give the reader a wider knowledge of the psychosocial aspects of physical disability. They suggest that successful rehabilitation requires more concern for the personality of the disabled, the psychological reaction to the disability, and one's relationship to the social environment.

REFERENCES

Abram, H. The psychology of chronic illness. *Journal of Chronic Disease*, 1972, *25*, 657–664.

Blacher, R. Loss of internal organs. In B. Schoenberg, A. Carr, D. Peretz, & A. Kutscher (Eds.), *Loss and grief: Psychological management in medical practice*, pp. 132–139. New York: Columbia University Press, 1970.

Cummings, J. Hemodialysis: Feelings, facts, fantasies. *American Journal of Nursing*, 1970, *70*, 70–83.

Fink, S. Crisis and motivation: A theoretical model. *Archives of Physical Medicine and Rehabilitation*, 1967, 592–597.

Kubler-Ross, E. *On death and dying*. New York: MacMillan & Co., 1969.

Levinson, D. *The seasons of a man's life*. New York: Alfred A. Knopf, 1978.

Moos, R. (Ed.). *Coping with physical illness*. New York: Plenum Medical Book Co., 1977.

Pearson, J. Behavioral aspects of Huntington's chorea. *Advances in Neurology*, 1973, *1*, 701–712.

Reichsman, F., & Levy, N. Problems in adaptation to maintenance hemodialysis. *Archives of Internal Medicine*, 1972, *130*, 859–865.

Sheehy, G. *Predictable crises of adult life*. New York: E. P. Dutton & Co., 1974.

Shontz, F. Reactions to crisis. *The Volta Review*, 1965, 364–370.

Shontz, F. Severe chronic illness. In J. Garrett & E. Levine (Eds.), *Rehabilitation practices with the physically disabled*, pp. 119–148. New York: Columbia University Press, 1973.

Shontz, F., & Fink, S. A method for evaluating psychosocial adjustment of chronically ill. *American Journal of Physical Medicine*, 1961, *40*, 63–69.

Weisman, A. *On death and dying*. New York: Behavioral Publications, 1972.

COPING WITH SEVERE ILLNESS

W. F. Kiely[1]

Illness, though one of the relatively certain and predictable facts of life, only recently has been the object of intensive study from the psychosocial standpoint. A comprehensive theory adequate to explain the many ways in which it is experienced and expressed by patients is now beginning to take shape. Intuitive physicians from time immemorial have sensed the meaning of individual responses to particular experiences of threat or loss in patients with serious illness or injury. A giant step forward toward understanding the *coping process* was provided by the variety of behavioral patterns exhibited during World War II by soldiers under the threat or the actual experience of serious injury.

The concept of *stress* came into vogue during and following the war years (Selye, 1950). Numerous monographs and journal contributions have dealt with fear, anxiety, anger, and somatic disorder, and the effects of these states on adaptive functioning. The term stress has been used with multiple meanings, while a variety of other terms have been used to refer to similar phenomena, namely conflict, frustration, extreme situation, and the like. Too infrequently have descriptive terms such as noxious, painful, or unpleasurable been distinguished from concepts of challenge, demand, or threat. Yet a careful analysis of *psychological threat* requires the distinction from *noxious injury*. In point of fact, there seems considerably less correlation between the nature and extent of physical injury or illness and one's adaptive response, than between certain psychosocial determinants of the individual and his coping pattern, adaptive or otherwise.

The recent expansion of psychiatric consultation services to all areas of medicine has provided broad experience in working with seriously ill patients for a growing group of psychiatrists. A variety of published studies dealing with facets of the coping process associated with serious illness have issued from such consultation services. The varieties of thought, feeling, and behavior exhibited by ill or injured persons have spurred a number of clinical investigators to publish studies dealing with the adaptive problems and mechanisms observed. Notable among these have been the contributions of Hamburg and a series of collaborators (Hamburg, Hamburg, & Goza, 1953; Visotsky, Hamburg, Gross, & Lebovits, 1961; Friedman, Chodoff, Mason, & Hamburg, 1963) who studied the psychological adapta-

Reprinted from *Advances in Psychosomatic Medicine 8,* pp. 105–118, © 1972, S. Karger AG, with permission.

[1]From Department of Psychiatry, University of Southern California, Los Angeles.

tions of persons with severe burns, with paralytic poliomyelitis, and the coping behavior of parents facing the prospect of death of a child with leukemia. Other important contributions have been those of Lindemann (1944) on grief, and Janis' (1958) observations on patients facing the threat of surgery.

THE CONCEPT OF THREAT

How persons experience the threat of illness or injury and how they cope with it, how they deal with hospitalization and the assumption of the sick role, the effects of these adaptive problems on family relationships and of family reaction upon the sick patient, are factors bearing upon the success or failure of therapeutic management. The nuclear concept unifying these multiple dimensions of experience is the notion of threat. Lazarus (1966) in a scholarly monograph deals with psychological stress and the coping process. He emphasizes the key role of *cognitive appraisal* and the *meaning* thereby attached to stress-stimuli in determining the type of adaptive or coping response pattern. Such appraisal depends upon two types of antecedent: 1) stimulus configurational features, for instance the degree of ambiguity in the significance of the perceived cue, and 2) personal psychological elements, for example one's self-estimate of capability or sense of competence. *Coping processes* are then set in motion whose function is to reduce, deflect, or eliminate the anticipated harm. These processes reflect cognitive function through which the degree of threat is assessed, the availability of options is scanned, and the strength of personal resources is brought to bear against the threat. Such appraisal determines the form of response, that is the particular *coping strategy,* adopted by the individual to deal with the challenge.

Engel (1962) has specified three principal categories of challenge which constitute human psychological stress:

1. Loss or threat of loss of psychic 'objects', that is personal relationships, body functions and image, social roles, and the like.
2. Injury or threat of injury to the body, involving notions of pain or mutilation.
3. Frustration of biological drive satisfaction, especially basic nurturant or libidinal needs and avenues for aggressive discharge.

Obviously, in the case of serious illness or injury these classes of stressful challenge overlap and often coexist to varying degrees. Engel emphasizes the highly individual character of what constitutes stress for particular individuals, allowing for the fact that separation may sometimes constitute welcome release, pain provide expiation for guilt, and sickness excuse the satisfaction of dependency needs.

COPING STRATEGIES

Coping, then, is seen to refer to strategies for dealing with threat and loss. Physical illness or disability may pose any or all the features of psychological stress defined by Lazarus from the standpoint of psychologic theory and by Engel from that of clinical practice. Coping strategies include the modes of dealing with challenges ranging from pain, prostration, or paralysis to the tasks of role redefinition, redirection of goals, and relationship alteration.

When the individual is threatened by the initial signs or symptoms of illness or disability, the process of cognitive appraisal is quickly or slowly followed by patterns of reaction which include thoughts, feelings, and behaviors, both visceral and somatic. These response patterns are partly conscious and partly unconscious. They reflect more or less enduring modes of stress-response characteristics of the individual, that is his *coping style*. A number of *intra-individual determinants* (Lipowski, 1970) are involved in shaping such a style. They include both biologic factors and early social experience. The individual's style is also influenced by the course of his life, and especially by his experience of psychological stress and successful ways of dealing with it.

The range of coping behaviors available to children obviously differs from that of a mature adult. Regressive behavior is more clearly expectable and permissible in the young than in the parent of the young. Confusion or crankiness in the old is common. The manner in which illness is experienced in the young, and the response patterns of significant others toward illness in the child, may set a pattern for future coping with illness by that individual. Other factors having to do with gender, level of intelligence, social and cultural background, value systems, and the cognitive and behavioral style of the person falling ill may importantly influence his coping pattern.

Disease-related factors likewise are important determinants of coping behavior. The type of illness, the nature and idiosyncratic meaning for the individual of the organ or system involved, the rapidity of onset and progression, the degree of potential reversibility of the process, and the extent of residual disability are features which help to shape the coping process and determine the degree of adaptiveness possible for the individual.

Life-setting is a very important influence both upon the likelihood of one's falling ill or incurring injury and upon the manner and resourcefulness of the coping with it. The particular importance of the 'giving up-given up' complex, both as a setting in which to fall ill and as a determinant of the coping efficacy of the individual, has been emphasized by the Rochester group under Engel's (1968) direction.

Hospital environmental factors complicate or add specific challenges to what are often already life-threatening illness demands. The particular coping problems posed for patients by hospital intensive-care units (McKegney, 1966), coronary care units (Hackett, Cassem, & Wishnie, 1968), and renal dialysis services (Abram, 1970) have been the subject of many reports. Whole organ transplantation (Cramond, 1967) poses both challenge and opportunity for an increasing number of persons otherwise doomed to death. The coping problems here are unique and often enormous.

If and when signs or symptoms are appraised by the ill or injured person as dangerous, *anxiety* is usually aroused. At times a dysphoric affect other than anxicty is noted or reported. Some individuals lack physiological response patterns indicative of anxiety. They may display emotional, behavioral or cognitive dysfunctional responses, such as depression, anger, delusional misinterpretation of environmental or bodily input, or hallucinatory experience. This conception views manifest anxiety as only one of the possible varieties of response. *Threat* is the intervening variable, perceived and appraised, underlying all the diverse and negatively toned affects. By thinking in terms of threat rather than anxiety, one is better able to understand the salient features of psychological stress theory; the nature and determinants of the cognitive activity that results in information being appraised as threat; the variable physiological concomitants; the degree of distortion or misinterpretation of information inputs; and adaptive, as well as maladaptive, coping behaviors.

COPING STYLES

Psychological 'style' (Shapiro, 1965) refers to a mode or form of functioning that is identifiable in an individual through a range of his specific behaviors. It refers to particular ways of perceiving, thinking, and feeling, and modes of activity. Coping styles may be considered in terms of their cognitive, affective, and behavioral aspects. A brief discussion of each of these is in order.

Cognitive Coping Styles

Individuals possess relatively stable cognitive tendencies that determine the form or kind of influence that wish or need exerts upon their perceptions, interpretations, and attitudes, as well as upon their manner of recall and report. Lipowski (1970) makes the useful and economical distinction of two general modes of cognitive dealing with the facts of illness or injury: 1) *minimization,* and 2) *vigilant focusing.* Minimization connotes the tendency to selective inattention, ignoring, denial, or rationalizing of the facts or the significance of the illness or its consequences. In overwhelming illness, especially early in its course, this style may be adaptive and allow the patient a more gradual acceptance of his condition. Where a distinct threat to survival exists, or there is the danger of permanent damage or disfigurement, the patient often refuses to acknowledge the full significance of disturbing facts. T. S. Eliot in his poem *Burnt Norton* observed:

...Human kind
Cannot bear very much reality.

A patient exemplifying the cognitive mode of minimization, one employing the denial, ignoring, and rationalization, was recently encountered.

C. W., a 58-year-old spinster, employed for many years as an office bookkeeper, having lived a socially isolated, pleasure-restricted, highly routinized life, was seen for gross hematuria many months after its initial and repeated occurrence. Only upon the insistence of her employer, who grew increasingly concerned about her pallor and evident fatigue, did she present herself at the Medical Center for advice and treatment. Urological work up disclosed carcinoma of the urinary bladder with metastases to surrounding soft tissue and bone. When advised of the nature of the problem and offered palliative treatment, Miss C. W. thanked the consultant coolly, said there must be 'some mistake', affirmed that in her view the problem was a residue of unresolved 'flu' and declined further hospital care, stating that what she needed was nourishing broth and more vitamins. She dealt with a consulting psychiatrist calmly and equally firmly, and declined the offer of follow-up consultation.

In many instances of acute illness or injury, the sensorium is cloudy due to the effects on cerebral metabolism of toxicity, fever, blood loss, reduction in cerebral blood flow, or sometimes brain injury or disease. In such instances the distinction of pathophysiological from psychological mechanisms is difficult or impossible. One sees delusional denial of disability, so-called anosognosia, in certain hemiplegic patients, who sometimes actually disown the paralyzed side of their body. Ranging from such organically determined deficits in cognitive awareness, one observes a spectrum of instances from selective misinterpretation of facts, through rationalization, to outright psychotic·delusion and hallucination, all serving in some sense to ease the burden of acceptance of reality. In the latter connection, we have more than once erred on the side of forcing heavy phenothiazine therapy upon floridly delusional and hallucinating patients in our intensive care unit for severely burned patients only to have the quiet, non-hallucinating individual promptly die. A case example comes to mind.

A. R., a 62-year-old widowed woman, suffered extensive mixed second and third degree burns of the face, neck, trunk, and forearms in an accident while igniting a gas stove. While being treated in the intensive care unit for burns, she was noted to be grossly delusional, exhibiting auditory hallucinations, and was markedly agitated especially at times of debridement and dressing of her wounds. Her memory and orientation were not impaired. Vigorous therapy with chlorpromazine over a 4-day period was associated with remission of the delusional and hallucinatory symptoms and a replacement of her agitation by seeming apathy and disengagement from her surroundings. Her cognitive function remained unimpaired. Without evidence of a basic change in the level of toxic stress upon the patient, she quietly died during the sixth night of treatment.

Likewise, as psychiatric consultant to medical-surgical wards, one not infrequently sees the hopelessness and helplessness of patients with inoperable or incurable, but not imminently critical, disease whose defensive denial and rationalization has been broken through by well-intentioned, but imprudent, spilling of 'the truth' on the part of their physician or surgeon. One also will occasionally encounter patients whose denial is so durable as to result in invincible incomprehension of such 'facts' and prompt forgetting, by repression, of any memory of such an unfortunate incident. Instances such as these, not uncommon in the experience of psychiatric consultants, bear witness to the truth of Eliot's poetic line.

The psychological defensiveness involved in attention deployments, distortional interpretation of stimulus significance, and wish-fulfilling delusion is an important coping strategy. Depending upon the other resources available to the patient, these techniques may be adaptive or maladaptive in terms of survival value. Only when and if they are seriously interfering with other available measures to deal with crisis, should they be frontally challenged. Given time, a supportive environment, and effective treatment for the underlying illness or injury, such emergency adaptive mechanisms generally yield to the light of reality.

On the other hand, there are many individuals, particularly hysterical personalities, for whom repression, denial, forgetting, and a fuzzy, impressionistic type of cognitive style are habitual modes of coping and not simply an emergency response to current calamity. Such persons characteristically experience and interpret illness after the manner in which they experience life in general, often with a dramatic emphasis.

At the pole opposite from the above is the cognitive style of *vigilant focusing*. This mode is characteristic for the obsessional character. Hypervigilance, sharply focused attention to detail, narrowing of interest to matters relevant to self, rigidity of opinion, and inflexibility in adaptation to the unexpected are features common to such persons. When ill, such individuals are compulsively observant to details of therapeutic management, often quick to criticize lapses or delays in carrying out of planned orders, and frequently somewhat doubtful or skeptical of the reliability of medical and paramedical professionals' competence or concern. They usually need meticulous explanation of all diagnostic or therapeutic procedures, and are sometimes caustic in their criticism of delay or inefficiency in the conduct of their care. Uncertainty or lack of clarity of intention on the part of medical and nursing personnel are quickly noted by such patients. Confidence, trust, and easy acceptance of dependency can be achieved with such a patient by repeated explanations and discussions of his illness and its management. Failure to observe such measures may result in the patient's heightened anxiety, hostility and, occasionally, paranoid psychosis. This latter development may complicate the course of serious illness, or postoperative care, as illustrated by the following case.

> M. B., a 44-year-old, divorced, unemployed electronics technician complained repeatedly of substernal chest pain which rarely occurred during the daytime but seemed regularly to occur while recumbent and asleep at night during the period of hospital study. The pain was unresponsive to nitroglycerine and usually required an injection of meperidine for relief. For many days the diagnostic studies, including resting electrocardiograms, failed to disclose evidence of coronary or other heart disease. The patient's rigid attitude and obvious lack of confidence in the medical house-officers responsible for his care provoked bristling, caustic verbal interchanges on several occasions. A night-nurse, refusing to provide a narcotic injection in response to the patient's complaint of pain, was reported as having told him that she believed he was feigning distress. Subsequent to these events clearcut coronary artery blockage was demonstrated by coronary arteriography, and a vascular by-pass procedure was performed surgically in an effort to improve coronary circulation. Three days postoperatively the patient was floridly psychotic, hallucinating voices calling him a 'dope-addict' and threatening to send him to a hospital 'for the criminally insane'. He had the delusion that the intravenous fluid being administered contained drugs to drive him insane, and that the pre-cordial *insitu* electrocardiographic monitor lead was designed to implant electricity to twist his mind. Three months postoperatively, while still under phenothiazine drug therapy, the patient continued to have lingering paranoid suspicions about the operative experience.

Affective Coping Responses

Unpleasant affects, often changing in variety through the course of illness or disability, are nearly uniformly predictable. Some degree of fear is an expectable component of most illness or injury and may approach panic proportions, depending upon features previously mentioned related to age, sex, personality, state of awareness, intelligence, and specific disease-related or situational features in the life of the patient. Cognitive coping style may significantly influence the nature and intensity of his emotional reaction, as outlined above. Generally speaking, however, anxiety and/or depression of some degree are to be found in the severely ill or injured during the acute phase. The patient's personal interpretation of his illness or injury in terms of its consequences to himself or to his important relationships, social role activities, and goals is responsible for emotional responses ranging from anxiety, depression, anger or resentment through shame, disgust, guilt, to a state of helplessness and hopelessness. On rare occasions one sees manic elation, euphoria or excitement triggered by illness or injury.

The particular quality of emotional response to illness or injury is often reflective of the threat or loss experienced by the individual by reason of his personality characteristics and his particular life history. The illness or injury may pose a threat to the capacity to be loved by others. In general, women will be more concerned about their physical attractiveness or sense of feminine integrity. Disease, injury, or surgery upon face, breasts, and sexual organs are especially important to them.

> H. T., a 50-year-old widowed woman, presented with a stony-hard mass in the left breast with palpable lymphadenopathy in the axillary space. Her mood was noted to be affable and her behavior during the physical examination somewhat seductive. A lymph node biopsy disclosed metastatic adenocarcinoma. When the facts of the examination were quietly and soberly presented to the patient by the house-officer the patient laughed gaily and remarked that probably the young doctor didn't know how else to justify his repeated examinations of her breasts. When seen in psychiatric consultation the following day, the patient was hypomanic, exhibited pressure of speech, flight of ideas, and grandiose delusions involving sexual themes. This manic psychotic decompensation responded dramatically to therapy with lithium, and a radical mastectomy was accomplished three weeks later.

Men are most threatened by physical helplessness and the prospect of limitation in their capacity for active, instrumental function. A sense of powerlessness is especially threatening to the type of individual who has characteristically denied or minimized dependency needs. Profound psychological effects are often observed in traumatic paraplegic patients, victims of cervical or thoracic gunshot wounds or other injury to the spinal cord, and also in those suffering from cerebral vascular hemorrhage or thrombosis with hemiplegia. The transformation, nearly instantly, of a healthy, functional individual into an invalid nearly totally dependent upon others poses a combination of coping challenges wherein catastrophic loss is the central stress—loss of power, autonomy, self-esteem, sexual potency, and the sense of being loveable—above all of the sense of an open future. In injuries of this type, as well as in a wider variety of severe illness, radical alteration of body-image often occurs (Orbach & Tallent, 1965). The sense of a whole, integrated, functional unitary person must be altered to take account of changes in one's capacity to stand, move, initiate and carry through independent action.

Affects ranging from fear and grief, on the one hand, through the gamut previously mentioned to deep depression, or to manic excitement, have been noted in our consultative work with patients coping with particular varieties of stress, for example: the isolation and loneliness enforced by communicable disease; the massive mutilation to face, extremities, and trunk of the severely burned patient; the near suffocating labor of the patient with chronic obstructive pulmonary disease; the doubt and concern mobilized by possible technical failures in patients with organ transplants, chronic renal dialysis, respiratory and cardiac support equipment; the prolonged monotony and enforced immobility of patients with bone-traction for fracture, or Stryker-frame bedding for spinal disease. These examples can be multiplied many times over in busy general hospital consultative psychiatric practice.

Behavioral Coping Patterns

The cognitive appraisal of threat in any cue stimulus, including that of perceived illness or injury, prompts action tendencies adaptive to the challenge. These action tendencies have elementary biological roots, which in the human person are capable of radical modification, suppression, or deflection in the face of situational constraints. Lipowski (1970) in his discussion of such behavioral coping refers to three principal styles: 1) tackling, 2) capitulating, and 3) avoiding.

The 'tackling' posture refers to a disposition toward active, energetic engagement with the tasks imposed by the illness or injury. It ranges from realistically modulated effort designed to minimize the direct and indirect effects of the injury or illness upon general strength or local functional capacity, on the one hand, to imprudent, driven over-activity, reflective frequently of the degree of stress generated by the prospect of powerlessness or helplessness implicit in acceptance of the sick role. Examples are the kind of compulsive busyness encountered in certain patients with dangerous hypertensive vascular disease, or the driveness seen in many victims of progressive rheumatoid arthritis who continue to stay 'on their feet' in the face of increasing disintegration of weight-bearing joints.

'Capitulating' behavior is characterized by passivity, inactivity, and often helpless dependency upon care-taking others. This type of patient too often stimulates dislike, resentment, and withdrawal on the part of caretaking hospital staff whose reactions frequently elicit even more pronounced dependency and sometimes demandingness from the patient. Such patients resent anyone's 'making light' of their illness. They seem often to mind less the actual injury or illness than not being cared for tenderly or devotedly enough. The resistance of such patients to measures designed to foster independent status is a very frequent source of origin for psychiatric consultation requests.

'Avoidance' is a behavioral style characterized by active effort to free oneself of the constraint implicit in the acceptance of illness or injury. It differs from the 'tackling' posture where, for the most part, the fact of the illness is cognitively accepted and dealt with by behavior aimed at mastery of the threatening features posed by the illness or injury. Avoidance behavior is nearly always accompanied by the cognitive mode of minimization referred to previously. Fear, usually denied and often perhaps only dimly perceived or recognized, prompts this form of behavioral reaction-formation. The writer recalls vividly the case of a man in his early forties admitted on six previous occasions to a medical service with symptoms and signs of coronary disease and fresh myocardial injury, only to sign out 'against medical advice' within a few days. On each occasion he admitted to his resumption of ocean surfing, a physically taxing sport, within a day or so of his release from hospital. The threat posed by dependency and physical disability for this individual lay behind his driven flight into over-activity.

CONCEPTS OF COURAGE, WILL, AND GROWTH

When a definitive stress theory is finally achieved it will need to account for strength as well as weakness, courage as well as fear, and for psychological growth as well as for failure. The literature dealing with the coping process in the face of challenge, including that of serious illness or injury, is really quite adequate in explicating such defensive adaptive maneuvers as psychological constriction, suppression, repression, and denial. Cognitive distortions in the form of illusion, delusion, and hallucination are recognized as having strategic value in certain overwhelming situations. Infantile behavioral regression with rocking, soiling, and sucking are not without adaptive function at times. Dependent clinging and isolated withdrawal serve certain persons at times.

The biological rootedness of animal courage is better understood by ethologists and veterinarians than by psychologists and psychiatrists. Splendid examples of 'the courage to be' encountered in individuals in crisis have perhaps been more adequately understood by certain poets, novelists, and philosophers than by those physicians and psychiatric consultants, whose work in general hospitals has revealed such coping strength, often in individuals whose unillustrious earlier lives had never suggested their possession of such potential. That the subhuman animal would appear to possess such inner fortitude more reliably and predictably than the human and may well prove to be a reflection of healthier early social learning experience, on the whole, than is the case for too many humans, paradoxical as this notion might seem. Patterns of mothering leading to firmly established trust, confidence, healthy autonomy, and a sense of mastery would seem less easy to provide to humans than are their counterparts for many infrahuman species. The sense of self-control without loss of self-esteem leading to a lasting sense of autonomy and competence is a transition all too unpredictable for many humans. The hidden sense of defective self-control, of clumsy or unpredictable mastery of one's body and one's self, and at a deeper level the impressions of having been deprived, divided, or of having been abandoned—leaving a residue of basic mistrust—these are the roots of powerlessness and hopelessness that the psychiatric consultant encounters in sick or injured persons. Where such early life experiences have been richer and more vitalizing one finds trust, confidence, and hope. The 'courage to be' of which Tillich (1952) spoke would appear to be founded upon such strength-inducing socialization experiences.

Such fundamental growth experiences would likewise appear to be the psychobiological underpinnings of the specifically human freedoms of decision and choice. Overly deterministic views of human psychology have for too many years tended to regard the person, in Houseman's words, as

> ...a stranger and afraid
> In a world I never made...

wherein individuals are seen as wholly controlled and directed by forces outside themselves which they cannot alter. The firm grip of necessity has been regarded as determinative. While this is exceptional, experienced consultants to the seriously sick and injured see examples of such magnificent courage and unambivalent decision as to make one proud to be human.

Wheelis (1970), an extremely perceptive psychiatrist as well as novelist, challenges the all too common rigid determinism in an impressive statement:

> Throughout our lives the proportion of necessity to freedom depends upon our tolerance of conflict: the greater our tolerance the more freedom we retain, the less our tolerance the more we jettison; for high among the uses of necessity is relief of tension. What we can't alter we don't have to worry about; so the enlargement of necessity is a measure of economy in psychic housekeeping. The more issues we have closed, the fewer we have to fret about...Tranquility, however, has risks of its own. As we expand necessity and so relieve ourselves of conflict and responsibility, we are relieved also, in the same measure, of authority and significance. When there arises then a crisis which does not fall within our limited routine we are frightened, without resources, insignificant.

To further paraphrase Wheelis, too often we regard patients as without freedom, note only constraint, label them victim. Yet in the consciousness of that patient, it makes great difference whether or not he experiences choice. If he knows the constraint and nothing else, then he lives his necessity. But if upon self-appraisal and situational assessment, perceiving the constraint he turns from it to a choice between two possible alternative courses, then however he chooses he is living his freedom, which may extend to his last breath. On the other hand, one can win the struggle to avoid responsibility for one's life, but if one does what is lost is one's life.

SUMMARY

Coping with severe illness or injury encompasses both psychological and biological adaptiveness. The development of psychiatric consultation services in general hospitals and clinics has provided rich experience in working with and coming to understand men under stress. The concept of threat is the key variable with its connotation of expected harm and its dependence upon cognitive appraisal including perception, memory, learning, and thought. The notion of meaning is defined as central to the coping responses produced by the threat of illness or injury. Coping strategies are seen to reflect intra-personal determinants as well as others that are disease-related, reflective of life-setting, and hospital environment. Various coping styles are discussed under cognitive, affective and behavioral types. The positive, as well as negative aspects of coping challenge are discussed, including the basis of courage, hope, and choice.

REFERENCES

Abram, H. S. Survival by machine: The psychological stress of chronic hemodialysis. *Psychiatric Medicine,* 1970, *1,* 37–51.

Bibring, G. L. Psychiatry and medical practice in a general hospital. *New England Journal of Medicine,* 1956, *254,* 366–372.

Cramond, W. A. Renal homotransplantation—Some observations on recipients and donors. *British Journal of Psychiatry,* 1967, *113,* 1223–1230.

Engel, G. L. *Psychological development in health and disease.* Philadelphia: Saunders, 1962.

Engel, G. L. A life setting conducive to illness: The giving up-given up complex. *Bulletin of the Menninger Clinic,* 1968, *32,* 355–365.

Friedman, S. B., Chodoff, P., Mason, J. W., & Hamburg, D. A. Behavioral observations on parents anticipating the death of a child. *Pediatrics,* 1963, *32,* 610–625.

Hackett, T. P., Cassem, N. G., & Wishnie, H. A. The coronary-care unit: An appraisal of the psychological hazards. *New England Journal of Medicine,* 1968, *279,* 1365–1370.

Hamburg, D. A., Hamburg, B., & Goza de, S. Adaptive problems and mechanisms in severely burned patients. *Psychiatry,* 1953, *16,* 1–20.

Janis, I. L. *Psychological stress.* New York: John Wiley & Sons, 1958.

Lazarus, R. S. *Psychological stress and the coping process.* New York: McGraw-Hill Book Co., 1966.

Lindemann, E. Symptomatology and management of acute grief. *American Journal of Psychiatry,* 1944, *101,* 141–148.

Lipowski, Z. J. Physical illness, the individual, and the coping process. *Psychiatric Medicine,* 1970, *1,* 91–102.

McKegney, F. P. The intensive care syndrome. *Connecticut Medicine,* 1966, *30,* 633–636.

Orbach, C. E., & Tallent, N. Modification of perceived body and of body concepts. *Archives of General Psychiatry,* 1965, *12,* 126–131.

Selye, H. *The physiology and pathology of exposure to stress.* Montreal: Acta, 1950.

Shapiro, D. *Neurotic styles.* New York: Basic Books, 1965.

Tillich, P. *The courage to be.* New Haven: Yale University Press, 1952.

Visotsky, H. M., Hamburg, D. A., Gross, M. E., & Lebovits, B. Z. Coping behavior under extreme stress. *Archives of General Psychiatry,* 1961, *5,* 423–448.

Wheelis, A. *The desert.* New York: Basic Books, 1970.

THE CONCEPT OF
THE DISABILITY PROCESS

Morton R. Weinstein[1]

In the early 1960s, Behan and Hirschfeld (1963, 1966; Hirschfeld & Behan, 1963, 1966) began a study in Detroit of what they called "the accident process," a study which grew out of their often frustrating experiences with several hundred industrial accident victims. Initially, their attention was directed to the same two points that had earlier preoccupied many others concerned with industrial injuries: they looked first at the accident, and then they looked at the outcome states of fixed and often disproportionate disability. As many had been before them, they were puzzled about the relationships between accident and outcome. How did one lead to the other?

In contrast to their predecessors, Behan and Hirschfeld attempted to answer this question by looking first at events preceding the accident and at the larger human and social context in which the accident occurred. They then searched for ways to understand the problem of chronicity through the assumption that a life of disability or of invalidism, with its constricted activity and reduced autonomy, would be chosen and maintained only if it resolved some extremely powerful and disturbing conflicts.

THE ACCIDENT PROCESS

Behan and Hirschfeld (1963; Hirschfeld & Behan, 1963, 1966) demonstrated that many of the most perplexing and resistant examples of chronic disability in the wake of industrial injuries were actually the late stages in a sequence they termed "the accident process." The four key features of this process were thought to be:

Tension and stress. In almost every instance, the accident is preceded by the development (not necessarily in the working area of the patient's life) of tension and stress, leading to feelings of inadequacy and depression. These unwelcome dysphoric states are often associated with a powerful sense of being insufficiently appreciated, with having too much demanded or expected of one, and with disappointments and frustrations about promotion, security, advancement, and competence.

Dependency denial. Essential to the initiation of the accident process is a personality configuration that makes the patient unusually sensitive to

---

Reprinted from *Psychosomatics,* 1978, *19*(2), 94–97, with permission.

[1]Associate professor of Psychiatry at the Langley Porter Institute, University of California, San Francisco.

perceptions of increased expectations and of reduced support and approval, and which also makes it very difficult for the patient to acknowledge or to ask for help directly and explicitly for the tension-depression state he is experiencing. The personality styles of these people (mostly men in the Behan-Hirschfeld series) have prominent dependent and passive qualities, along with an inability to accept or acknowledge such dependent wishes or passive strivings—a complex commonly found in the working blue-collar population of our industrial centers and still (but of recent date less strenuously) widely considered to be normal or even ideal for American men in general.

The injury. The coupling of increasing subjective distress with an attitude that makes it difficult to ask for help sets the stage for the next phase of the accident process—the occurrence of an injury that transforms the employee into someone whose distress and impaired performance can be understood by him and others as the result of an externally generated event, something that "could happen to anyone," understandable to all and compatible with an image of tough self-sufficiency. In brief, the accident transforms an "unacceptable disability," equated with weakness and failure, into an "acceptable disability," neither dishonorable nor shameful. None of this requires us to assume that the accident happens *because of* the need for an acceptable disability, but of course the concept of the accident-prone person is an old and recurrent one and would seem to have one of its bases here.

Disability as a way of life. The remainder of the accident process has to do with the crystallization and stabilization of disability as a way of life, energized by the patient's ongoing personality characteristics, by the rapid accumulation of reinforcing social and financial responses to the initial disability and, sometimes, unfortunately, by the consequences of diagnostic and therapeutic interventions of physicians and health-care agencies.

THE DISABILITY PROCESS

Our concern with the contributions of social agencies and social systems (including medicine) to the stabilization phase of the accident process, and later our realization that the initiating event could be a non-industrial illness rather than a work-related accident, led us and our associates to publish studies of our own (Ruesch & Brodsky, 1978; Weinstein, 1968, 1969), extending Behan and Hirschfeld's concepts, under the titles "The Illness Process" and then "The Disability Process."

Figure 1 is a graphic summary of the "disability process." This process can be initiated not only by industrial injuries, but also by episodes of illness. Figure 1 shows the contributions of agencies and public programs to the development of states of fixed disability.

At two points in the disability process the line representing work competence and the line representing self-esteem diverge. Both these divergence

Stages in the Disability Process

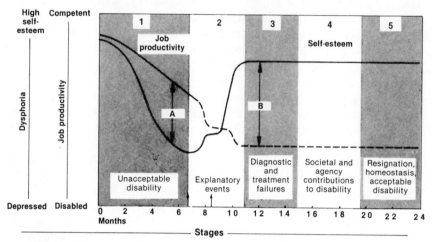

Figure 1.   The disability process.

points (A and B) are important; their components are set out in the disability equations A and B, shown in Figure 1.

At point A, in the phase of crisis build-up, a rapid decline in self-esteem and a rise in dysphoric feelings such as depression or tension are shown to begin before the occurrence of the symbolic event (the job-related accident or the non-vocational illness). The historical primacy of this initial dysphoric state—and, of course, of the vulnerable personality on which this state impinges—may not be apparent to the observer and is often fully outside the patient's awareness. However, careful evaluation, especially the inclusion of family members in the reconstruction of the evolution of the disability process, will often confirm the presence of a troubled mental state *before* the triggering event. This troubled state leads to the later slow decline in competence; it is perceived by the patient, and often by the patient's family and co-workers as well, as the unacceptable disability.

The second divergence of mood state and job performance (point B) follows the event (the accident or illness). The occurrence of this event transforms the unacceptable state of being disabled because of "feeling bad" into the more acceptable state of being disabled because of what has befallen one—the acceptable disability. The consequences of that transformation are represented by the crossing and second divergence of the two measures—restoration of self-esteem concurrent with a decline in the patient's work capacity.

How can the realization that work disability is commonly the end result of a complex process rather than the direct consequence of a discrete accident or illness help in the prevention, evaluation, and rehabilitation of such tenacious syndromes as the "industrial low back"? First, such realization helps us to predict and appreciate the tenacity with which some disabilities may be sought and maintained: whenever self-esteem is elevated, change is difficult and unlikely; when it is low, change is actively sought by the patient and can be facilitated by others. Second, our contemporary cultural valuations of depression and anxiety as being unworthy, shameful, and unacceptable—valuations that often seem to initiate the disability process—appear to be changing. To the extent that we can further soften the cultural polarization of some kinds of suffering as honorable and other kinds as unacceptable, especially for men, we will reduce the energy that makes the disability process operate. Third, in view of their prominence as ingredients of the disability process, we could re-examine some of the social and programmatic reinforcements and supports for ongoing disability: we can slow the crystallization and stabilization phases of the disability process by promoting public policies that reduce the reinforcement of disability by monetary and other rewards. Finally, but more nearly at hand to health-care providers, we can re-examine our own activities to see whether our diagnostic efforts, our treatment interventions, our participation in the establishment of awards, even our covert messages about hopelessness or the rightness of the patient's "claim" against society, contribute to the disability process (Weinstein, 1967).

The task of inducing changes in cultural values and societal patterns is enormous, but the disability process is, after all, only a statement of what our society believes to be good and what it holds to be bad about people and their behavior. In the final analysis, the disability process is not likely to change unless the values that energize it are themselves changed.

REFERENCES

Behan, R. C., & Hirschfeld, A. H. The accident process. II. Toward more rational treatment of industrial injuries. *Journal of the American Medical Association,* 1963, *186,* 300.

Behan, R. C., & Hirschfeld, A. H. 1966. Disability without disease or accident. *Archives of Environmental Health,* 1966, *12,* 655.

Brodsky, C. M. Social psychiatric consequences of job incompetence. *Comprehensive Psychiatry,* 1971, *12,* 526.

Hirschfeld, A. H., & Behan, R. C. The accident process. I. Etiological considerations of industrial injuries. *Journal of the American Medical Association,* 1963, *186,* 193.

Hirschfeld, A. H., & Behan, R. C. The accident process. III. Disability: Acceptable and unacceptable. *Journal of the American Medical Association,* 1966, *197,* 85.

Ruesch, J., & Brodsky, C. M. The concept of social disability. *Archives of General Psychiatry,* 1968, *19,* 394.

Weinstein, M. R. A program for the rehabilitation of socially disabled psychiatric patients through retraining. *Comprehensive Psychiatry,* 1967, *8,* 249.

Weinstein, M. R. The illness process. *Journal of the American Medical Association,* 1968, *204,* 209.

Weinstein, M. R. The disability process. Contributions of service agencies to client disability. *Comprehensive Psychiatry,* 1969, *10,* 398.

CHAPTER 3

IMPACT OF DISABILITY/ ILLNESS ON THE CHILD

Paul W. Power and Arthur E. Dell Orto

In the two articles that follow in this chapter there is an extensive discussion of the psychological aspects of chronic illness in children. Both provide a thorough explanation of the determinants of the child's emotional response to disability, the problems specific to certain illnesses, and the effect of the illness on the child's development. Management suggestions are also given that can be most helpful for health professionals. Consequently, the material presented before these articles only briefly identifies some of the highlights or general principles that are important to understand when working with disabled children and their families.

Children have specific, emotional reactions to their own chronic illness or disabling condition. The unique fear of the medical procedures, the severe peer pressure encountered by young persons who are handicapped and attempting to establish an identity, and the very young children's lack of understanding of what is happening to them suggest that disabled children's responses are usually different from those of disabled adults. Often it is necessary for the health professional to interpret or explain these reactions to the adult family members. This may be part of the helper's intervention approach. Many families need this information before they can assist their child to adjust to the illness or disability. The following pages present in summary form some of the information that is elaborated upon in the articles by Steinhauer and Hughes, knowledge that can become a basis for effective family intervention.

DETERMINANTS OF REACTION

When analyzing why children react as they do to a chronic disease or handicap, some of the following causes should be considered:

1. *Nature of the disability or chronic illness* The course of the child's illness may be stable or rapidly deteriorating, may require constant or in-

frequent medical treatment, cause permanent disfigurement, and necessitate many hospitalizations. These conditions or effects will influence the child's emotional response. Long hospitalizations, for example, may prevent a child from developing necessary socialization skills to play with peers, or disfigurement may cause the afflicted child to seek social isolation.

2. *Age of the child at the onset of the disease* What illness means to children at the time it occurs and the impression it leaves on their personality are largely affected by their stage of development (Travis, 1976). Freeman (1968) believes that congenital defects are more likely to produce personality alterations than acquired handicaps. Chronically ill children of 1 to 3 years of age may have separation anxieties and fears of hospital strangers; as they grow older and their self-image becomes better established, they may begin to react to disease and handicaps with added fears, such as those of painful procedures and perceived harm to their body.

3. *The pain experience* Children generally do not understand the origins of the pain associated with illness or disability. A child with juvenile rheumatoid arthritis, for example, will be harrassed by almost constant pain and will usually show continued anxiety. Pain can cause a child much confusion and generate frustrations at not being able to control it. Pain may also be viewed as a punishment.

4. *Previous experience with loss* Children who have been made insecure by previous separations from the mother will usually enter a hospital with more fright and become more distressed by treatment (Travis, 1976). If children have encountered earlier, painful experiences, a similar experience, such as the medical procedures associated with treatment, will remind them of those earlier experiences. If the family system has had many losses, such as family deaths or the separation or divorce of mother and father, the meaning of the disability or illness may be all the more severe for the child. Young persons might believe that their illness can cause close family members and friends to leave them.

5. *Parental attitudes* Davis (1975) reports that one major factor in poor child personality adjustment to a physical disability is the impact of parental attitudes. Overprotectiveness, for example, which is a natural response of parents to a child's disability, may harm the child's adjustment. Children may also demand more and more attention and refuse to do even the simplest things for themselves or others. Pity can harm children by causing them to feel sorry for themselves. This attitude can defeat the treatment efforts that particularly encourage the child to accept bravely a disability situation. Parental anxiety over the disability could also have a serious effect on the children, causing them to become

constantly tense. Parents with hemophiliac children, for instance, very frequently show overanxiety for the ill child (Travis, 1976). The child picks up this cue and, in turn, becomes very fearful when approaching daily tasks.

EMOTIONAL REACTION AND COPING METHODS OF THE CHILD

Unlike the stages of adult psychological reaction to illness that have been reported in the literature and outlined in the previous chapter, similar responses have not been widely identified with children. Because of the variety of environmental influences on the child, and the many patterns of emotional needs, it is difficult to catalogue the different emotional reactions to disability or illness that could take place. Yet in describing the child's emotional reactions, many authors (Freeman, 1968; Steinhauer, Mushin, & Rae-Grant, 1974; Hughes, 1976; Travis, 1976) have used familiar concepts and these are explained briefly. Some examples of the child's reactions are:

Anxiety   This is a feeling of fright, not only of medical procedures but also of the unknown future and the possibility of losing parents and family members. Separation from parents during hospitalizations may aggravate anxiety.

Depression   This is frequently characterized by sadness, which, in turn, is often expressed by boredom or restlessness. Children with kidney disease, for example, limited in their activities with peers and forced to undergo frequent medical procedures, may become unhappy and express this in periods of restlessness at home or by anger at other family members.

Feeling different from others   Children who are congenitally disabled must begin at an early age to deal with their difference from others (Johnson, 1979). Such acknowledgment may cause them to become passive and apathetic and experience doubt about their bodies. Older disabled children may feel at a distinct disadvantage regarding physical attractiveness and harbor deep feelings of inferiority.

With these emotional reactions, however, there are certain coping methods that are used by many children to deal with the physical and emotional implications of being disabled. The different ways of coping will depend on the developmental level of the children and their experience with earlier traumas. A few coping mechanisms that can be utilized by children are:

Regression   Life-threatening illnesses, such as asthma, heart disease, or nephrosis, may bring the danger of infantilization and heighten dependency needs (Travis, 1976). In this state, the child refuses to do anything himself and demands constant attention from others. In becoming the center of attention the child finds a way to deal with the disability/illness.

Denial   Many young people simply deny that they have the disease. This occurs often with juvenile diabetics who will ignore dietary restrictions and a treatment schedule in order to take part in the activities of their peers.

Compensation   Many young people will become very accomplished at certain endeavors, e.g., music or school work, in order to make up for their perceived deficits. One woman known to the authors became a champion ice skater during adolescence because she wanted to overcome feelings of inferiority caused by a congenital facial disfigurement. Maria, whose personal statement begins this section, has drawn many people to her because of her socialization skills. She is compensating for her many physical limitations by emphasizing friendliness and concern for others.

Although emotional reactions and coping mechanisms have been identified, there is no general agreement regarding the incidence of emotional disturbance with each type of disability, nor is there any reason to believe that a specific personality type or reaction pattern is inevitable for a child with a particular handicap. Multiple factors, such as the climate of the family environment, the attitude of health professionals, and the emotional stability of the child, are operative. However, an understanding of these emotional reactions will assist the helping professional to enlighten the family members on the disability-related feelings of the child.

FACTORS CONDUCIVE TO GOOD ADJUSTMENT

Freeman (1968) has identified several factors that are important to understand when utilizing the family for the child's rehabilitation. They are viewed as conditions for successful restoration, and these five factors are stated in summary form:

1. There is a stable family situation, in which the parent-child relationship is predominantly positive and siblings have the awareness they are basically trusted by their parents. The relationship between parents is also positive and parental anxiety toward the disabled child is generally kept under control.
2. There is realistic information about the disability/illness available to the family and child. Accurate information can reduce uncertainty and allay many feelings of anxiety. This knowledge should stress the child's capabilities.

3. There are adequate opportunities for the disabled child for peer contact and play. If a child is restricted unnecessarily, he will often act out or regress to a more unacceptable, infantile state. This restriction may be caused by unwarranted overprotectiveness.

4. There is open communication between the involved professionals and parents, so that they are working cooperatively, rather than at cross purposes. Johnson (1979) found, when working with spina bifida children and their families, that open communication among the parents, siblings, and the disabled child communicates to the child that the abnormalities is an acceptable topic for discussion. It tells handicapped children that their body is acceptable, and facilitates speaking about their unexpressed fears and frustrations. A lack of communication suggests shame to these children.

5. There is preparation of the child and parents for hospitalization and painful or complicated procedures. Such preparation alleviates many fears of the child, especially the fear of the child that the parents may abandon him.

CONCLUSION

For the child to adapt to an illness or disability means that the family must first adjust. This adaptation requires that the family members be aware of what the ill child is going through emotionally. Such a recognition is often difficult for family members if they are caught up with their own anxiety and sadness over the illness experience. Often these feelings will have to be identified, understood, and accepted before the family can reach out to help their child.

The following two articles give a comprehensive treatment of the child's emotional reactions to disability. In particular, Dr. Hughes's article is directed to the health professional who is seeking the reasons why many ill children react as they do to the chronic disease or handicap. He provides suggestions, as does Dr. Steinhauer, on how to study the child with a severe illness in order to prevent or minimize the emotional impact.

REFERENCES

Davis, R. Family of physically disabled child. *New York State Journal of Medicine,* 1975, June, 1039–1041.

Freeman, R. D. Emotional reactions of handicapped children. In S. Chess & A. Thomas (Eds.), *Annual progress in child psychiatry and child development,* pp. 379–395. New York: Brunner/Mazel, 1968.

Hughes, J. The emotional impact of chronic disease. *American Journal of Disabled Children,* 1976, *130,* 1199–1203.

Johnson, A. *A case study of developmental achievement in latency-aged, spina bifida children: Implications for social work practice.* Unpublished doctoral dissertation, Smith College, 1979.

Steinhauer, P., Mushin, D. N., & Rae-Grant, Q. Psychological aspects of chronic illness. *Pediatric Clinics of North America,* 1974, *21*(4), 825–840.

Travis, G. *Chronic illness in children—Its impact on child and family.* Stanford, Cal.: Stanford University Press, 1976.

THE EMOTIONAL IMPACT OF CHRONIC DISEASE
The Pediatrician's Responsibilities

James G. Hughes[1]

I am deeply honored in having been selected as the recipient of the Abraham Jacobi Award for 1975. In view of the great pediatric pioneer for whom this award is named, and the list of distinguished pediatricians who have preceded me in being accorded this honor, I feel humble on this occasion.

The recipient of the award is permitted to choose his own subject and to discuss it in the way he deems most appropriate. Indeed, from the awardee's standpoint, this is one of the nice features of the occasion—to have a captive audience and the opportunity to harp on a favorite theme!

During my professional years I have always maintained a lively interest in pediatric psychiatry, especially from the practical viewpoint of what the physician can do to prevent or minimize emotional tensions in the child and his family, and if present, to relieve them.

I intend to share with you my views of how the physician should analyze the child with a chronic illness and his family milieu, and to discuss the deliberate actions he should invariably take to prevent or minimize the emotional impact. A systematic approach, based largely on personal experience will be presented.

FUNDAMENTAL OBJECTIVE OF PEDIATRICS

The fundamental objective of pediatrics is to guide children safely and happily through childhood so that they will become healthy, well-adjusted, normal young adults—to enable them to achieve their maximum potential physically, intellectually, psychologically, and socially.

Since physical, mental, emotional, and social growth and development proceed simultaneously, the understanding physician recognizes that a threat to any one of these fields is a threat to all the others. This is especially true of the child with a chronic disease or handicap.

The basic concept is that there is no such thing as a purely organic illness or a purely emotional disorder. We do not become sick in the flesh or

Reprinted from *American Journal of Diseases of Children 130*, pp. 1199–1203, © 1976, American Medical Association, with permission.

Read before the Section on Pediatrics at the 124th annual convention of the American Medical Association, Atlantic City, NJ, June 16, 1975.

[1]From the Department of Pediatrics, University of Tennessee, and Le Bonheur Children's Hospital, Memphis.

in the spirit alone. Every organic illness is invariably associated with some degree of psychic disturbance, not only of the child himself but of his parents and others to whom he is dear. Similarly, every emotional disorder is to some degree accompanied by a disturbance in body function, ranging from the trivial and inconsequential to psychosomatic manifestations of such intensity as to mimic organic diseases.

One may visualize illness, then, as a spectrum in which the almost purely organic conditions are at one end and the almost purely psychic at the other, with all possible combinations and variations between. Ordinarily, one of these factors predominates, but it is always a combination, and it often takes a perceptive physician to determine the extent to which each participates.

COMPREHENSIVE ANALYSIS

In the comprehensive analysis of a child with chronic disease or handicap, the following factors should be taken into consideration.

1. Nature of the chronic disease or handicap.
2. Age of the child at the onset of the disease.
3. Parental attitudes and emotional balance.
4. Emotional adjustment of the child at the onset of the disease.
5. Threats to the basic emotional needs of the child.
6. Availability of special facilities and programs.

1. Nature of the Chronic Disease or Handicap   Chronic diseases and handicaps range from those that are minimal to those that are severe, even life-threatening. Therefore, the physician needs to ask himself the following questions: 1) Is the diagnosis accurate? 2) What is the prognosis? 3) Is the condition disfiguring? 4) Will it greatly restrict the activities of the child and his participation in school and social contacts with his age group? 5) Is there a treatment that gives hope of success? 6) Is excellent treatment easily available to this particular child? 7) How will the cost of treatment be borne?

Accuracy of Diagnosis

An accurate diagnosis, early established, does much to emotionally stabilize the parents and the child who is old enough to appreciate medical uncertainty. Nothing exceeds fear of the unknown in creating anxiety and tensions. Therefore, diagnostic measures should be planned intelligently, executed promptly, and should be so well-coordinated that the result is known as soon as possible. A poorly planned, piecemeal diagnostic approach may be completely upsetting. Unfortunately, all chronic diseases are not easily diagnosed. When there continues to be doubt, appropriate consultants are called in, and the fact that they *are* called in is, in itself, a stabilizing factor.

CONSULTATIONS

Let me interject a comment concerning consultations. A physician should request a consultant under the following circumstances: 1) when he does not know what he is dealing with and needs another opinion; 2) when he *does* know the diagnosis, but the treatment is out of his field; 3) whenever he makes the accurate diagnosis of a chronic disease of major importance or a disease with an invariably fatal outcome; and 4) when the family is anxious because of uncertainties in diagnosis or treatment and is about to request a consultant.

In the case of major chronic disease or uniformly fatal disease, parents invariably feel better when a second physician has also certified the diagnosis and approved the treatment.

Requesting a consultant when one senses that the parents are about to suggest one is not done to save face. It is done for the child's sake—specifically, to permit the suggestion of a consultant who could really be of help.

Once an accurate diagnosis is established, one is able to analyze the other items regarding the nature of the disease or handicap.

Prognosis

Chronic diseases range from those that are easily controlled to those that may become progressive, or may eventually cause death. Armed with the right diagnosis, the physician is, of course, able to predict the probable outcome of the illness, at least in general terms. Nevertheless, in view of unpredictable variations in certain chronic diseases (rheumatoid arthritis, for example), determining the outlook is often far from exact. The best that can be done in most instances is to adopt an optimistic attitude and to emphasize that the child may well fall into the group that makes good progress.

Is the Disease or Handicap Disfiguring?

It makes a great difference whether the disease or handicap is disfiguring—whether it is visible or invisible. One might even say whether it is audible, as in children with severe cleft palate who may never speak perfectly despite skillful operations. If the defect is disfiguring, it will have a more profound emotional impact on the child and parents than if it is invisible, as in diabetes. It will also be essential to correct the disfiguring defect surgically, where this can be done, and as early as possible in order to lessen the period of maladjustment of the child and the parents.

Restriction of Activities

The degree to which a chronic disease or handicap restricts a child's activities has great bearing on his emotional, social, and intellectual growth and development. At one end of the spectrum are bed-ridden invalids and at the other those whose chronic disease or handicap interferes only slightly with their activities.

If the child's activities must be greatly restricted, special attention should be given to affording contacts with other children, within the limits of his clinical condition. Thus, his friends should be encouraged to visit him in the hospital or home, and as close a contact as possible should be maintained with his social world.

Does Treatment Give Hope of Success?

The parents and the child old enough to understand will be much comforted, and therefore better adjusted, if there is a treatment that offers hope of success. Diabetes, with all its difficulties, may be well controlled. Epilepsy may be perfectly controlled. The child with celiac disease may blossom under proper treatment. Not so the child with severe scoliosis, advanced renal insufficiency, sickle cell disease, and a host of other permanently difficult problems.

Is Excellent Treatment Easily Available for This Child?

Unfortunately, not all children have excellent treatment facilities easily available. There are innumerable children in our nation who are geographically remote from medical centers. This includes those who must cross the asphalt jungles of metropolitan complexes to reach medical facilities. They are remote in the sense of the time and effort necessary to attend special clinics for the chronically ill or handicapped. Fortunately, much effort is being made to reduce these geographic and temporal barriers to good medical care. The psychologic burdens of the child and his parents will obviously be reduced if good longitudinal care is easily available.

The Cost of Treatment

Chronic diseases and long-term handicaps are notably expensive. Federal, state, and city medical programs for children are often available, and voluntary health agencies and medical insurance include more and more of the nation's population. Yet these programs do not always cover the entire cost of care, and family finances often suffer.

2. Age of the Child at Onset of Disease   The age of a child at the onset of a chronic disease or physical defect strongly influences the degree of emotional impact. The simplest example is the very young infant who is, of course, psychologically oblivious to the fact that his illness or defect makes him different from others. However, an infant less than 6 months of age may react to hospitalization with what has been called a "global" reaction—alterations in patterns of feeding, sleeping, and elimination. In the second half of the first year, he may react to prolonged hospitalization by what has been termed "stranger anxiety" and "separation anxiety."

The child 1 to 3 years of age may also have anxiety based on separation and on fear of hospital strangers, and may show regressive behavior. Under the emotional impact of regimentation and hospitalization, he may become detached, withdrawn, fail to eat well, and may even become permanently blighted emotionally if lack of sensory stimulation and warm affection lasts too long.

As the child grows older and his self-image becomes better established, he begins to react to disease and hospitalization not only with separation anxiety, but many fears—fears of painful procedures and fears in regard to harm to his body. Deeper anxieties now flood his mind—the thwarting of achievement goals, worry over loss of independence, concern over future occupation, fear that he will not be accepted socially, and damages to his self-image. Small wonder he so often becomes withdrawn, embittered, and reacts with aggressive overcompensation.

3. Parental Attitudes and Emotional Balance   Adjustment of parents and, in turn, the child depends to a great extent on parental attitudes and the degree of emotional balance of the parents prior to the onset of the child's illness.

Thus, one is especially interested in evaluating whether the parents have the normal love and affection for the child, whether they actually reject him, whether they are overprotective, or whether they are domineering. We need to know whether they can give him the warmth of love and affection that every child deserves and the chronically ill child specifically requires.

Every parent initially rejects the diagnosis of a chronic disease in his child. This is a normal impulsive flight from the truth, through self-protective denial of the diagnosis. Once the diagnosis has been accepted, the child himself may be rejected, although the converse is usually true; afflicted children usually call forth great parental love and sympathy. Nevertheless, there are undoubtedly secret moments of rejection. But these transitory rejection thoughts, born of the burden of the disease and the dashed hopes of the parents, are usually quickly overcome by the much greater love for the child. However, when parents catch themselves thinking this way, they have deep guilt feelings.

Indeed, parents invariably have guilt feelings when the diagnosis of a deformity, chronic illness, or a fatal disease is made. The physician should always recognize this fact and attempt to relieve the parents of false thoughts that they contributed to the child's condition. It is amazing how gratified parents are for this open approach, and how obviously relieved they are for the absolution of their presumed sin.

Overprotectiveness is another parental attitude that needs evaluation. It may have been present before the onset of the chronic disease, and it understandably flourishes during the management of the condition. There is ordinarily a surge of sympathy for any afflicted person, most of all one's own child. This is so normal and so therapeutic for the parents that it is often difficult to hold in check. But, if it is overdone, it will harm the child's adjustment to his handicap. He may feed on overprotectiveness, demand more and more attention, resign from doing even the simplest things for himself or others, and become insistent and even domineering and tyrannical.

Overprotectiveness may also impair treatment. Having given in to the child on so many fronts, parents may also give in on strict adherence to the home treatment schedule.

Pity often accompanies overprotectiveness. Pity is, of course, invariably and understandably present. However, the parents should not openly pity the child. He will then begin to pity himself, and this will defeat efforts to encourage him to accept his situation bravely and make the most of his remaining capacities.

Though fortunately in the minority, one does encounter self-willed, domineering parents—often with strong feelings of rejection—who make it all the more difficult for the child to adjust to his illness. They sometimes give the physician a rough time: questioning the diagnosis, debating the treatment, concentrating on the minutiae of home treatment, holding the child to a superstrict schedule, and expecting a Spartan bravery with little consolation.

We also need to know something of the personal relationships between the parents. Marital discord may have been present all along, but the burden of a chronically ill child often accentuates it. Parents may blame each other for the child's illness. One may accept the diagnosis and the other may not. They may debate the treatment and whether the physician is capable. Their families may pit them against each other. One may want to shop for an optimistic diagnosis and the other may not. Disagreements centering about the chronically ill child may also lead to divorce.

FRANK DISCUSSIONS ARE ESSENTIAL

For the above reasons, it is important once the diagnosis is established to have a series of gentle but frank talks with the parents, not only about the many other things mentioned above, but also about how the chronic illness conceivably might impair their marriage.

They should be encouraged to maintain their normal business and social life insofar as possible; if they can get away from the child at times, their strength to carry on may be renewed.

When their families insist on them showing the physician newspaper clippings or magazine articles concerning miraculous cures or a uniformly successful treatment, the physician should not act in a condescending manner. He should accept the article and write the author, asking him to send an immediate reply. Almost invariably, the author writes back that he was badly misquoted and really has nothing new. When these letters are shown to the parents, pressure on the physician is diminished as he stands in the proper position of having been quite willing to pursue any conceivably hopeful lead.

The physician should identify other individuals in the family circle who are close to the parents and the child and who therefore exercise an influence on how the parents adapt to the illness, and who play prominent roles in the family dynamics.

With the knowledge of the parents, the physician should properly orient these influential relatives concerning the nature of the disease, what they can do to help minimize emotional impact, and how they can best help the parents. They should be so well informed that they understand the situation as well as the parents. They should be particularly cautioned against blaming one or both parents for the child's illness, and they should be told that the physician has strongly recommended that the parents continue to be as active as possible in their usual activities outside the home.

4.   Emotional Adjustment of the Child at the Onset of the Disease Just as the parents react to the child's disease against the background of their prior emotional adjustment, so does the child respond from his own emotional baseline. A happy, secure, sociable, sufficiently independent, achieving child who feels warmly accepted by parents, siblings, and associates is, of course, best prepared to weather the emotional storms of a chronic disease or handicap. An unhappy, insecure, overly dependent, socially inept child without a strong self-image, and who already feels unloved, is the least prepared.

One of the physician's chief responsibilities is to determine what sort of a child he is dealing with from the standpoint of emotional balance. Having determined this, the physician can plan more intelligently for the care of the child.

5.   Threats to the Basic Emotional Needs of the Child One might list the basic emotional needs of children (and of adults) as follows: 1) love and affection;   2) security; 3) acceptance as an individual; 4) self-respect; 5) achievement; 6) recognition; 7) independence; and 8) authority or discipline. Knowing how these basic needs are threatened by a chronic disease or handicap helps the physician in his efforts to minimize the emotional impact.

Love and Affection

The child may feel that he is being punished or deserted by his parents when he is hospitalized and has to undergo extensive and sometimes painful tests. He may feel guilty and rejected. Now that he has a chronic illness or a handicap, he may feel himself to be a burden on the family and that they will now prefer his brothers and sisters.

Security

The chronically ill child has a multitude of threats to his security. Among them are fear of the unknown when the diagnosis is in doubt; fear of the known when the diagnosis is certain; fear of being abandoned; fear of pain; fear of death; worries about the destruction of his self-image; anxiety about possible mutilation, as from operations; long thoughts about his future (social acceptability, vocation, marriage); and, high on the list, concern that he is different from his fellows.

Acceptance as an Individual

A feeling of being accepted for what he is is a basic emotional need of every child. But now the illness has changed him. He is different, feels the difference, and knows that others know he is different. He magnifies the importance of this and he may well imagine that, since he has changed, his parents and friends may no longer accept him as they once did.

PARENTAL ADJUSTMENT TO CHANGED CHILD

The parents, too, have to adjust to the changed child. Perhaps their expectations for him are now thwarted, or blighted. His appearance may have been permanently changed for the worse, as when severe facial burns are suffered. Perhaps he has nephrosis and is taking corticosteroids that in a high dosage can change him into a fat caricature of the beautiful child they formerly had. A 6-year-old child in our city screamed and wanted to "go to God" when she saw her steroid-bloated face for the first time in a mirror. How casually we talk of "moon faces" but seldom tell the child that his appearance will be changed while the dosage is high. Why do we not take photographs of his face before the therapy is begun so that we can remind him that his appearance will return to that of the photograph when the drug dosage is decreased or treatment discontinued?

Self-Respect

The chronically ill child, or the child with a severe handicap, may suffer a loss of self-respect. He may think the disease is a punishment for his wickedness, or for his hostile thoughts toward his parents, or a personal weakness. His inability now to achieve his goals may weaken his self-respect. His changed body image and self-concept may make him feel inadequate.

Achievement

The maturing capacities of the growing child must find their outlet in achievement. But achievement may be blocked by the chronic disease or handicap. The athletic boy can no longer excel in sports. The popular girl may not even be able to attend social events. The sense of success in life is gone, and the child lies in bed or sits in restriction amidst his broken dreams. Of all the bitter pills to swallow, the worst may be this thwarting of dynamic achievement.

WHAT POTENTIALITIES REMAIN?

The physician should take not only the usual negative inventory—what is wrong with the child—but also a positive inventory—what potentialities remain. Unfortunately, too many physicians are content if they pin down the diagnosis in all its details and ramifications, satisfied that they have catalogued all the defects. Too few carefully evaluate the remaining capacities of the child and specifically seek to develop his strong points.

As an example, a 12-year-old boy had severe rheumatic carditis, with aortic regurgitation and mitral insufficiency of such a degree as to permit him to walk only a block or two slowly. Formerly a fine athlete, now he could not compete. He refused to ride to school in the family car, preferring to go on his own, however slowly. Participation in social activities was greatly limited.

The physician arranged for him to be trained by a radio-television repairman, and soon the boy was the idol of his group because of his ability to repair radio and television sets. The town photographer then accepted him for special instruction. He learned rapidly, set up his own darkroom, and began developing prints for his friends. His father interested him in collecting stamps. His continued sense of achievement helped immeasurably to maintain his emotional adjustment and he remained, as he was before his illness, one of the most secure and popular boys in his town.

On the other hand, a 14-year-old girl with mild rheumatoid arthritis was converted into a confirmed hypochondriac by an overly protective mother and a doting aunt. They sympathized too openly over her most minor complaints, waited on her hand and foot, encouraged her to remain at home in bed when resumption of activity had been advised, and in other ways adopted an overly lenient attitude toward the prescribed home management. She retired from the world—dropped out of school, drifted away from her friends and soon did not want them to visit her, lost ambition to achieve, and accepted the role of martyr to an illness that was never more than mild and by no means incapacitating.

We should remember that we are not only responsible for the prevention of disease where that is possible, and the prompt diagnosis and adequate treatment of it when it does occur, but also for comprehensive rehabilitation of those who are left with residual impairment. Rehabilitation means much more than improvement in the mere physical aspects of the disease. It also means detailed attention to the emotional impact, and a positive approach in order to minimize the impact.

Recognition

All children need recognition of their achievements and approval of their parents and associates. Yet in many instances there is such a concentration on the chronic disease itself that only the disease is recognized—the child is important only because he has the problem. The child should know that others realize the impact of the illness on him, and sympathize, but that they also notice his good qualities and approve of him and the way he bravely faces his handicap. He needs to feel that he amounts to something, even though he is ill or handicapped.

Independence

Chronic illness or handicap thwarts to a variable degree the acquisition of independence. Indeed, the illness often requires the child to be dependent on others at the very time he most needs a greater degree of independence.

Small wonder that many children who become chronically diseased or handicapped go through a period of denial of the diagnosis and reject the idea that they will have to suffer limitations, have to depend more on others. Small wonder also that they often overcompensate with a rebellious attitude—sometimes a virtual defiance of the disease and its treatment—and a hostility to all connected with it—parents, physicians, and nurses.

Authority or Discipline

In the complex and sometimes chaotic world of the child, there is a vital need for the steady exercise of kindly yet firm parental discipline and authority. When the child is ill, there is a great tendency to diminish, or even to abandon, authority and discipline. The ordinary, sensible rules and restrictions break down. This road leads to tyranny by the child, who takes over the family in a domineering manner, using his illness as a lever to get what he wants.

The physician should encourage parents to maintain a sensible degree of authority and discipline. Even the chronically ill child must learn to accept the restrictions on behavior that the civilized world demands of its inhabitants. Of what avail is it to rehabilitate him physically if he then emerges as a headstrong, self-willed, impetuous person who later tramples on the world?

    6. Special Facilities and Programs   Space does not permit consideration of all the ways in which the environment can be arranged to improve the outlook for the chronically ill child—improved hospital construction, motel-hospital arrangements,, rooming in for parents, playroom, recreational programs, hospital teaching programs, homebound instruction, special education, medical foster homes, and parent group discussions. But it is clearly apparent that the objective of minimizing the emotional impact of chronic diseases can best be achieved when proper facilities, programs, and personnel well-experienced in the management of such children are available.

CONCLUSIONS

The approach to the chronically ill or handicapped child should be thoroughly comprehensive.

The objective is to enable the child, insofar as possible, to achieve his maximum potential physically, mentally, emotionally, and socially.

Chief factors that govern the emotional impact of a chronic disease or handicap include 1) nature of the chronic disease or handicap, 2) age of the child at the onset of the disease, 3) parental attitudes and emotional balance, 4) emotional adjustment of the child at the onset of the disease, 5) threats to the basic emotional needs of the child and how they are met, and 6) whether special facilities and programs are available.

Viewed in this manner, the management of a child with a chronic disease or handicap becomes intellectually challenging, exciting, and personally rewarding.

PSYCHOLOGICAL ASPECTS
OF CHRONIC ILLNESS

Paul D. Steinhauer,[1] *David N. Mushin,*[2] *and Quentin Rae-Grant*[3]

When parents bring a sick child to a physician, they come with a number of questions and one overriding request.

The questions, in their language, are simple. What is the matter with my child? What has caused it? What can the physician do to help? What can the parents do? How long will it last? Will he be completely cured? But the hope is that, by medicine or by magic, the child will be rapidly, uneventfully, and successfully returned to complete health. This is frequently asking, however, more than the physician can deliver.

With improvements in the treatment of the infectious disease and our ever-increasing ability to sustain life even when we cannot restore health, the practicing pediatrician is increasingly relied upon to aid in the management of the child who is severely and chronically ill. Here, contrary to parental expectations, he cannot cure. But there are a number of things, all of them important, that he can do. He may be able to control the rate of progression or the frequency and severity of complications of the disease. He may do a great deal to help the child compensate for some of the more destructive effects of his illness. Finally, and equally important, he may be able to help child and family face the limitations, anxieties, and discouragements which accompany the disease, to develop a plan of management which can serve as an antidote to feelings of utter helplessness, and to rise above the feelings of resentment and despair which could otherwise crush and overwhelm them (Garrard & Richmond, 1963; Pakes, 1974).

Any illness of a child represents a crisis for the family. The degree to which this crisis can be sustained or resolved depends on the answers to the above questions and on the pre-existing strengths of the family unit. Even an acute and rapidly responsive illness may lead to further decompensation in an already precarious family situation. It requires on the other hand great strength, stability and support to sustain a severe chronic illness in one family member.

Reprinted from *The Pediatric Clinics of North America 21*, pp. 825–840, © 1974, W. B. Saunders Co., with permission.

[1]Senior Staff Psychiatrist, The Hospital for Sick Children, and Associate Professor, Department of Psychiatry, University of Toronto.

[2]Staff Psychiatrist, The Hospital for Sick Children, and Assistant Professor, Department of Psychiatry, University of Toronto.

[3]Psychiatrist in Chief, The Hospital for Sick Children, and Professor of Child Psychiatry, University of Toronto.

Table 1.   Emotional responses to acute and chronic illness

	Acute illness	Chronic illness
Onset	Sudden	Sudden or insidious
Duration of illness	Brief	Prolonged
Treatment	Often effective	Palliative or none
Outlook	Frequently excellent	Generally poor
Crisis identity	High	High
Crisis duration	Brief	Prolonged
Family reactions	Anxiety	Denial and disbelief, anxiety, depression, guilt and respon-
	Relief	sibility, resentment
Physician's reactions	Relief	?

This article deals with the emotional responses to chronic illness (Table 1), the responses of patients, their parents, and their siblings to the hardships imposed by the disease. It also deals with our role as physicians, and the contribution we can make toward helping the family minimize the destructive effects of these responses (Pakes, 1974).

Since the child is a developing individual with different needs and capacities depending on his stage of development, the nature and extent of disruption occurring during illness will vary according to the stage at which it occurs. Either the illness itself or restrictions imposed during its management may affect the child's function and disrupt normal living. By and large, the common acute illnesses of childhood leave few major or lasting emotional sequelae. Although their behavior while in the hospital may present problems, few children show long-term effects following short-term hospitalization unless they previously showed evidence of maladjustment (Vernon, Schulman, & Foley, 1966).

Chronic illness, however, is associated with defects and ongoing problems. The prolonged disruption in life experience may have lasting effects on the cognitive and emotional development of the child. To manage chronically ill children and their families, one must understand the child's premorbid personality and needs, his stage of development and its vulnerabilities, his perception of the illness and its management, the nature of the illness itself and its potential effects on child and family, the nature of management procedures, and the potential for support of the child from family and medical staff.

PREMORBID PERSONALITY AND NEEDS

A child's development and adjustment prior to becoming ill will influence his responses during the illness. The child who has difficulty separating from parents may have problems coping with hospitalization. The previously phobic child is likely to develop inordinate fears of minor procedures, while the hyperactive child will have difficulty tolerating forced immobilization. The child who already fears and resents authority figures can be expected to rebel against doctors and nurses, whereas a previously shy and withdrawn child whose illness involves some deformity is prone to extreme self-consciousness which may seriously interfere with his relationships. A child from a previously depriving environment may, through the demand for enforced isolation, fall even further behind in his intellectual development.

Circumstances at the onset of illness may influence the child's adjustment to his disease. Thus a young child who was severely burned during a phase of jealousy following the birth of a new sibling might ascribe infrequent parental visits to the parents being more interested in the new sibling than in him. He might interpret the burn as a punishment for hostile and rivalrous feelings toward the sibling. An independent and secure child would probably cope better with a chronic illness than one who is immature, insecure, and inhibited. There is some evidence, at least in acute illness, that certain children's emotional adjustment may be improved with successful handling of their illness.

NATURE OF THE ILLNESS AND MANAGEMENT AND POTENTIAL EFFECTS ON THE CHILD

The child's adjustment will be affected by a number of factors which, separately or in combination, may be present during the course of an illness. Consider the following:

General Factors in Chronic Illness

Separation from Parents   This is particularly upsetting for children between 6 months and 4 years of age, but may also cause problems for older children who have had prior separations. Three stages are described in the child's adverse reactions to separation (Bowlby, 1973). First is the stage of protest where the child demands the parents, and tearfully and angrily resists attempts to care for him. When the child has lost hope of forcing the return of the parents, he withdraws and loses interest in his environment and even in food. Following this stage of despair the child may become more alert, regain appetite, and relate to people, but avoid attachment to any one person and ignore the parents if they visit. This is called the stage of detachment or denial. While the first two stages are reversible on being reunited with parents under appropriate circumstances persistent defects in the ability to form relationships and in intellectual functions may result if the third stage is reached. The child who is institutionalized for long periods is particularly vulnerable to these complications of separation. Repeated actual or threatened separations may produce frequent and irrational anger and anxiety in the child, which will cause difficulty in his management.

Separation problems can be alleviated by regular, predictable visiting by the parents, and by ensuring that the child is looked after by a small number of staff whom he gets to know. Infrequent and sporadic visiting by parents and care from many adults with only superficial contact increase the traumatic effects of separation.

Restriction, Sensory Impairment, and Isolation   Some illnesses may require that the child experience periods when mobility is restricted, or that he be isolated from familiar people and objects. In addition, certain illnesses can impose sensory restrictions upon the child: blindness, deafness, and the decreased tactile stimulation that accompanies the treatment of the burned child. Cognitive development, particularly in young children, depends partly on physical exploration of the environment. All children require stimulation from the environment and an ability to take in such stimulation. From the emotional point of view, restrictions on play may remove the safety valve a child needs to drain off anxiety and unpleasant feelings, while sensory impairment may interfere with explaining proceedings to the child, as well as interfere with his relationships with parents and medical personnel. When such avenues are blocked, the child may withdraw into excessive fantasy as a means of coping, this tendency being enhanced by isolation. This may lead to an escalation of fears and unrealistic expectations regarding the illness and management.

Dependency and Lack of Consistency   In dealing with sick children, adults tend to gratify dependency needs in an attempt to help the child feel more secure and to comfort him (Maddison & Raphael, 1971). While to some extent this additional support is needed, prolonged and excessive gratification of these needs may prove so satisfying that the child may resist giving it up. This may interfere with the normal striving toward mature independence, thus blocking the development of self-confidence and initiative. Such problems are more marked in children who for any reason (including congenital illness where parental guilt fosters overprotection) have prior dependency problems. Rehabilitation and the achievement of maximal functioning in spite of residual physical problems may be impeded. The aim in management is to maintain a balance between allowing dependence during the acute phase and gradual encouragement toward independence whenever possible.

Pain and Deformity   A child's response to pain will vary with the way he perceives the pain as well as with the amount of pain accounted for on a physiologic basis (Freud, 1961). Pain interpreted as punishment or maltreatment (e.g., reaction to injections) may be accompanied by anxiety, which will intensify the pain. Other children may perceive pain as pleasurable, leading to passive devotion to the medical staff who inflict it. The young child who imagines adults are all-powerful and capable of removing all pain may interpret their failure to do so as an expression of anger toward him. This may be reinforced if the adult becomes angry at the child's persistent complaints or apprehensions regarding procedures.

The threat of surgery and deformity is greatest in the late preschool and early adolescent years. Toddlers see surgery as a punishment with potentially dire consequences, for in this age group the least scratch is blown up to the proportions of a major wound. In the adolescent, deformity and fears of mutilation are the result of an increased concern with body image, a need to be the same as peers, and fears of being a defective and hence inadequate person.

Threat of Death   A full discussion of this topic is beyond the scope of this article and is discussed by writers such as Kubler-Ross (1970). It is not until age 9 or 10 that the child fully understands death as being both universal and permanent. Prior to that, he views death as similar to sleep or as a separation. Parents' feelings about imminent or threatened death may interfere with their ability to relate to the child. This will increase the child's anxiety. The child may interpret his parents' depression as anger, leading to a feeling that he is letting the parents down. Similar problems may occur between the child and medical staff, for example, when the surgeon avoids his dying patient after an unsuccessful operation (Kubler-Ross, 1970).

Medication   Certain forms of medication may affect the child's alertness (e.g., barbiturates) and behavior (e.g., corticosteroids). Such effects should be considered in prescribing these durgs. Drugs having physical side effects (e.g., cytotoxic drugs) may cause anxiety through disturbance of body image. Prolonged and regular use of drugs (e.g., insulin) or diets may be accepted at younger ages but rebelled against in early adolescence where it is seen as an imposition by authority figures. Acceptance of such regimens may be seen as a sign of weakness, a constant reminder of the illness, and a symbol of dependence and inadequacy which the child would often rather forget.

Absence from School   Multiple absences not only may contribute to the child's falling behind in school work, but also may seriously interfere with his peer relationships. These may be of crucial importance to the older child and adolescent. Relaxed visiting privileges and provision for continuing his schooling while in hospital or at home may do much to minimize the seriousness of these potential complications.

PROBLEMS SPECIFIC TO CERTAIN ILLNESSES

Certain illnesses may directly influence behavior and cognitive development. Various causes of mental retardation affect intellectual development.

Certain forms of brain damage may be associated with hypersensitivity, poor impulse control, and poor attention span. These may affect perception, and thus learning, in a child with normal intelligence. Children with temporal lobe epilepsy may exhibit a wide range of psychological problems ranging from behavior disorder through episodes of depersonalization to hallucinations, and it is feasible that some psychoses in children, for example, types of autism, have at least in part a physiologic basis. In such conditions, the specific effects of the illness interact with the general problems described above.

THE EFFECT OF THE ILLNESS AND DEVELOPMENT

Illness may impair the child's ability to overcome the problems which occur during normal development. Thus the toddler who is learning to walk and to develop bowel control will have this movement toward normal independence disrupted by forced confinement to bed and chronic diarrhea. Such a child, in seeking mother's help during the illness, may substitute the gratification this brings for the advantages of autonomy. At a later age, the danger is that the child will remain overly dependent rather than learning to rely on his own resources. Unresolved problems at an early stage of development (e.g., separation problems) can affect development at later stages (e.g., development of an independent identity as an adolescent).

FAMILY REACTIONS

Faced with the diagnosis of a severe and chronic illness, the entire family is confronted with a series of stresses and demands that will tax relationships both within and beyond the family unit. The degree and nature of the stress will vary, as will a particular family's ability to meet it. The following factors will influence the family's response to the illness.

The severity of the illness, the likely prognosis, and the availability of an effective treatment. The more debilitating the illness and the poorer the prognosis, particularly in a previously healthy child, the greater the stress on the family. This is especially true if the clinical course is one of relentless progression. In such cases, the parents face the constant threat of losing their child. The resulting strain is intensified if sudden death is a possibility (e.g., some forms of congenital heart disease, Riley-Day syndrome, some severe asthmatics).

Whether the disease is congenital or acquired. Illnesses in which congenital factors have been implicated (e.g., fibrocystic disease, the muscular dystrophies, congenital heart disease, some forms of mental retardation) are likely to intensify parental feelings of guilt and responsibility.

The age of onset of the illness, and of diagnosis. If the diagnosis is made at birth, the family will never have experienced the child as normal. Their concept of him will always have included expectations altered because of his illness. If, however, the illness appears or is diagnosed after the child's personality has developed and his place in the family is established, family members will have had time to think of him as a normal child, so that an even greater sense of loss and depression will be experienced when they are forced to scale down their hopes and expectations in view of the illness. Illness striking first in adolescence is resented by both child and family as a particularly painful cheating of someone about to experience all the supposed freedoms and opportunities that go with adult status.

One must also consider the effects of parental expectations on the ongoing process of development. The more the child is able to be seen and treated like a normal child, the less his development will be interfered with. However, the earlier the diagnosis is made—and the more the parents see the child as fragile, handicapped, or limited—the more likely the parents are to grossly overprotect and overindulge the child, thus distorting the parent-child relationship and the normal process of development.

Presence of pre-existing emotional disturbance within the family. The greatest psychological or social problems are likely to develop when serious chronic illness occurs within an already disturbed family situation. While the entire family will inevitably affect—and be affected by—severe, chronic illness in any family member, there are two situations in which this poses a particular threat to the family's emotional equilibrium: One occurs when chronic disease develops in a child whose relationships are already disturbed. The other is seen when the parents' marriage is already strained almost to the limit of tolerance.

The nature and effect of the illness itself. Pain or malaise resulting from the child's illness, or a resented treatment program may cause the child to be cranky, irritable, unpleasant, or demanding. These same traits will present additional pressures and evoke feelings of resentment, guilt, and inadequacy in the parents, especially the mother. If the illness is clearly apparent and frequently elicits reactions of disgust or aversion from others (e.g., congenital amputations or deformities, severe scarring from burns, conspicuous mental retardation) the continued confrontation with the discomfort of others will prove a serious blow to the normal parental desire to have an attractive, healthy child who will reflect well on them. This may also be so if failure to thrive secondary to the disease rather than a more obvious deformity deprives the parents of the beautiful, healthy child they long for (Maddison & Raphael, 1971).

Effects of program of home management and restrictions on family life. Some illnesses involve a demanding program of home management and restrictions, e.g., fibrocystic disease, with its daily regimen of inhalations, positive pressure, postural drainage, and frequent medications, and juvenile diabetes with its dietary restrictions, regular testing, and daily insulin injections. These demands, despite their absolute medical necessity, may be resented and vigorously resisted by the child they are intended to help. Even with appropriate explanations of the purpose and importance of the regimen, the child may not be able to accept the need for unpleasant restrictions or treatments. Indeed, excessive compliance on the part of the child is more likely to indicate pathologic passivity and depression than mental health. Even normal resistance, however, will result in additional work and emotional strain for the parents who are struggling to administer the prescribed regimen. If they respond with excessive impatience, resentment and guilt—or, alternatively, if they back off and provide only inconsistent care—both physical health and emotional relationships are bound to suffer.

A moderate amount of self-assertion and opposition to parental authority is an essential feature of the normal child's progression toward independence. In the child who is chronically ill the oppositional behavior may become concentrated around opposing the unwanted treatment regimen, which will then become a daily battleground, resulting in developmental disorders and resentment and guilt in both parents and child that may spread to contaminate not only their relationship but the emotional tone within the family as a whole.

Presence or absence of other affected siblings. The parental reaction may be very much affected by whether or not this is the first child to have been affected by the illness. The presence of other healthy children—especially in situations in which a congenital factor has been demonstrated—may serve to mitigate the parents' feelings of inadequacy and distress. Alternatively, parents who have more than one afflicted child—or who have lost a child to the disease—can be expected to have even more than usual difficulty adjusting to the illness of a subsequent afflicted child.

Repeated hospitalizations and surgical procedures. Should the disease be one requiring frequent hospitalizations, painful treatments or repeated surgery (renal failure, severe burns) additional pressures will be brought to bear on the parents. Children, especially toddlers, often find coming into the hospital upsetting. They may not understand why they have to leave the family or the reason for frightening or painful procedures. As a result they may feel punished or abandoned by their parents, whose uncertainty and guilt will be intensified if the child is miserable and resentful. At times (e.g., the severely burned child) parents may see their child suffering but be totally unable to comfort him. Even worse (e.g., the parents of a child with congenital heart disease) they may be forced to make decisions which can literally determine whether their child lives or dies, without any assurance that they are deciding correctly.

Cost of the illness. In estimating the cost of the illness, there is no avoiding, even in the state-underwritten systems, the hidden dollars-and-cents costs (e.g., doctor and hospital bills, medications, special diets,

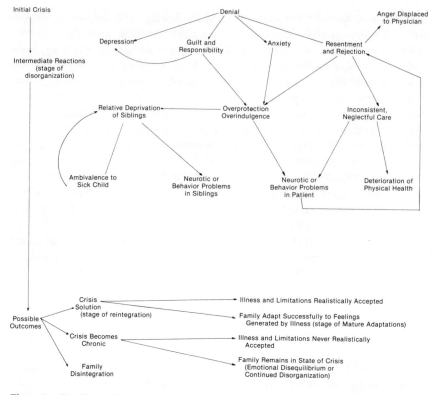

Figure 1.   Family reactions to severe chronic illness.

needed equipment and appliances, etc.). For families with limited incomes, these expenses may prove additional sources of pressure and anxiety. They may necessitate the mother going out to work or the father having to take on a second job to make ends meet. Drained and exhausted, the parents then come home to the demands of administering or supervising a vigorous and unpopular program of management or restrictions. The cycle is vicious. Emotional needs of both parents and children frequently go unmet. The rate of family breakdown in families with severe chronic illness is high (Solnit & Green, 1959; Freud, 1961; Pakes, 1974).

Specific Emotional Reactions

These include the following (Figure 1).

Denial. All parents to some extent react with denial in response to the shock of their child's illness. While denial may help the parents through the initial trauma and subsequent disorganization, normally—but by no means always—their use of denial should gradually decrease as the family's ability to come to grips with the reality of the illness increases. Denial is probably never completely abandoned, certainly not at any single point in time. Persistent massive denial in the face of obvious illness will interfere with the family's learning to live with their reactions to their child's illness, and with their successfully meeting the day-to-day needs of the child, thus perpetuating the crisis precipitated by the illness. It is this denial, closely related to their need for hope, that may lead parents to misinterpret what their physician is saying, or to go from doctor to doctor in an attempt to find one who will give them the diagnosis—and prognosis—they want to hear.

Anxiety. To a greater or lesser degree, the parents are chronically anxious about the health—or the very survival—of their child. If the parental anxiety is excessive, either because of realistic possibility of sudden death or because of a neurotic overreaction, it may lead to overprotection, overindulgence, and difficulties in disciplining the child.

Feelings of guilt, responsibility and self-blame. Some parents see their child's illness as a punishment from God for their sins, while others will feel victimized by Fate. Still others, particularly if the disease is a congenital one, may feel that the child's illness is proof of their inadequacy (i.e., their inability to bear a normal child). Although these feelings of responsibility are totally irrational, attempts to use logic to argue parents out of them are likely to fail. Each of us has his or her own secret sins and personal inadequacies, and these (e.g., an unwanted pregnancy, an abortion attempt, unacceptable feelings toward the sick child) may be seized upon and elaborated in a manner that grinds the depressed parent ever deeper into the rut of despondency.

Depression. Basically, the depression experienced is a mourning for the child who, but for the illness, might have been. It is a stage in coming to terms with the reality of the child's illness. In some cases, the parents may have come to accept the child's illness or handicap and its implications for their family. Other parents may never be able to do so and their family's life —and possibly its continued existence—will be dominated by their unresolved depression.

Resentment and rejection. The parents' resentment, a reaction to their disappointment and despair, may be converted to bitterness directed toward each other, family and friends, physicians, the community at large, or the child himself. The child may be overtly or covertly rejected. Covert rejection may be expressed via inadequate or inconsistent care, by unnecessary demands for hospitalization, by avoidance of the child through overinvolvement in work or other activities. It may be masked by its opposite, overprotection, that leads to failure to discipline the child appropriately, resulting in misbehavior that the parents then use to rationalize their rejection.

Reactions to the extended community. Shame, embarrassment, or sheer exhaustion may lead to decreased interest and involvement in recreational and other extrafamilial activities and alienation and bitterness toward relatives, friends and neighbors just when they are most needed for support. The burden of a child's illness is sometimes used as the reason for failure to advance vocationally or professionally.

Sibling reactions. The sibling of the sick child has no easy task to handle. He will frequently react with jealousy and resentment toward the child who draws off so much of the attention and energies of the family. The parental preoccupation with the sick child and their own reactions to his illness may result in the other children experiencing a moderate to severe degree of emotional deprivation. But, in some families, it is not "right" to feel jealous of a sick or dying child. If the parents cannot allow the other children to express openly their resentment toward the sick child or their feelings of being shortchanged, the guilt they feel secondary to their resentment will be intensified. This will frequently result in their hostility going underground, to be expressed covertly by pathological withdrawal, underachievement in school, behavior problems or delinquency, or neurotic reactions.

> Ten year old Nina had one younger brother who, almost a year before, had been left hemiplegic and aphasic following a sudden and dramatic illness. Needless to say, this had deeply upset the entire family. Every day after work, both Nina's parents would rush down to the hospital, leaving Nina in the care of her aged grandmother. Nina too was very upset about her brother's illness, but she also deeply resented it. She felt her parents no longer had time or love for her, but if she complained, she was called selfish and punished. She stopped complaining, but developed pain and a persistent limp in her left knee which defied repeated investigation. During her third appearance in emergency, an intern noted that the brother was paralyzed on his left side and wondered if her symptoms represented a hysterical reaction. On inquiry, Nina told of a series of repeated dreams. In some of these, her brother had died and was going to heaven. In others—and she broke down and sobbed as she told of these—she had killed him. Further investigation suggested that Nina's intense conflict between feelings of love, hate and guilt had been converted into the leg pain and stiffness which to her symbolized (unconsciously) an identification with the ambivalently loved brother.

Cain, Fast, & Erickson (1964) have studied children's disturbed reactions to the death of a sibling which they found related to factors such as the nature of the death; the child's preexisting relationship with the dead sibling; the immediate and the long-term impact of the death upon the parents; the child's cognitive ability to understand death; the parents' handling of the immediate impact of the death on the surviving child; the impact of the death upon the total family structure. Pathologic reactions, when they occurred, took the form of excessive and prolonged guilt reactions; depressions; blaming the parents for the death of the sibling; distorted concepts of illness and death; disturbed attitudes toward doctors, hospitals, and religion; death phobias; and identification with the dead child. The need to recognize the impact of a child's death on the surviving siblings if these disturbed reactions are to be avoided cannot be overstressed.

PHYSICIAN'S REACTIONS TO CHRONIC ILLNESS

Physicians and other attending staff may react emotionally to chronic fatal illness in a child. The physician who is unable to tolerate being unable to provide a cure may feel increasingly helpless, hopeless, and guilty. This may lead him to withdraw from patient and family, leaving them to face the stress of the disease without his support. He may overidentify with the parents, or in his anxiety may say too much too soon, i.e., before the parents have overcome their initial shock and denial to the point where they can hear what he is saying. Physicians may resent parents, sometimes in response to parental hostility but at other times in reaction to parental dependence which merely underlines the physician's feeling of helplessness. Garrard and Richmond (1963) have stressed the importance of the physician maintaining an awareness of his own separateness from the family, while recognizing just how difficult this may prove to be. They stress that what families need is empathy, not sympathy; detachment rather than avoidance. Pakes (1974) has drawn attention to the extent to which physicians' reactions to their chronically ill patients often parallel those of their parents.

MANAGEMENT

1. Successful management of the emotional aspects of chronic illness is based on a recognition that illness in one child will have major implications on mental health, relationships, and possibly even the continued existence of the family.
2. The more successful family members (especially parents) are able to resolve the feelings of anxiety, depression, responsibility, and resentment aroused by the illness the more able they will be a) to meet the physical and emotional needs of the child and b) to resolve the crisis created by the diagnosis and the additional strains imposed by their child's illness with minimal damage and disruption to the family as a whole.

   On the other hand, failure to resolve the emotional sequelae of the illness will substantially diminish the family's ability to satisfy the emotional needs of all its members and will increase the likelihood of family breakdown.
3. Only when parents have been given a clear and definitive diagnosis can they begin to deal with reality first at the level of practical planning. Only then can they begin the arduous but no less important task of emotional acceptance.

4. The diagnosis of a severe chronic illness will precipitate a state of crisis in the family. If the physician recognizes the potential for disorganization this will inevitably produce in both instrumental and emotional functioning, he may play a major role in minimizing the destructive effects and aiding in the reintegration and mature adaptation of the family as a whole.

    Often if one looks for them, the family's past history of adjustment will give clues that will allow one to anticipate the nature of potential difficulties. An assessment of previous family responses to stress is helpful. An awareness of marital problems would indicate the need to communicate with both parents to help them face problems together. Prior peer, school, and behavior problems may indicate possible difficulties for the child and staff during management. Observed interaction between the child and his parents is a guide to possible reactions to medical staff.

5. It is essential that the attending physician recognize that what the family *hear* and *understand* may differ considerably from what they have been *told*. Parents can assimilate only what they are emotionally ready for. In their distress, they may hear what they need to hear, selecting or distorting what has actually been said either to obtain false reassurance or to confirm their worst fears. Be simple and direct, avoiding unwarranted optimism or excessive pessimism. Timing may be important here. While saying too much too soon may cause unnecessary anxiety, more commonly too little is said too late, and in too ambiguous a manner. One important reason for maintaining regular contact with the family is to explore with them what they *have* heard regarding diagnosis, prognosis, and management, and how they are coping, in terms of both day-to-day management and emotional adjustment.

6. It is desirable that the physician review periodically with the parents their concept of the child and his overall management. Severe overprotection and unnecessary restrictions on activity, failure to provide age-appropriate expectations and to supply discipline, the presence of obvious behavior or academic problems in a sibling or mounting tension within the marriage, and a major and continuing discrepancy between physician and parents around what the child can do may be as serious an indication that the family is in trouble as is evidence of inadequate or inconsistent care.

7. Similarly, through his ongoing contacts with the child, the physician is in a position to explore the child's understanding of the nature of his illness and help him deal with his feelings about it. By asking questions about how the child sees himself and his illness, the child can be encouraged to express his concerns. Often the parents in their anxiety cannot allow the children, including the sick child, to raise openly any

of their anxieties. Helping the parents face and master their own anxieties, thus preparing them to tolerate and deal with the concerns of the children, can be crucial in minimizing serious and long-lasting emotional damage. What is spoken and acknowledged is often less threatening than that which is known but not talked about. The conspiracy of silence which leads to avoidance of any mention of consequences of the illness—including hospitalizations, operations (especially when they involve mutilation, e.g., amputations) or approaching death—is usually a pretense, trying for all, but especially for the child, who is the central character. This topic deserves far more discussion than is possible here, and is discussed in more detail by Cain et al. (1964), Patterson, Denning, & Kutscher (1973), and Kubler-Ross (1970).

8. School and peer relationships are extremely important in the life of the child. In chronic illness there may be significant absence from school, requiring tuition during hospitalization. The assistance of the child's teacher should be sought in coordinating schooling. Despite hospitalization, the child should be encouraged to maintain contact with peers either through visits or by mail. The child's embarrassment and shame regarding illness and deformity may in fact contribute to an alienation from the peer group which, under the right circumstances, could be a source of support for the child. With the older child, alertness on the part of the physician to a refusal to contact peers may help him to discuss the child's worries regarding his friends.

9. Physicians are frequently the undeserving objects of hostility. This is not intended as, and should not be construed as, an attack on them personally even though it may be expressed in very personal terms. Rather, it is a displacement of the parents' resentment that this (the child's illness) has occurred, and a reaction against the one who, out of necessity, confronts them with painful realities they would rather not hear. If the physician responds with hostility or by withdrawing from and rejecting the family, he will lose the opportunity to provide needed services at this time of great distress. If the feelings are too intense to be resolved right at the moment, it is probably advisable to have the parents back in to discuss the situation again in the near future. Some parents may need a chance to vent their emotional reactions before they will be able to listen and take hold, make the necessary practical decisions, and cooperate regarding management. If the physician can approach the parents with continued empathy and objectivity, he may be able to help them deal with their distress more appropriately and move on to the problems of practical management.

10. The management of the chronically ill child and his family requires the resources of a team of professionals. Adequate paths of communication should exist between team members for coordination of manage-

ment. A frustrating family, by increasing demands and creating tension between team members, may cause friction and breakdown of team coordination. Disagreements among team members may be taken out on the patient. Under such circumstances, team meetings can help place problems in perspective, and will allow team members to support each other at times of stress.

11. Restrictions on activity are often inevitable. While preschoolers generally limit their own activities, older children, because of their need to conform and to prove their social adequacy, may tend to overtax themselves. The physician may be helpful in defining and explaining necessary activity restrictions, as well as in arbitrating between parent and child about them. Realistic restrictions because of illness, however serious, may not be as crippling as those constructed or fantasied by parent or child. By highlighting areas of satisfactory function and potential strengths, the physician may do much toward helping the family toward an acceptance of the child's real strengths along with his realistic limitations.

Children need and use play as an avenue for expressing their feelings and as a vehicle for resolving conflicts. Young children require play materials for such purposes, and puppets, painting materials, and toy medical equipment can be used. Such play also provides a means of activity and an area of independence for the immobilized child. Occupational therapy and play therapy are important in this regard for all such children.

12. Any major decision (around surgical intervention, around whether or not to hospitalize) or any necessary but disappointing statement regarding prognosis may unleash a severe and unpleasant emotional reaction, or may be greeted with docile passivity. In either case, one should realize that the obvious parental reaction may be very different from what the parents are struggling with within themselves. Some parents may need active encouragement if they are to express feelings which have been held in but are tearing them and their family apart. In making important decisions, the family needs help in recognizing and weighing the facts of the situation, and reassurance and encouragement once a decision has been made.

13. Physicians differ in their ability to help families cope with their emotional reactions to chronic illness. While each family needs on an ongoing basis someone who can help them with their emotional responses to the illness, this might or might not be their physician. Should the demands of meeting the emotional needs of the families of chronically ill patients seem excessive (i.e., extending beyond what the physician is in a position to provide) there is always the alternative of referring the family to someone geared to helping them deal with the

emotional sequelae of the illness. A child psychiatrist, a social worker, a pastoral counsellor, or an association of parents who have experienced a similar problem could be of major assistance to the family and to the physician. In making such a referral, it would be important to distinguish clearly between whether the physician is planning to continue to play a major role in helping the family with their emotional difficulties and is seeking a consultation, or whether he prefers the referral agent to take over the management of the emotional aspects of the case in continuing consultation with regard to overall management.

14. Episodes of hospitalization may represent acute or chronic crisis situations. When hospitalization is necessary, hospital staff may be at the receiving end of parental criticism or over-involvement. Parents may indeed be demanding, critical and competitive with nursing staff. But hospital staff may need reminding that *their* patient is *still* the parents' child and that the parents' reactions are a response to anxiety and a displacement of their resentment at having a seriously ill child. This may help hospital staff maintain some understanding and empathy for parents, instead of responding with hostility and rejection. This serves only to aggravate the parental distress as friction and antagonism between parents and hospital staff escalate. By anticipating, recognizing and mediating such conflicts as they appear to arise, the physician may be of great help to all in avoiding or breaking the vicious circle of recrimination.

REFERENCES

Bowlby, J. *Separation—Anxiety and anger: Attachment and loss* (Vol. II), pp. 3–24. New York: Basic Books, 1973.

Cain, A. C., Fast, I., & Erickson, M. E. Children's disturbed reactions to the death of a sibling. *American Journal of Orthopsychiatry,* 1964, *34,* 741–752.

Freedman, A. M., Helme, W., Havel, J., et al. Psychiatric aspects of familial dysautonomia. *American Journal of Orthopsychiatry,* 1957, *27,* 96–106.

Freud, A. The role of bodily illness in the mental life of children. In R. S. Eissler et al. (Eds.), *The psychoanalytic study of the child* (Vol. 7). New York: International Universities Press, 1961.

Garrard, S. E., & Richmond, J. B. Psychological aspects of the management of chronic disease and handicapping conditions in childhood. In H. I. Lief, V. F. Lief, and N. R. Lief (Eds.), *The psychological basis of medical practice,* pp. 370–403. New York: Harper & Row Publishers, 1963.

Glaser, H. H., Harrison, G. S., & Lynn, D. B. Emotional implications of congenital heart disease in children. *Paediatrics,* 1964, *33,* 367–369.

Kubler-Ross, E. *On death and dying.* New York: Macmillan Publishing Co., 1970.

Lefebvre, A. *Problems of patients with cystic fibrosis in adapting to adolescence and adulthood,* pp. 15–17. Unpublished dissertation prepared as part of requirement for Diploma in Child Psychiatry, University of Toronto, 1974.

McKay, R. M. Coping with a family-shattering disease. In P. R. Patterson, C. Denning, & A. H. Kutscher (Eds.), *Psychosocial aspects of cystic fibrosis.* New York: Columbia University Press, 1973.

Maddison, D., & Raphael, B. Social and psychological consequences of chronic disease in childhood. *Medical Journal of Australia,* 1971, *2,* 1265–1270.

Meyerowitz, J. H., & Kaplan, H. B. *Familial responses to stress: The case of cystic fibrosis. Social science and medicine* (Vol. 1), pp. 249–266. London: Pergamon Press Ltd., 1967.

Natterson, J. M., & Knudson, A. G. Observations concerning fear of death in fatally ill children and their mothers. *Psychosomatic Medicine,* 1960, *22,* 456–465.

Pakes, E. H. Child psychiatry and pediatric practice: How disciplines work together. *Ontario Medical Review,* 1974, *41,* 69–71.

Patterson, P. R., Denning, C., & Kutscher, A. H. (Eds.). *Pyschosocial aspects of cystic fibrosis.* New York: Columbia University Press, 1973.

Rosberg, G. Parental attitudes in pediatric hospital admissions. *Acta Paediatrica Scandinavica,* 1971, *210* (Suppl.).

Solnit, A. J., & Green, M. Psychological considerations in the management of deaths on pediatric hospital services. I. The doctor and the child's family. *Paediatrics,* 1959, *24,* 106–112.

Turk, T. Impact of cystic fibrosis on family functioning. *Paediatrics,* 1964, *34,* 67–71.

Van Leeuwen, J. J. Dialysis transplantation. *Ontario Medical Review,* 1974, *41,* 71–73.

Vernon, D., Schulman, J., & Foley, J. Changes in children's behaviour after hospitalization. *American Journal of Disabled Children,* 1966, *3,* 581–593.

CHAPTER 4

GENERAL IMPACT OF ADULT DISABILITY/ ILLNESS ON THE FAMILY

Paul W. Power and Arthur E. Dell Orto

The disability or chronic illness of a family member challenges family adaptation. The family is required to accommodate the reality of the disability within the family group. The occurrence of disability or illness touches each family member. It is essential that the family continue to maintain a sense of membership for the disabled person by re-grouping its members, its resources, and its functions in order to continue existing as a unit. How the family reorganizes depends upon its emotional response to the trauma.

In this chapter the authors review many existing theories and identify the varied ways that family members react to a disability or illness in an adult family member. Bringing these reactive patterns into sharper focus can enhance the helper's understanding of the different influences the family can have on the rehabilitation of the patient. Family members, for example, who deny the existence of a chronic disease, e.g., heart disease or hypertension, are not going to assist the patient in treatment concerns. At the same time, a family that has adapted to the implications of a chronic illness could be a constructive force on the patient's residual capabilities. However, each family is unique, so the family responses may be diverse.

DETERMINANTS OF FAMILY REACTION

There are many causes for why the family reacts as it does to disability trauma. A knowledge of these factors not only can indicate why a family is behaving in such a way, but it also suggests what may be done by health professionals to assist the family to adjust, and, in turn, how they can be used to help the patient.

145

How the Family Has Dealt with Previous Crises

When a severe illness represents a totally unfamiliar event, the family will usually display confusion and have a more difficult time marshalling its resources. When previous crises have identified family resources, and even helped to establish coping patterns, then often the impact of the disability will be softened. Shock and a feeling of helplessness will still be present after the initial diagnosis, but they may be managed more readily if the family has successfully handled other serious traumas. A family that has weathered the experience of having a husband/father out of work for many months because of a back injury, for example, has had an opportunity to assess its resources. When the wife/mother in the same family is diagnosed with a severe illness a few years later, the family will often adapt successfully if its resources were used effectively during the previous illness. If coping patterns have been effective in the past, then these will usually be adopted again in the new crisis.

The Meaning the Illness Has to the Family

How the family understands the illness will depend on the kind of information that has been imparted to family members and when it has been given. Early and appropriate communication of information by health professionals will generally diminish much unnecessary anxiety and allow the family to start working toward adjustment goals. If the family is very much in doubt about the nature of the disease and its implications for the affected family member, this uncertainty will create continued family tension and inhibit the formulation of realistic plans.

The Family Life-style

If a family, for example, is assessed as one that is nurturing, well structured, organized, and in which there is free, easy, and warm communication with ample opportunities for the expression of feelings, this family will have the potential to more readily develop effective coping mechanisms for the illness/disability situation. In contrast, in a family where there are often indications of indecisiveness and contradictory types of behavior, family members will generally display much anxiety and have a difficult time reaching out to each other for mutual support. A disability or illness for this family will usually bring protracted periods of confusion and much avoidance behavior in confronting the realistic implications of the disease.

Coping Resources

Coping resources include various emotional strengths that family members may possess to deal with a crisis. Satisfying work activity, the support from extended family, the availability of necessary community resources, anticipation of planned activities, and self-help groups can be helpful in times of continued stress. Included in these resources are financial means and the ability of family members to use community agencies. A family that has financial protection and will not suffer severe economic hardship because of the disability will theoretically cope much better than one for which the disability represents a financial disaster.

Who Is Ill and the Status and Role of the Ill Family Member

It may make more of a difference to the family if the wage earner or homemaker is seriously affected by a deteriorative illness than an elderly parent living in the home. If the wife has performed many of the home responsibilities and suddenly becomes disabled, this could also have a decided impact on family functioning.

The Stage of the Family Life Cycle

Each family stage brings the necessity of accomplishing certain tasks, i.e., raising children or building financial security for the family. The presence of a disability in a mother of young children who has been married for a few years could have a different impact on the family than if she were older, the children had left home, and the parents were starting to plan their retirement years together.

If the health professional understands the reasons why the family members are responding in a certain way to a disability, this awareness can form the basis for intervention. For example, when the health professional learns that the family has inadequate knowledge about a severe disease, and ascertains that the family members are emotionally receptive to further understanding and could profit from this communication, then helping efforts might be directed mainly to imparting appropriate information.

PATTERNS OF FAMILY REACTION
TO CHRONIC ILLNESS/SEVERE DISABILITY

A review of the literature (Christopherson, 1962; Bray, 1977; Epperson, 1977; Giacquinta, 1977) indicates that during the past 17 years there have been contributions from researchers on family reactive patterns to disability. Those that have been highlighted in the literature are now outlined and described briefly. The different authors' formulation of what happens to a family under stress of illness provide useful concepts for the health professional. The conceptualization of each stage that the family may be experiencing indicates a particular need the family has at that particular time in their adjustment to disability. For example, family members who have found that denial of the implications of a disease enables them to have some hope for the future may have a need to have that denial respected, or families who harbor much guilt about the occurrence of an illness need someone with whom to share that guilt and to provide them with more realistic feedback. Families who are still in grief over the loss of a family member usually need extra emotional support from others.

Christopherson (1962)

Acute stage ⟶ Reconstruction ⟶ Plateau ⟶ Deteriorative

Having worked for many years with different disabled clients, Christopherson (1962) outlines four stages that both the patient and family members experience. Following a period of initial anxiety (acute stage), and then a time when the patient attempts to regain as much residual strength as possible (reconstruction stage), the family members begin to perceive the patient's condition realistically. They become aware that the patient's rehabilitation has reached a point of diminishing returns. This is the plateau stage, and possibly the most difficult time for the family members. They realize that hope for improvement has diminished and perhaps a long period of care faces both the patient and family. It is a time when the family needs realistic objectives. Following this stage, the ill family member may suffer a setback. Grief and anger among the family are aggravated, and constant anxiety may pervade the family (deteriorative stage) unless selected resources, i.e., coping mechanisms, involvement from extended family, and support from community agencies alleviate this tension.

Bray (1977)

Anxiety ⟶ Acceptance ⟶ Assimilation

After observing 180 families of severely disabled individuals at the Georgia Warm Springs Hospital and Georgia Rehabilitation Center, Bray (1977) believes that family members progress through developmental stages that parallel the adjustment process of the client. A more extensive discussion of this research is reported in his article in this chapter. With the onset of the disease, the family experiences fear. As this fear diminishes and the family realizes that the patient is going to be severely disabled, roles are redefined among the family members. However, as the disabled person is incorporated again into family life, and new family experiences are shared, family members gradually develop more positive expectations for the patient. These expectations foster reintegration, but this may take place over a period of many years.

Giacquinta (1977)

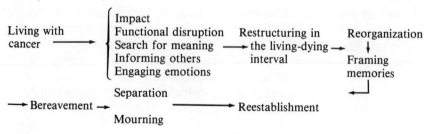

Based on an analysis of 100 families, Giacquinta (1977) presents a sequential pattern that becomes stages for the family to overcome in order to reach rehabilitation goals. Her article, which carefully elaborates on these stages, follows in Chapter 10. She focuses on cancer; its diagnosis can cause the entire group to become disorganized. A sense of despair invades the family, which becomes the main hurdle, but even then the family members begin to confront the illness situation. They seek a meaning for the purpose of the trauma—"Why did it happen to us?"—and also have a need to inform others about the disease. However, as the family members slowly recognize the losses they feel, they gradually reorganize themselves. While family duties are redistributed, they show a need to recapture the past through shared memories with the ill family member. As the patient becomes worse, however, renewed mourning occurs, which is accompanied by guilt. After successful resolution of their grief, the family will reenter the social environment that extends beyond the family. Life for the family then takes on a new dimension.

Epperson (1977)

High anxiety ⟶ Denial ⟶ Anger ⟶ Remorse ⟶ Grief ⟶ Reconciliation

In observing 230 families of multiply injured accident victims, Epperson (1977) viewed families in sudden crisis and formulated a series of stages that the family members undergo in adjusting to the trauma. These are explained in her article in Chapter 10. She believes that the family goes through six distinct phases, although families will differ in both the sequence of phases and how long the phases will last. She identified different emotions that family members will experience as they slowly adjust to the trauma, and each phase highlights a focal point for intervention. For example, during the time of anger the helper may encourage the ventilation of angry feelings, and at the time of grief the health professional may provide an effective contribution by giving silent support.

All of these reactive theories describing how the family responds to a chronic illness/severe disability are not intended to reduce the complexity of human behavior nor to stereotype emotional reactions. The stages are not sharply defined, and often they are not experienced in any particular order. Rather, their formulation constitutes a framework for the helping professional, providing a guideline for appropriate intervention. The reactive patterns may be cyclic or may overlap, depending on the nature of the disease. When an adult experiences a remission of a disease, as often happens with multiple sclerosis, family members may feel that adaptive patterns once achieved will be maintained continually. However, an exacerbation could cause a new beginning to a reactive pattern if the family members feel intense anxiety and renewed grief. Bray (1977) calls this occurrence "reflux," and the emotions accompanying it are explained in his article in Chapter 6.

When an adult experiences a remission of a disease or disability, family members may feel that the illness will not reappear, but an exacerbation only causes a new beginning to a reactive pattern.

CONCLUSION

Each reactive stage identifies a distinctive need of the family members and suggests a particular influence by the family on the patient. If the family members are still harboring much anger because of their perceived losses due to the disability, this emotion might prevent them from encouraging the ill family member to achieve rehabilitation goals. Resentment can cause family members to isolate themselves from the patient and to neglect treatment responsibilities. In contrast, a family that reached some form of disability adaptation would be more capable of assisting the patient to form appropriate, productive objectives. An understanding of each stage helps the health professional to plan an intervention approach. Intervention involves both describing what is happening to the family and suggesting what needs to be done to help the family assist the patient.

The three following articles discuss the family as a unit with its own emotional reactions to a disability or chronic illness trauma. John Bruhn explains the effects of chronic illness on the family and emphasizes that illness becomes an agent of family change. It can modify the attitudes and behaviors of all the family members. He explains how families usually cope with a chronic illness and offers suggestions for effective intervention. Grady Bray reports that the family experiences many of the same emotions, concerns, and conflicts as the patient. He believes that family members progress through developmental stages that parallel the adjustment process of the client. Yen Peterson reviews the literature concerning marital adjustment among couples with a physical disability. The particular value of her article is her precise identification of the many family influences that could determine the adjustment of the patient, and how the patient's behavior affects the life-style of other family members. All three articles show that there is a relationship between family dynamics and the presence of a physical handicap in the marital relationship. When this connection is understood by the health professional, family helping approaches can become more effective.

REFERENCES

Bray, G. Reactive patterns in families of the severely disabled. *Rehabilitation Counseling Bulletin,* 1977, March, 236–239.
Christopherson, V. The patient and family. *Rehabilitation Literature,* 1962, February, 34–41.

Epperson, M. Families in sudden crisis. *Social Work in Health Care,* 1977, *2-3,* 265-273.
Giacquinta, B. Helping families face the crisis of cancer. *American Journal of Nursing,* 1977, October, 1585-1588.

EFFECTS OF CHRONIC ILLNESS ON THE FAMILY

John G. Bruhn[1]

Our personal experiences tell us that illness is a potent agent of change. Chronic illness especially disrupts the usual ways in which family members behave toward one another and then hampers their ability to overcome the effects of this disruption. The effects of chronic illness on families are more often disintegrative than integrative; indeed, they change the attitudes and behavior of both sick and well family members, as individuals and as members of a family unit. Tasks and responsibilities must often be reassigned and this creates a period of disequilibrium. The duration and outcome of family disequilibrium is influenced by the clinical manifestations and management of the illness as well as how well the family adapts to the changes created by the illness.

The purpose of this paper is to examine some common effects of chronic illness on the family and to indicate how the family physician can assist families in adjusting to chronic illness.

CHRONIC ILLNESS CREATES ROLE CHANGE

Short-term changes in the role structure and task allocation in families as a result of illness are similar to the permanent or long-term changes caused by loss of one parent (Roghmann, Hecht, & Haggerty, 1973). When duties and responsibilities are taken away from one family member and assumed by another, often one will feel a sense of loss and the other feels burdened. Role change and task reallocation is perhaps easier to accept in short-term illness. In chronic illness, the ill person and other family members assume or hope at first that role change will be temporary. Indeed, if the clinical course of the illness stabilizes, or there is improvement, the ill person may regain some of his former family functions. If the clinical course of the illness declines, however, and duties and responsibilities must be removed from the ill person rather abruptly, he or she may feel a real sense of personal loss. The patient, especially one with a long-term illness, is sensitive to his dependence upon others and if his former duties and responsibilities within the family are completely removed, he will feel unneeded. Roles must be changed and reallocated in ways which minimize a sense of personal loss

Reprinted from *The Journal of Family Practice* 4(6), pp. 1057–1060, © 1977, Appleton-Century-Crofts, with permission.

[1]Associate Dean of Medicine and Coordinator for Community Affairs at the University of Texas Medical Branch, Galveston, TX 77550.

and prevent the ill person's social and psychological withdrawal from the family. We are familiar both with chronically ill persons who "gave up" living and became resigned to their illnesses and with ill persons who attempted to overcome the effects of their illness with determination, hope, and a "will to live." The latter group have usually retained a role within the family and feel wanted and needed.

Thus, it is important that the physician realistically convey to the family what the ill person can and cannot do with respect to duties and responsibilities. Discussions with the physician, the ill person, and the family members should be held periodically as the course of the illness changes. The ill person should be a part of these discussions so that his expectations can be geared to the clinical progress of his illness and possible paranoia about "what they know that I don't know about my illness" can be avoided.

THE SEE-SAW EFFECT OF ILLNESS

The chronic illness of one family member may create new, or revive former, symptoms in other family members, especially as roles are changed. The interactive effects of illness on marital pairs was studied by Klein and his associates in chronically ill outpatients and their spouses (Klein, Dean, & Bogdonoff, 1967). They found that the development of physical illness by one marital partner was accompanied by his failure in his role, which led to tension and physical symptoms in both partners. Klein observed that spouses reported new or increased symptoms during the illness of their partners. In addition, there was increased role tension between patients and their spouses and a reduction in work activity of both partners. Some spouses showed more symptoms than their ill partners. This latter finding led Klein to ask, "how does one family member become defined as 'the patient'?" The researchers speculated that some spouses are symptomatic before the patient is treated and may be waiting in the wings to become patients themselves. Thus, alternating illness between partners may be related to changes in roles rather than to the development of a new illness.

Vincent has suggested that there may be "familsomatic" ailments that accidentally or purposefully, real or imagined, are developed to avoid certain tasks, since the illness of one spouse increases the tasks of the other spouse (Vincent, 1963). Indeed, the development of symptoms is one way of sharing attention and concern, especially if the illness of a family member has diverted attention away from the "well" members of the family.

It is possible for a person disabled by illness to achieve secondary gains for himself as well as to behave in a manner that will increase gains for others. It has been found, for example, that when some husbands lose their capacity to earn a livelihood they attempt to compensate for this inadequacy by becoming more considerate of their wives, helping around the house, and changing their usual role behaviors in the family (Komarovsky, 1940). It may be that the value the person places on his various life activities helps to determine how disability in one role affects his performance in others. If the disability occurs in a role which is only one of several which are important and satisfying to the person, disability will be less destructive to his identity than if there are no role options.

In the clinical management of chronic illness, it is important to recognize that a sick member may become sicker in response to role changes in the family and "well" members may become "sick" to call attention to themselves or to the need to reallocate tasks, especially if they feel overshadowed or overburdened by the ill family member.

PREDISPOSITION TO CERTAIN ROLES AND ILLNESSES

There is some evidence to indicate that illness does not just "happen" to people and that individuals and families do not just "react" to the occurrence of illness. Lewis has observed family patterns of illness or a tendency in some families for illnesses to cluster. He raises the question, "Is there a way of being a family which influences the vulnerability of family members to all disease processes?" (Lewis, 1976).

A study conducted at the University of Michigan found substantial social effects of rheumatoid arthritis that are perpetuated between parental and conjugal families (Cobb et al., 1969). Women with rheumatoid arthritis make marriages which resemble those of their parents; there is a high degree of status stress (great discrepancies between their own and their husband's status on several factors measuring status), and they are more likely to be married to men whose status variables are incongruent. Women with rheumatoid arthritis feel and express a good deal of anger and aggression toward their husbands as well, which is reciprocated by the husband. This mutually directed anger-aggression was shown to relate significantly to the appearance of peptic ulcer in the husband. Men with rheumatoid arthritis were found to be low in feelings of anger and aggression and their rather benign attitude was reflected in the low level of marital hostility in marriages to healthy women. Thus, there is some indication that roles are carried from parental to conjugal families and that the interaction between certain types of roles over time may create a setting in which certain chronic illnesses may occur. For example, Sampson and his colleagues found that a family member is likely to become defined as a mental patient when he tries to break out of a chronic pattern of either intense dependency or of disinvolvement with other family members (Sampson, Messinger, & Towne, 1962). In essence, the person is labeled a mental patient when he tries to change his longstanding role in the family and disrupts the family organization.

It is important for the physician to determine the role that the ill person occupied both in his parental and conjugal families, as this information will tell a great deal about the expectations that family members hold of the ill person with respect to his future role and responsibilities. For example, there is evidence that a family member who is mentally ill is less likely to be hospitalized or rehospitalized if living with his parents (Freeman & Simmons, 1958). In the setting of the parental family, the mother especially is more likely to tolerate deviant behavior and there are few, if any, pressures to be independent. Therefore, role shifts among one or more family members can signal the onset of illness. Role shifts among "well" family members may also be necessary to fill voids created by a sick member. Although sources outside of the family are often available and helpful in filling voids, neighbors and friends supplement, rather than compensate for, family sources of aid. Hence, members must act to restore equilibrium within the family; sources outside the family can assist in this endeavor, but they alone cannot hold a family together (Croog, Lipson, & Levine, 1972).

FAMILY BREAKDOWN—FAILURE TO ADAPT

The rate of breakdown in families with severe chronic disease is high. It has been shown that the combined effects of poor health and unfavorable family situations are cumulative over time (Pless, Roghmann, & Haggerty, 1972). Diabetes mellitus, hemophilia, and epilepsy are examples of chronic illnesses with high rates of family breakdown. Family breakdown in these instances often results because family members would not or could not change roles and reallocate tasks.

The presence of a diabetic child is associated with lower marital integration and greater conflict among parents. Although a new equilibrium can be established in the family, it is often less stable and integrative than before the chronic illness (Crain, Sussman, & Weil, 1966). The families of diabetic children show a variety of psychological structures (Treuting, 1962). Since diabetes enforces a certain way of life, the child and his family react according to preexisting yet unspecific patterns. Diabetes seems to reinforce existing patterns. Childhood diabetes present numerous difficulties because of the susceptibility to other diseases, changing requirements of growth, unpredictable outbursts of physical energy, and emotional disturbances. The effects of the disease continue throughout adulthood, influencing the diabetic person's educational, marital, and occupational plans. Thus, as the diabetic person grows older, problems expand into other systems outside his immediate family.

The presence of a hemophiliac son can draw parents together. In the majority of families, however, hemophilia contributes to the withdrawal of the husband from family relationships and to the breakup of the marriage (Salk, Hilgartner, & Granich, 1972). Hemophilia limits family mobility, creates financial strain, generates feelings of guilt and resentment among the parents, and often strains the relationships between healthy sibs and the hemophiliac child.

The idea that epilepsy is a shameful disease is often foremost in the minds of the parents of an epileptic child. Many parents feel that epilepsy has a hopeless prognosis, especially if a cause cannot be discovered for their child's convulsions. Parents may become protective of the child with respect to emotional excitement and physical activity. Young children sense any type of restraint and soon learn that others, even family members, do not see them as normal. The actions of others help to mold the epileptic's self-image which, in turn, influences his educational, marital, and occupational plans (Livingston, 1957).

Chronic disease in a child or adolescent is perhaps more difficult for the physician to manage clinically for several reasons. 1) Parents often protect the chronically ill child or adolescent from learning adult roles and responsibilities. 2) The chronically ill child or adolescent may learn to use his illness as with, for example, control over diet and insulin in diabetes to "get his way," learning, possibly, that manipulation of others is a successful way to solve problems of living. 3) The chronically ill child or adolescent is permitted by society to have more freedom in the expression of feelings and behavior regarding his illness than adults. So, when he becomes an adult, he may have to learn new and more socially acceptable ways of expression and behavior. 4) The chronically ill child or adolescent usually lives with one or both of his parents or relatives who impose their perception of the type of life style or routine that the ill person should follow. Therefore, the young chronically ill person may not be able to adjust to his illness as he wants to. 5) The chronically ill child may be the "lightning rod" for marital and family problems, so his and his family's adjustment to the illness is further complicated.

These issues, which must be discussed with the parents, present problems for the physician in the clinical management of chronic illness. Parents often think they are being thoughtful and helpful in removing tasks and responsibilities from a sick child completely, especially from a child with a chronic illness. Indeed, such action may foster feelings of hopelessness and helplessness and work against good clinical management of the illness. Chronically ill persons, irrespective of age, must retain their integrity as human beings and be given the opportunity to participate in their families and society as their social and clinical circumstances permit.

ROLE EXPECTATIONS AND ADJUSTMENT TO CHRONIC ILLNESS

What others expect of the ill person will influence how he adjusts to his illness as well as the degree of success in the clinical management of the illness.

Davis studied the social-psychological impact of spinal paralytic poliomyelitis on the families of 14 children, ages four to twelve (Davis, 1963). He observed that when the child made significant strides in his physical capacities, there was an aura of achievement in the family and often unrealistic parental expectations regarding recovery. In those families in which the child showed little or no functional improvement, family members hoped for a spontaneous cure, and rehabilitation gains were neglected or only half-heartedly pursued. As might be expected, the adjustment period was more difficult, prolonged and pervasive in families where the child remained handicapped. However, many of these families appeared to be coping also with other longstanding problems that tended to merge with those created by the chronic illness. Thus, it is not surprising that the families leaning toward dissociation from the chronic illness tended to isolate themselves from others, whereas families tending toward normalization denied the social significance of the handicap rather than the handicap itself. So, the degree of success in the rehabilitation of youthful polio victims was intimately tied to the social climate and outlook on life of their families.

Ezra, in a follow-up study of 50 men who had heart attacks and their families, found interesting discrepancies between the interpretations of family difficulties by husbands and wives (Ezra, 1961). The problems most frequently mentioned in interviews with the husbands were: 1) financial problems, 2) depression, 3) curtailment of activities, and 4) fear of recurrent attack. The wives, however, responded that stress and tension as a result of their husbands' illness, financial problems, and the adjustment of their husbands were more crucial concerns. The wives of these disabled men believed that their husbands had more serious problems of adjustment than they would admit, and a high percentage of the wives believed that the family could have benefited from counseling. Respondents were also asked how they felt about the way responsibilities were handled in the home as compared to the way they were handled before the disability. A complex relationship between financial stress and changes in role relationships was found. The greater the financial difficulty resulting from the disability, the more negative were family reactions to the disability and the changes it produced.

Landsman has observed that patients with chronic renal failure all share in a desperate effort to determine for themselves a realistic set of expectations and goals (Landsman, 1975). After the initial impact of illness dissipates they tend to find themselves adrift somewhere between the worlds of the sick and the well. Marginal men, in effect. According to societal expectations the patient with renal disease is not sick, for unless he is severely impaired he is expected to pick up where he left off at the time of hospitalization and resume his former obligations. The marginality between what society defines as healthy and the fact that every aspect of life is altered by his dependence on dialysis is responsible for the renal disease patient's inner struggle to arrive at an appropriate self-image.

The physician also has his own expectations of the ill person regarding his motivation, his compliance with clinical regimen, and his cooperation in controlling the illness. The ill person must sometimes balance the expectations of family members with those of his physician. Thus, it is important that the physician, the family, and the patient discuss expectations jointly so all will arrive at realistic expectations regarding adjustment.

HOW FAMILIES COPE WITH CHRONIC ILLNESS

Families with greater family strain seem to have more illness than families with less strain. Yet, badly functioning families are not less ready to cope or to seek help. How families cope with chronic illness and whether or not they seek help to adjust is tied to how they cope with other problems of living. If the family has ways of coping that work for them, they are less likely to see the need for help. To others outside the family, these coping patterns may be seen as maladaptive or as conflicting with the effective clinical management of the illness. Families have been found to feel less threatened by illness for which they have well-established coping rituals than for other types of life problems for which there are no rituals (Roghmann et al., 1973). Many individuals and families feel comfortable in coping with acute illness. But chronic illness is insidious in onset, difficult to treat and contain, and its clinical course is often unpredictable. Therefore, chronic illness may not fit the ways a family has established for coping with acute illness. Any suggestion that a family's way of coping with chronic illness is ineffective would create much anxiety and imply that the family does not cope effectively with problems of living. So it is important that the physician ascertain the family's way of coping with life problems previous to the diagnosis of the chronic illness before he makes judgments about their effectiveness in coping with the chronic illness.

Since chronic illness is progressive in onset the family may have been told earlier of the gradually debilitating effects of an illness diagnosed in a family member, but they may have chosen to deny or ignore this until the effects were undeniable. In addition to denial there is a variety of feelings such as guilt, anxiety, shame, embarrassment, depression, resentment, rejection, alienation, self-blame, and bitterness which are a part of a family's armamentarium in coping with chronic illness. The family must be assisted in resolving the emotional antecedents and sequelae of the illness before it will be able to satisfy the emotional needs of its members. Unless a family's emotional baseline is reestablished, role change and task reallocation will be emotionally painful, if not impossible, to carry out. This reestablishment is necessary for minimization of the negative effects of poor family dynamics on clinical management of the illness.

Family members have been found to go through stages associated with cancer similar to those the patient experiences. There is shock and anger at the diagnosis, guilt for missed past appointments, and a period of anticipatory grief and hope, at first for curative drugs and later for one more remission (*The question of coping: Coping with cancer,* 1974). For families coping with cardiovascular disease, a key factor is that the family members be given information routinely along with the patient. How well the family is organized can be a crucial factor in how well the patient follows a therapeutic regimen. But a crucial way for families to cope with cardiac illness is to work together and communicate freely, especially during the period of convalescence. What heart patients need most is emotional support and guidance towards a realistic style of work and home life (*The question of coping: Coping with cardiovascular disease,* 1974).

IMPLICATIONS FOR PHYSICIANS

The doctor-patient and doctor-family relationships are critical ones for chronically ill patients. For some chronic illnesses, such as cancer, there is little patients can do to alter the disease once treatment has begun. For other chronic illnesses such as diabetes, patients can control their disease through diet and insulin. Whatever the degree of individual control over the illness, the physician is seen as a symbol of hope by chronically ill persons. The key to coping with chronic illness is having and maintaining hope. Although the patient and his family have to cope somehow with changes in life style and roles, few people can make these adjustments without periods of discouragement, anxiety, and resentment. The family physician is in a key position to enhance the changes for successful clinical and psychosocial adjustment to chronic illness by using his knowledge of the family and its dynamics to create strong family support for the ill person. Physicians, like their patients, are not immune to feelings of discouragement in treating chronic disease. Many physicians prefer not to tell their patients and families the truth about the clinical course of a chronic illness. Direct two-way communication between physician and the family is essential because it builds confidence and rapport. This is often the most effective treatment available for chronic illness.

REFERENCES

Cobb, S., Schull, W. J., Harburg, E., et al. The intrafamilial transmission of rheumatoid arthritis: An unusual study. *Journal of Chronic Diseases,* 1969, *22,* 193–194.

Crain, A. J., Sussman, M. B., & Weil, W. B. Effects of a diabetic child on marital integration and related measures of family functioning. *Journal of Health and Human Behavior,* 1966, *7,* 122–127.

Croog, S. H., Lipson, A., & Levine, S. Help patterns in severe illness: The roles of kin network, non-family resources and institutions. *Journal of Marriage and the Family,* 1972, *34,* 32–41.

Davis, F. *Passage through crisis: Polio victims and their families.* New York: Bobbs-Merrill Co., 1963.

Ezra, J. *Social and economic effects on families of patients with myocardial infarctions.* Denver: University of Denver, 1961.

Freeman, H. E., & Simmons, O. G. Mental patients in the community: Family settings and performance levels. *American Sociological Review,* 1958, *23,* 147–154

Klein, R. F., Dean, A., & Bogdonoff, M. D. The impact of illness upon the spouse *Journal of Chronic Diseases,* 1967, *20,* 241–248.

Komarovsky, M. *The unemployed man and his family.* New York: Dryden, 1940.

Landsman, M. K. The patient with chronic renal failure: A marginal man. *Annals of Internal Medicine,* 1975, *82,* 268–270.

Lewis, J. M. The family and physical illness. *Texas Medicine,* 1976, *72,* 43–49.

Livingston, S. The social management of the epileptic child and his parents. *Journal of Pediatrics,* 1957, *51,* 137–145.

Pless, I. B., Roghmann, K. J., & Haggerty, R. J. Chronic illness, family functioning and psychological adjustment: A model for the allocation of preventive mental health services. *International Journal of Epidemiology,* 1972, *1,* 271–277.

The question of coping: Coping with cancer. The fifth of an ongoing series by Hoffmann-La Roche Inc., Nutley, N.J., 1974.

The question of coping: Coping with cardiovascular disease. The sixth of an ongoing series by Hoffmann-La Roche Inc., Nutley, N.J., 1974.

Roghmann, K. J., Hecht, P. K., & Haggerty, R. J. Family coping with everyday illness: Self reports from a household survey. *Journal of Comparative Family Studies,* 1973, *4,* 49–62.

Salk, L., Hilgartner, M., & Granich, B. The psychosocial impact of hemophilia on the patient and his family. *Social Science and Medicine,* 1972, *6,* 491–505.

Sampson, H., Messinger, S. L., & Towne, R. D. Family processes and becoming a mental patient. *American Journal of Sociology,* 1962, *68,* 88–96.

Treuting, T. F. The role of emotional factors in the etiology and course of diabetes mellitus: A review of the recent literature. *American Journal of the Medical Sciences,* 1962, *244,* 93–109.

Vincent, C. E. The family in health and illness: Some neglected areas. *Annals of the American Academy of Politics and Social Science,* 1963, *34,* 109–116.

REACTIVE PATTERNS IN FAMILIES OF THE SEVERELY DISABLED

Grady P. Bray[1]

The prognosis for the severely injured client includes a long hospitalization, discomfort, pain, and alterations in self-concept. The number of these patients increases annually, with at least 10,000 new patients each year (Fitzpatrick, 1963). This increase in the number of severely disabled clients, along with the demand for implementation of current federal legislation, has caused the disabled to become the focal point of the activities of an allied health and rehabilitation team. However, in their haste to provide services for severely injured clients, many teams overlook the necessity of strengthening the clients' natural bulwark—their families (Carpenter, 1974).

The client's family is often exposed to long and grueling hours at the hospital. During this time, they experience the added tensions of financial strain, extended absence from familiar surroundings, and changes in family roles.

Rehabilitation and psychological investigation into the adjustment process for severely injured clients and their families has evolved more slowly than research into the medical aspects of severe disability. In her studies with terminally ill patients, Kubler-Ross (1975) identified five stages that the patient experiences prior to death. Similarly, developmental stages have been observed and reported by Wright (1960) for clients experiencing general physical disability. However, only limited research has been conducted on the impact of family involvement in the rehabilitation process or the developmental stages experienced by families with a severely disabled member.

The family of the severely disabled individual experiences many of the same emotions, concerns, and conflicts as the client. They progress through developmental stages that parallel the adjustment process of the client. These stages are not envisioned as mutually exclusive with separate and easily identified boundaries. Interfaces may occur between aspects of any or all states; however, a natural and logical progression has been observed in 180 families studied at the Georgia Warm Springs Hospital and Georgia Rehabilitation Center.

Reprinted from *Rehabilitation Counseling Bulletin,* March, pp. 236–239, © 1977, American Personnel and Guidance Association, with permission.

[1]Director of Psychological Services, Georgia Warm Springs Complex, Warm Springs, GA.

ANXIETY STAGE

The initial reaction of the severely injured person's family is fear. They are fearful of death, and they express relief when they are informed that their family member has not died. The residual anxiety produces an obsession with the care of the injured family member since the threat of death, although diminished, remains a reality. Anxiety is heightened by new and strange medical terminology compounding the frustration produced by ignorance of injury and prognosis.

During this phase, families generally question the competency of the staff and the quality of patient care. Family members are frequently fearful that discussing their criticisms with the staff will result in less treatment and inferior service for the client. They seldom realize that they are expressing their own feelings of inadequacy, frustration, and despair.

To reduce family anxiety, team members can reinforce and clarify information, explaining the physiology and prognosis of the injury. The flow of regular information does much to ease the acute distress precipitated by ambiguity.

The demonstration of good communication skills both within the team and between team and family members can serve as a model for families. When families receive conflicting information, increased stress and unrealistic expectations may occur. The information transmitted to the family embraces divergent opinions by team members but primarily reflects the attitudes and beliefs of the entire team.

As the fear of death diminishes, the family is confronted with the reality of a prolonged, extensive recovery period and the possibility of a permanent handicap. Most families cannot readily assimilate such a prognosis. The denial of this reality takes many forms. Some (9 percent of our study group) become angry and initially refuse to deal with staff members who confront them with the realities of paralysis, brain damage, or loss of function. Greater than 60 percent of our study group turned to religious beliefs for succor; the clinical chaplain is a most beneficial person at this time. Exposing the family to other clients who have sustained similar injuries and have experienced the recovery process can demonstrate to the family the future of their patient.

The most noticeable behavior of families with a severely injured family member is depression. The foundation of their depression is impotent anger. To reduce the feelings of impotence, family members are involved in a family education program, which emphasizes the needs of the client and family, problem-solving skills, goal setting, and behavior contracting, and it helps the family plan for the patient's return home. The anxiety stage lasted an average of nine months for our study families.

ACCEPTANCE STAGE

During the acceptance stage a second presentation of meaningful and realistic information by members of the rehabilitation team can have a reassuring and motivating effect. This review of information can aid the family in developing a new operational structure. During this period of stress, the family's beliefs about each other are in a state of flux, and the psychological moment exists for the rehabilitation team to assist the family through a process of reconstruction and acceptance.

As the family moves to complete the final aspect of acceptance, they develop systems of accommodation. The client is once again an active part of the family but is only that and not the focal point of life itself. It is not unusual for family members to express hidden and often guilt-ridden feelings. For the first time, anger and hostility can be expressed openly toward the severely injured person. These feelings need to be expressed, discussed, and resolved. Such feelings are generally repressed and express themselves in devious ways, thereby creating a hidden agenda for family members. It is with the resolution of such hidden agenda issues that the family is able to move to the final stage in the development process.

ASSIMILATION STAGE

In our study group, the acceptance stage usually lasted from the tenth month into the second year. By the second year most recovery for the person has occurred and new experiences provide an additional source of positive data for the family's perception of the injured person. These experiences allow the family to live through the injured person, as well as through other family members. Total reintegration into the family structure does not happen in one spontaneous reaction, but rather over a period of years. The process is retarded by the physical absence of the injured family member from the family during hospitalization, treatment, evaluation, or training. Many times such absence requires the family to work through problems they felt had been previously resolved. They fail to realize that extended absence often results in emotional insulation and isolation similar to reactions associated with death. To assist in understanding and resolving these issues, the rehabilitation team should include follow-up personnel to work with the families from the acute through the chronic phases. The continuity of staff aid and information remains a vital aspect of the comprehensive rehabilitation program and serves as a source of reference and encouragement to families of the severely disabled.

SUMMARY

Current legislation and increasing numbers of clients require that greater emphasis be placed on services to the severely disabled. The involvement of families of the severely disabled involved in the comprehensive rehabilitation program has been minimal, and utilizing them as a positive force in the rehabilitation process has been largely neglected.

REFERENCES

Carpenter, J. O. Changing roles and disagreement in families with disabled husbands. *Archives of Physical Medicine and Rehabilitation*, 1974, *55*, 272-274.
Fitzpatrick, A. J. Family myth and homeostasis. *Archives of General Psychiatry*, 1963, 457-463.
Kubler-Ross, E. *Death: The final stage of growth*. Englewood Cliffs, N.J. Prentice-Hall, 1975.
Wright, B. A. *Physical disability—A psychological approach*. New York: Harper & Brothers, 1960.

THE IMPACT OF PHYSICAL DISABILITY ON MARITAL ADJUSTMENT:
A Literature Review

Yen Peterson[1]

Contemporary American culture has assumed that physical handicaps are stress factors in marriage. Illness becomes a handicap of both a physical and a social nature from Parsons' (1972) view that somatic illness may be defined in terms of incapacity for relevant task performance. Parsons and Fox (1970) have noted the particular difficulties which small isolated nuclear families faced in these circumstances and their tendency to rely on outside institutions for care of the seriously physically ill. The question has arisen whether or not such an assumption has unconditional affirmation in empirical studies. To this end, this review of literature sought to assess the presence or absence of marital stress due to physical handicaps and to identify factors contributing to the stress. Between 1960 and 1970 over one hundred empirical studies on marital interaction were published (Hicks & Platt, 1970). The present literature review is focused on only those works which address marital adjustment in the context of physical disability.

MARITAL STRESS AND PHYSICAL ILLNESS

Research findings suggested that physical and psychological health were associated with marital happiness regardless of marital history (Renne, 1971). Also physical disability was related to marital dissatisfaction (Renne, 1970; Palmer, 1971).

In a study of hemodialysis patients and their spouses Steele, Finkelstein, and Finkelstein (1976) concluded that there was a substantial discrepancy between the global ratings (overall ratings of marital problems) by the pair and assessment of specific aspects of the marriage. Global ratings indicated relatively little discord while more detailed investigation of specific areas revealed substantial marital discord. Their findings suggested that the variable, depth of analysis, may interfere with comparability among studies and account for some discrepancies in results. At the same time, the above

Reprinted from *The Family Coordinator*, January, pp. 47–51, © 1979, the National Council on Family Relations, with permission.

[1]Associate Professor, Department of Sociology and Anthropology, Saint Xavier College, 3700 West 103rd St., Chicago, IL 60655.

study concluded that there is a significant relationship between marital stress and illness.

Some factors were more predictive of stress in physically handicapped populations than others. A comparison of post-polio patients (Nagi & Clark, 1964) revealed sex differences between those still married and those divorced or separated. Women who have had polio "...are slightly more likely..." (Nagi & Clark, 1964, p. 215) to be divorced than men, with the divorce or separation occurring most frequently within five years of the onset of the disease. There was also greater likelihood of divorce among the younger, compared to older persons, consistent with findings among the United States population as a whole (United States Bureau of the Census, 1971, p. 1).

MARITAL ADJUSTMENT AND SOCIOECONOMIC LEVELS

Another factor consistent with findings among the total American population was the tendency for an inverse correlation between divorce rates and socioeconomic level (Goode, 1956). This trend was supported by the work of Renne (1970), Palmer (1971), and De La Mata, Gingras, and Wittkower (1960).

It would be an oversimplification to say that the major variables which determined social status, namely education, income and occupation were functioning independently of one another in their effect on the marital satisfaction of couples in which one partner was physically handicapped. Marriages in which a spouse was handicapped were likely to encounter a number of problem solving areas for which society has not provided adequate socialization. Problem solving ability and access to resources for solving problems are enhanced by higher socioeconomic status.

Family income, however, is not directly related to who goes home from the hospital among the severely disabled (Deutsch & Goldston, 1960). The latter study concluded a relationship between partial fulfillment of the instrumental role which the person had prior to disability and the likelihood of returning home. The Deutsch and Goldston (1960) study strengthened the argument that socioeconomic level was not a sufficient explanation for marriages remaining intact among the physically handicapped, emphasizing as it did, the importance of role performance.

ROLE FLEXIBILITY AND INTERACTION

A variable expected to be related to marital satisfaction was the degree of mobility on the part of the physically handicapped spouse. Fink, Skipper, and Hallenbeck (1968) concluded this was not the case for either spouse in their study of disabled wives. They concluded that need satisfaction and marital satisfaction were correlated while role ambiguity was more likely to occur in marriages in which the wife was less rather than more disabled. The importance of clear role definitions was further supported by De La Mata et al. (1960). In spite of a disability-induced disruption of roles, the more severely disabled were no more likely to be found in extended marital relationships than the less disabled (Gibson & Ludwig, 1968).

Role flexibility operated differently among men and women in American culture. In a study of disabled breadwinners, Collette (1969) concluded that there was greater marital disharmony with greater dependency needs of the disabled. On the surface this finding militated against the earlier assertion that the degree of disability was not directly related to marital satisfaction. These findings were generated from a sample of disabled husbands while the previously mentioned study (Fink et al., 1968) examined a sample of disabled women. These findings, therefore, supported the conclusion that both role ambiguities and a wide discrepancy between performance of the generally sanctioned roles for men and women in the larger culture were conducive to marital discord. Role intactness rather than role flexibility was advanced by Livsey (1972) as the important variable. She pointed out that a bedridden mother may continue homemaking decisions and perform the mother role for her children. Only when these roles were lost, as when the husband adopted the homemaker or mother roles, did stress occur in the family. Many of the roles were no longer intact in Livsey's examples. It can, therefore, be asserted that she was speaking about role flexibility.

Role flexibility in marriages in which one spouse is physically handicapped was more likely to have a deleterious effect on marital adjustment if the disability affected cognitive and psychological functioning. Additional confirmation of this conclusion was the finding that impairments resulting in loss of communication skills were disabling in interpersonal relationships (Zahn, 1973).

MARITAL ADJUSTMENT AND DEPENDENCY

A physical handicap did affect the daily living of marital partners. In a study of diabetics' wives, Katz (1969) found conflict between the dependency needs of the wives of diabetic men and the requirements of caring for their husbands. Disabled females were more likely to find it acceptable to have the family take care of them than disabled males (Thomas & Britton, 1973). Neither chronological age nor age at the onset of the disability were significantly related to the acceptability of having the family take care of the woman.

In determining the effects of disabled breadwinners on the daily activities of the marital pair, Ludwig and Collette (1969) found dependent husbands had more role flexibility and less role rigidity than husbands who were not so dependent. Dependent husbands, those needing assistance in bathing, dressing and moving around the house, also spent more time with their spouses than less dependent husbands. This suggests that the degree of marital satisfaction was related to time spent together, offsetting perhaps some of the lowered marital satisfaction due to the handicap (Marini, 1976). The direct relationship of dependence to marital adjustment has not been examined for men. Additional support for influence of marital satisfaction and physical handicap was offered by Skipper, Fink, and Hallenbeck (1968). The husband's companionship satisfaction was found to be correlated with the degree of physical disability of the wife while the degree of marital satisfaction did not correlate with the degree of handicap. Husbands who were dependent on their spouses for daily living activities had less decision-making power in the marriage than less dependent husbands (Ludwig & Collette, 1969). The latter finding was consistent, regardless of the degree of handicap, suggesting the relationship between variables was due to the degree of dependency of husbands on their wives. Stone and Shapiro (1968), however, found family roles of post-hospital patients redistributed and reorganized with the sick spouse often retaining decision-making functions while relinquishing other domains. From non-handicapped samples it is known that wife-dominant marriages, in terms of decision making, are less satisfactory for both partners than husband dominated marriages (Blood & Wolfe, 1960). However, in marriages where the husband was handicapped, the increased marital power of the wife may not have the same social meaning for the partners and, therefore, may not adversely affect the relationship.

MARITAL ADJUSTMENT AND
RELATIONSHIP TO FAMILY AND FRIENDS

Support for an alteration in the social meaning of activities and expectation for the marital pair was documented by Peterson (1977). She claimed that for progressively disabled persons and their spouses marital interaction was sufficiently modified to constitute a specific life style. Such a life style was entitled "disability marriage" and was defined as the condition under which need fulfillment commonly associated with the roles of husband and wife were so significantly altered as to violate cultural prescriptions for these roles. Disability marriages did not appear at a particular point in time but gradually emerged over a period. The length of this period would be a function of the extent to which "normal" expectations from the marriage could function either because of the physical requirements of the handicap or the relative reluctance to redefine the situation or a combination of both.

More disabled husbands with employed wives devoted greater time to cooking and housework than those of non-employed wives (Carpenter, 1974). The husbands were least likely to do housework if they were highly disabled themselves and the wife did not work. Carpenter (1974) also found a high degree of agreement on household role performance between husbands and wives. There appeared to be the same proportion of working and non-working wives who handled the money. Overall, the required changes in role definitions were greater for the disabled husbands than for the disabled wives. Therefore, role flexibility on the part of husbands who were disabled was more crucial for marital satisfaction than for disabled wives.

Another facet of role behavior concerned ambiguities in the role of the handicapped, vis-a-vis family members and friends. According to Zahn (1973), characteristics of impairment which clearly indicated sickness or disability were also associated with better interpersonal relationships with both friends and family. A viable interpretation by Zahn was that with severe impairment, the sick role became acceptable and sympathetic; humanitarian responses became more likely. In addition, persons sufficiently handicapped to be unable to work had a better relationship to their spouses than those able to work. The reason appeared to be that clear-cut functional limitations required one family member to be cast into a new role. This disability role altered the expectations of the family members as a different family organization emerged. These research findings did not warrant the conclusion that the severity of the handicap was directly related to marital satisfaction. On the contrary, they affirmed the previous argument that role ambiguity had greater detrimental effects on the marital relationship. There were more negative consequences for handicapped individuals who were not working but who were judged capable of work by spouses and family. There were fewer negative consequences from co-workers and friends. The reason for more negative consequences from spouse and the family was explained by Croog, Lipson, and Levine (1972) as resulting from the sustained level of help required of the family; friends, though helpful, tended to respond only intermittently and situationally.

CONCLUSION

In conclusion, this literature survey has demonstrated that there is a relationship between marital stress and the presence of a physical handicap in the marital relationship. The stress factors appear not to be directly related to the severity of the handicap and to be differentially affecting the spouses, dependent on the integration between role performance and sex of the person. Cognitive and mental deterioration produce greater stress on marriage than physical disability. Clear and appropriate definitions with regard to role expectations related to the performance of the handicapped spouse appear to be related to higher marital satisfaction for the couple.

REFERENCES

Blood, R. O., Jr., & Wolfe, D. M. *Husbands and wives: The dynamics of married living.* Glencoe, Ill.: The Free Press, 1960.

170   Peterson

Carpenter, J. O. Changing roles and disagreements in families with disabled husbands. *Archives of Physical Medical Rehabilitation*, 1974, *55*, 272-274.

Collette, J. P. Disability as crisis: An analysis of the marital relationships of disabled breadwinners. Unpublished doctoral dissertation, Ohio State University, 1969.

Croog, S. H., Lipson, A., & Levine, S. Help patterns in severe illness: The role of kin network. *Journal of Marriage and the Family*, 1972, *34*, 32-40.

De La Mata, R., Gingras, G., & Wittkower, E. D. Impact of sudden, severe disablement of the father upon the family. *Canadian Medical Association Journal*, 1960, *82*, 1015-1020.

Deutsch, C. P., & Goldston, J. A. Family factors in home adjustment of the severely disabled. *Marriage and Family Living*, 1960, *22*, 312-316.

Fink, S. L., Skipper, J. K., Jr., & Hallenbeck, P. N. Physical disability and problems in marriage. *Journal of Marriage and the Family*, 1968, *30*, 64-73.

Gibson, G., & Ludwig, E. G. Family structure in a disabled population. *Journal of Marriage and the Family*, 1968, *30*, 54-63.

Goode, W. J. *After divorce*. New York: The Free Press, 1956.

Hicks, M. W., & Platt, M. Marital happiness and stability: A review of the research in the sixties. *Journal of Marriage and the Family*, 1970, *32*, 569-574.

Katz, A. M. Wives of diabetic men. *Bulletin of the Menninger Clinic*, 1969, *33*, 279-294.

Livsey, C. G. Physical illness and family dynamics. *Advancement of Psychosomatic Medicine*, 1972, *8*, 237-251.

Ludwig, E. G., & Collette, J. Disability, dependency, and conjugal roles. *Journal of Marriage and the Family*, 1969, *31*, 736-739.

Marini, M. M. Dimensions of marriage happiness: A research note. *Journal of Marriage and Family*, 1976, *38*, 443-448.

Nagi, S. Z., & Clark, D. L. Factors in marital adjustment after disability. *Journal of Marriage and the Family*, 1964, *26*, 215-216.

Palmer, S. E. Reasons for marriage breakdown: A case study in western Ontario. *Journal of Comparative Family Studies*, 1971, *2*, 251-262.

Parsons, T. Definitions of health and illness in the light of American values and social structure. In G. E. Jaco (Ed.), *Patients, physicians and illness* (2nd ed.). New York: The Free Press, 1972.

Parsons, T., & Fox, R. C. *Illness, therapy and the modern urban American family: Modern introduction to the family*. New York: The Free Press, 1970.

Peterson, Y. *Marital adjustment in couples of which one spouse is physically handicapped*. Unpublished doctoral dissertation, Walden University, 1977.

Renne, K. S. Correlates of dissatisfaction in marriage. *Journal of Marriage and the Family*, 1970, *32*, 54-67.

Renne, K. S. Health and marital experience in an urban population. *Journal of Marriage and the Family*, 1971, *29*, 338-350.

Skipper, J. K., Jr., Fink, S. L., & Hallenbeck, P. N. Physical disability among married women: Problems in the husband-wife relationship. *Journal of Rehabilitation*, 1968, *34*, 16-19.

Steele, T. E., Finkelstein, S. H., & Finkelstein, F. O. Hemodialysis patients and spouses. *Journal of Nervous Mental Disorder*, 1976, *162*, 225-237.

Stone, O. M., & Shapiro, E. Posthospital changes in role systems of patients. *The Social Service Review*, 1968, *42*, 314-324.

Thomas, K. R., & Britton, J. O. Perceptions of family dependence by the physically disabled. *Rehabilitation Counseling Bulletin*, 1973, *16*, 156-161.

United States Bureau of the Census. Social and economic variations in marriage, divorce and remarriage: 1967. *Current population reports* (Series P-20, No. 223). Washington, D.C.: U.S. Government Printing Office, 1971.

Zahn, M. A. Incapacity, impotence, and invisible impairment: Their effects upon interpersonal relations. *Journal of Health and Social Behavior,* 1973, *14,* 115–123.

CHAPTER 5

GENERAL IMPACT OF CHILD DISABILITY/ ILLNESS ON THE FAMILY

Paul W. Power and Arthur E. Dell Orto

The personal statements of Maria and Karen reveal the many difficulties that a family encounters in living with a severe disability. The condition has a devastating impact on the family members. In reality, the family is called upon both to react and to employ actively coping behaviors within the family system and in relationship to the community. Treatment responsibilities for the child demand a long-term commitment, and over many months and years family members may find it difficult to master their feelings, especially anger, guilt, and grief. Their reactions can be complex and as diverse as the personalities of the family members.

This chapter contains brief discussions of the different family reactions to child disability, and the following articles present a more comprehensive explanation of the family's emotional responses. The materials in this chapter also highlight the determinants of the family's reaction. An understanding of the reasons for the family's response to adult disability provides a basis for helping approaches; the same is true for child disability. The health professional can become aware of the unique way family members are reacting to a handicapped child by understanding the causes for the reaction. A knowledge of these causes facilitates understanding the many sources of family influence on the child's rehabilitation. A family, for example, that acknowledges the underlying value of the community in the management of family stress will usually be able to utilize effectively community resources. This assistance could influence the family's reactive pattern to the disability, as well as enable them to share more productively in the child's disease-related treatment.

DETERMINANTS OF FAMILY REACTION

The reasons why a family copes in a particular way with a disabled child are varied. Some of the more important are:

1. *The age of the child*   The parental reactions to a handicapping condition that appears in an older child follow a course similar to that of responses to birth of a defective child (Poznanski, 1973), with one important difference. When an older child becomes handicapped "the parents have usually formed a strong attachment to the child; with the newborn, the mother's emotional attachment to the child is still highly tenuous" (Poznanski, 1973, p. 323).
2. *Family size and structure*   The chronically ill child needs two parents, because it takes two to cope with a child who is sick at home over a long period of time (Travis, 1976). The complete burden on one parent can be emotionally and physically devastating. If a family's life-style has become well established and the family members have settled into a pattern of living together, such an atmosphere may facilitate family adjustment more than a family life in which one of the parents has just remarried. This is not always true, but the new parent might have conflicting feelings about the expenses and inconveniences associated with a chronic illness. A large family might contain more possible resources for coping responsibilities. Siblings could assume an integral role in the child's treatment.
3. *How the sick child understands the condition*   Jordan (1963) believes that this perception is the key to the reaction of other family members. Any severe childhood disease makes the family more vulnerable to stress. Children who perceive that the illness can be controlled and that they can get better may express more optimistic feelings, which promote a better attitude in family members. Children with juvenile diabetes, for example, who follow their treatment regimen and believe that they can live normal lives, will allay much family anxiety. If a child ignores the necessary treatment, the family may react to this behavior rather than to the disease itself.
4. *The complexity of family demands*   Many diseases affecting children, e.g., asthma, cardiac disease, and muscular dystrophy, often mean severe disruption in the daily lives of family members. Frequent sleep interruptions or continued visits to the hospital for treatment can generate fatigue and leave an individual more susceptible to irritability and tension.
5. *The visibility of the defect*   Poznanski (1973) explains that, if the disability is visible, people more readily tend to view the child as handicapped. The visibility may create many questions from others, and

parents often feel ashamed under public scrutiny. Many families withdraw from social interaction because of the prejudice they perceive in others.

6. *The religious beliefs of the family*   Religion can play an important role in the family's ability to manage stress (McCubbin, 1979). Religious values may alleviate guilt or assuage grief. Spiritual support can contribute to maintaining the family unit and to preserve the family's feelings of adequacy.

7. *The degree of financial burden and availability of community resources*   All chronic illness creates great financial demands. Travis (1976) reports that hemophilia imposes the most catastrophic demands, since the cost of blood plasma is very high and often is not covered by insurance. If treatment costs result in severe financial deprivation for the rest of the family, often resentment is aroused. If the parents are willing to take advantage of homemaker services and day care, this might alleviate their physical and emotional burden and foster a more relaxed atmosphere in the home.

8. *The stage of the family life cycle*   Like adult disability, it can make a difference to a family if living patterns with each other are well established or if the couple has been married for just a year and their first child is born with serious defects. The reaction to the disability will often depend upon the development of the couple's own personal relationship. It may be a selfish one or the couple may have the ability to tolerate the supposed imposition of a disabled child. The presence of disability will demand tremendous sacrifices from the couple.

With an appreciation of the many determinants of a family's emotional reaction, health professionals can more completely understand what is needed for the family to help the child reach adjustment goals, although they must realize that there are many patterns of family reaction to a chronic illness / severe disability.

PATTERNS OF FAMILY REACTION

From his work with disabled children and their families Jordan (1973) reported that all patterns of reactions to disability pose some fundamental questions. For example, are patterns of reaction to disease specific? When the disease is visible do the parents and children react in the same way? The research (Poznanski, 1973; Travis, 1976) indicates that a given disease does not cause a definite pattern of family adjustment or style of reaction specifically different from other family responses. The theories that follow illustrate reactions that can occur with many different types of child illness or disability. Each theory provides the health professional with concepts to be used when interpreting a family's emotional response. Since each family may show a unique sequence of reactions, these concepts are helpful when attempting to describe the stages of family response.

Pearse (1977)

Shock ⟶ Denial ⟶ Guilt ⟶ Anger ⟶ Sense of normalcy

Having worked with school age children with a malignancy and their families, Pearse believes that grief underlies many of the family's adjustments. Grief is always present as family members attempt to maintain a "sense" of control in everyday life. She indicates that different emotions will occur among the family members, with denial being an important reaction. If used in realistic moderation, denial can stimulate hope that perhaps the disease can be controlled. She stresses that the adjustment patterns facilitate an eventual "sense of normalcy" within the family. For example, before a family returns to living with the harsh reality of cancer, their guilt and anger must be identified and be given an opportunity to be expressed. Otherwise, these emotions will inhibit any family adjustment.

Drotar, Baskiewicz, Irvin, Kennell, and Klaus (1975)

Shock ⟶ Denial ⟶ Sadness / Anger / Anxiety ⟶ Adaptation ⟶ Reorganization

From their study of the parents of 20 children with congenital malformations, Drotar et al. (1975) formulated a reactive pattern that showed the common themes of the parental reaction. An elaboration of their research is found in the article included in this chapter. Beginning with shock over the news of the child's disability, parents try to deny the information, not believing that it could occur to them. Then they have intense feelings of sadness and anger, which cause disruptions in family life. As these feelings slowly diminish, the parents discover a confidence in their ability to start caring for their infants. Parents may reach this stage of adaptation at different rates, but, once achieved, a time of family reorganization and long-term acceptance of the child follows. The authors believe that such acceptance demands the parents' mutual support of one another from the time of birth of the disabled child.

Gordon and Kutner (1965)

Shock ⟶ Anxiety and confusion ⟶ Denial ⟶ Rejection of the child ⟵⎯⎯⎯⎯⎯⏌

Criticism of the diagnosing physician

Gordon and Kutner (1965) reviewed varied family studies that had explored the reactions of parents to long-term and fatal illness of children. They then organized a sequential pattern of parental reaction. The pattern is concisely outlined in their article in this chapter. They believe that the initial reaction provokes a time of shock, confusion, and helplessness among parents, followed by a time of denial when the family attempts to pull together its own resources. Unfortunately, some parents are unable to accept the reality of the illness and reject the child, avoiding caring concerns and transferring them to other family members or the hospital staff. For the health professional they highlight the importance of understanding that many parents will show their anger by criticizing the diagnosing physician or related helpers. They found this to be true since parents were studied in a stress situation where feelings of helplessness dominated.

Steinhauer, Mushin, Rae-Grant (1974)

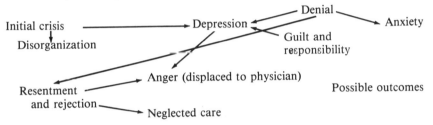

In their medical practice Steinhauer, Mushin, and Rae-Grant have worked extensively with children and their families, and their beliefs about how the family reacts are described in their article in Chapter 3. They view the illness of the child as a crisis situation for the family, and the nature of the illness is one among many strong determinants of the family reaction. They emphasize the importance of health professionals understanding the family reaction, because this awareness can facilitate successful disease management.

SYNTHESIS OF THEORIES OF FAMILY REACTION TO CHILD DISABILITY

All of the different theories outlined in this chapter have many reactive stages in common and they show the complexity of family behavior. When put together in a sequential pattern, the common phases represent a synthesis of the reactive patterns:

Trauma ⟶ Shock ⟨ Denial / Grieving ⟶ Depression ⟶ Adjustment

All family members usually experience shock, characterized by heightened anxiety and occasionally a sense of confusion and helplessness. As the family gradually learns more about the trauma or illness, denial and grieving occur. The family members realize there is a new loss in the family, which provokes grieving, yet at the same time they deny the implications of the trauma both to the patient and the family. This time of denial can be an important period for the family, because it helps them to manage their anxiety and to begin making the necessary changes in family life. There may be much hope in the family at this time; they believe that the patient will get better and perhaps return to a normal life. As time proceeds, and there is the realization that the disability/illness has brought definite limitations to the child, as well as certain restrictions on the family members because of caring concerns, family members tend to become depressed. Behind the depression is anger because this event has brought perceived losses or seriously disrupted family life. The anger may be suppressed or projected onto other family members or health personnel.

Slowly, however, the family restores its equilibrium while still harboring sadness and some anxiety over what eventually will happen to the patient. The authors of this volume believe that with most families there is really not a time of acceptance. The family learns to live with the disability, and their style of living constitutes their form of adjustment. The living may be characterized by sorrow, disappointment, readaptation of family roles, and the expression of positive coping mechanisms. Family members may also find their own outlets for coping responsibilities and these are resources for emotional replenishment. They may obtain part-time work or volunteer participation in charitable organizations. Coping behaviors will vary, but they assist the family to endure the daily reality of disability or chronic illness, divert the sources of stress, and strengthen its internal functioning.

It is important to note that because a family has a disabled child or adult, it does not mean a devastating experience. The authors have met many families who consider their disabled child not as a continued burden, but rather as a unique opportunity for family growth. The presence of the child brings the family members closer together as they unify their efforts to provide the child with a productive and satisfying life.

CONCLUSION

All the articles in this chapter provide the reader with directives to helping the family that is attempting to cope with a disabled child. The Drotar, Baskiewicz, Irvin, Kennell, and Klaus article analyzes the varied stages that parents may experience as they try to cope with the birth of a congenitally malformed infant. They give the reader suggestions on the type of questions to ask when assessing emotional reactions. Their article contains valuable and comprehensive information. Dr. Mattsson's article is a classic, containing many unique descriptions of the way parents and their children react to varied chronic illness. He explains the many related adaptational techniques used by the child and parents. Norman Gordon and Bernard Kutner describe the drastic effects that serious childhood illnesses can have on the stability of family life. They provide suggested approaches to parent counseling and identify many research implications. All of this material develops a broader base of family understanding for the health professional. To help family members assist a child to develop as normally as possible implies that they have largely come to terms with their own emotional responses. The health professional can help the family to accomplish this, and, in doing so, prepare the family to share in the child's rehabilitation.

REFERENCES

Drotar, D., Baskiewicz, A., Irvin, N., & Klaus, M. The adaptation of parents to the birth of an infant with a congenital malformation: A hypothetical model. *Pediatrics*, 1975, *56*, 710–717.

Gordon, N., & Kutner, B. Long term and fatal illness and the family. *Journal of Health and Human Behavior*, 1965, *6*, 190–196.

Jordan, T. E. Physical disability in children and family adjustment. *Rehabilitation Literature*, 1973, November, 330–336.

McCubbin, H. Integrating coping behavior in family stress theory. *Journal of Marriage and the Family*, 1979, May, 237–244.

Pearse, M. The child with cancer: Impact on the family. *The Journal of School Health*, 1977, March, 174–178.

Poznanski, E. O. Emotional issues in raising handicapped children. *Rehabilitation Literature*, 1973, *34*, 322–326.

Steinhauer, P. D., Mushin, D., & Rae-Grant, Q. Psychological aspects of chronic illness. *Pediatric Clinics of North America*, 1974, *21*, 825–840.

Travis, G. *Chronic illness in children*, Stanford, Cal.: Stanford University Press, 1976.

LONG-TERM PHYSICAL ILLNESS IN CHILDHOOD:
A Challenge to Psychosocial Adaptation

Ake Mattsson[1]

Robert Louis Stevenson, a victim of pulmonary tuberculosis, once wrote, "Life is not a matter of holding good cards, but of playing a poor hand well." Children with a chronic physical disorder who have successfully mastered the physical, social, and emotional hardships associated with their illness well illustrate his point. This paper intends to review the common forms of emotional stress experienced by the child with a long-term illness and by his parents. It also describes the major adaptational techniques enabling the sick child and his family to achieve a satisfactory psychosocial adaptation.

Long-term or chronic illness refers to a disorder with a protracted course which can be progressive and fatal, or associated with a relatively normal life span despite impaired physical or mental functioning. Such a disease frequently shows periods of acute exacerbations requiring intensive medical attention. Long-term childhood disorders may cause significant and permanent interference with the child's physical and emotional growth and development. This is in contrast to acute nonlife-threatening illnesses in which both physical dysfunctioning and attendant emotional upset usually are of a limited duration and do not as a rule interfere with the child's overall development (Mattsson & Weisberg, 1970; Carey & Sibinga, 1972).

The prevalence of chronic conditions in childhood is staggering if visual and hearing impairments, mental retardation, and speech, learning, and behavior disorders are included. Such a scope yields an estimate of 30% to 40% of children up to the age of 18 suffering from one or more longterm disorders. (Stewart, 1967). Even if only serious chronic illnesses of primary physical origin are included, American and British surveys still report that 7% to 10% of all children are afflicted (Pless, 1968; Rutter, Tizard, & Whitmore, 1968). The most common physical conditions are asthma (about 2% of the population under age 18), epilepsy (1%), cardiac conditions (0.5%), cerebral palsy (0.5%), orthopedic illness (0.5%), and diabetes mellitus (0.1%). Less frequencies pertain to cleft palate, bleeding disorders, anemias, blindness, and deafness.

Reprinted from *Pediatrics 50* (5), pp. 801–811, ©1972, American Academy of Pediatrics, with permission.
[1]From the Departments of Pediatrics and Psychiatry, University of Virginia School of Medicine, Charlottesville.

The following classification of long-term childhood disorders is based on consideration of ontogenetic stages and nature of pathogenic factors:

1. Diseases due to chromosomal aberrations (e.g., Down's syndrome, Klinefelter's syndrome, Turner's syndrome),
2. Diseases as results of abnormal hereditary traits (e.g., spherocytosis, sickle cell anemia, hemophilia, cystic fibrosis, muscular dystrophy, osteogenesis imperfecta, diabetes mellitus, inborn errors of metabolism; certain forms of "congenital malformations" such as microcephaly, clubfoot, cleft palate, dislocation of the hip, blindness, and deafness),
3. Diseases due to harmful intrauterine factors (e.g., infections such as rubella, congenital syphilis, and toxoplasmosis with their attendant malformations; damage from massive radiation, various drugs, prenatal hypoxia, and blood type incompatibilities),
4. Disorders resulting from perinatal traumatic and infectious events including permanent damage to central nervous system and motor apparatus, and
5. Diseases due to serious postnatal and childhood infections, injuries, neoplasms, and other factors (e.g., meningitis, encephalitis, tuberculosis, rheumatic fever, chronic renal disease; physical injuries with permanent handicaps; tumors and leukemia; orthopedic diseases; convulsive disorders; atopic conditions; mental illness and mental retardation of organic etiology).

PSYCHOLOGIC IMPACT OF LONG-TERM ILLNESS

Children with long-term physical disorders are subjected to a multitude of emotionally stressful situations, often of a recurring nature. Acute illnesses pose similar psychologic threats which usually prove less harmful due to their shorter duration (Freud, 1952; Langford, 1961; Prugh, 1963; Shrand, 1965; Apley, 1968; Mattsson & Weisberg, 1970; Carey & Sibinga, 1972). The common causes for emotional stress associated with long-term illness are:

Malaise, Pain, Various Physical Symptoms, and Reasons for Illness

Uncertainty as to why pain and suffering occur is a psychic stress to anyone. The preschool child in particular has little ability to comprehend the causality and nature of an illness and tends to interpret pain and other symptoms as a result of mistreatment, punishment, or "being bad." In a child's mind nothing happens by chance, and he looks for reasons for an event such as an illness in the immediate past (Jessner, 1959; Freeman, 1968). Children up to the ages of 8 to 10 often attribute illness and injury to recent family interactions, e.g., they got sick because of their disobedience or because the parents failed to protect them. They might then blame themselves or other family members for causing the disease. These distorted interpretations of their bodily changes often become perpetuated by their reluctance to ask questions and vent their irrational fears about why they became ill. Other examples of children's crude cause-and-effect reasoning relative to illness are: a young colitis patient blamed his illness on having "eaten something dirty"; a child with cardiac disease had "run too much"; a diabetic girl had "eaten too much candy"; a hemophilic boy developed a hematoma because his "skin was so thin."

Young patients afflicted with a hereditary illness will usually learn of the likely genetic transmission before or during adolescence. Under whatever circumstances this knowledge is obtained by the child, it is potentially traumatic to the child-parent relationship. Many such children voice hostile accusations against their parents, as they try to master the anger, sadness, and anxiety aroused by their recognition of the hereditary nature of their disability.

Hospital Admissions, Nursing, and Treatment Procedures

The often frequent and lengthy hospital admissions for the chronically ill child involve separations from his family, school, and set of friends. He is expected to adjust to an unfamiliar, regimented hospital environment, with a confusing array of health specialists and frightening, often painful medical procedures (Robertson, 1958; Langford, 1961; Vernon, Foley, Sipowicz, & Schulman, 1965). Again, it is the preschool child that tends to suffer most from these stressful separations from the trusted family setting. Such repeated episodes can be destructive to the child unless a strong "therapeutic alliance" between his parents and the medical staff provides him with a plenitude of visiting and care by the mother, a homelike ward setting, and ample information and preparations regarding procedures (Robertson, 1958; Prugh, 1963; Mason, 1965; Apley & Mackeith, 1968).

Any ill person who receives nursing care at home or in a hospital experiences feelings of helplessness, embarrassment, and irritation. To be "treated like a child" during an illness is often more upsetting to a young patient than to an adult (Freud, 1958; Jessner, 1959; Langford, 1961). A bedridden child, unable to dress and feed himself and to use the bathroom without help, resents the loss of such recent gains in his development. The less ill he feels, the stronger his resentment. Anger, humiliation, and anxiety about the backward pull toward a state of helpless dependency are frequently observed, and the hospital staff and the parents may become targets of defiant protests. Some children regress to more babyish behavior without much protest and need considerable help to regain achievements in motor and social functioning after an illness.

Injections, infusions, immobilization, surgery, and other procedures arouse anxiety beyond the discomfort involved, because they reactivate the universal childhood fears of bodily mutilation and disfigurement and the illogical views of medical procedures as a punishment for actual or imagined misdeeds. Such fantasies generally cause less problems for the older grade school child, because his strides in cognitive development enable him better to comprehend the causal and temporal relationship of an illness or injury (Freeman, 1968). Most sick children find immobilization and restriction of activity emotionally stressful. They rely on freedom of movement to discharge tension, to express dissatisfaction and aggression, and to explore and master the environment. Sudden or prolonged motor restraint of a young child can cause him to panic, develop temper tantrums, and become a serious management problem. At other times, he might show the opposite reaction of withdrawal into an apathetic, depressed state. The child with poor ability or lack of opportunity to verbalize his feelings is more prone to show marked behavioral reactions to forced restraints.

Changes in the Emotional Climate

Family members tend to change their attitudes toward their sick child and usually become more loving and indulgent, letting up on discipline and rules (Freud, 1952). Changes in the opposite direction are rare but potentially more dangerous: some parents reject their ill child, criticize him for causing much inconvenience, and even neglect his care. Any of these changes in family attitudes can be confusing to the child as for instance, when he has to relinquish the secondary gains of being sick.

Stress Factors Related to Special Chronic Syndromes

Certain aspects of causation, symptomatology, and medical care of many long-term illnesses pose special problems and fears to the child and his family. Some common examples of such situations follow.

Fluctuations in the control of *juvenile diabetes* frequently seem related to emotional factors (Swift & Seidman, 1964; Tietz & Vidmar, 1972). The diabetic child, along with his family, may worry about attacks of hypoglycemia or acidosis as a result of highly emotionally charged family interaction. Some adolescents in rebellious, hostile, or depressed states abandon their diabetic regime as angry and self-destructive means to threaten or retaliate. This abandonment is often conscious, which indicates a far more serious maladjustment than the chronically ill person's common use of his ailment as an escape or a defense.

Similar to the young diabetic patient, the child with a *convulsive disorder* frequently fears loss of consciousness or uncontrollable strange behavior while suffering from a seizure. Seizures are socially stigmatizing especially when they take place at school and among peers. The epileptic teen-ager feels uniquely frustrated, as he cannot obtain a driver's license until after several years without seizures. This prolongs his dependence on the parents for providing transportation in regards to many school and leisure activities.

Children with *serious respiratory disease*, such as asthma (Dubo, McLean, Ching, Wright, Kauffman, & Sheldon, 1961; Purcell, Brody, Chai, Muser, Molk, Gordon, & Means, 1969; Purcell & Weiss, 1970) and cystic fibrosis, (McCollum & Gibson, 1970), commonly harbor fears of suffocation, drowning, or dying while asleep. The asthmatic child often finds that his wheezing will evoke anxious, indulgent, and sympathetic responses from his family, whose members may feel responsible for contributing to his attacks of labored breathing and discomfort.

The child with cystic fibrosis has to cope with such embarrassing symptoms as flatulence and stool odor, with the complex management of postural drainage and nebulization, and with the growing awareness that his illness is hereditary and progressive, carrying a poor prognosis.

Chronic bleeding disorders, such as hemophilia, often cause the young child to be concerned about fatal bleeding resulting from physical trauma and certain medical procedures, e.g., venous puncture. Emotional distress might increase the likelihood of bleeding in face of minor physical trauma or even lead to "spontaneous" bleeding episodes without apparent trauma (Agle, 1964; Mattsson & Gross, 1966a).

The child with a *chronic heart disease* of infectious or congenital nature often has minimal signs of a serious condition and may find it difficult to comprehend the nature of his illness and the reasons for restrictions, extensive work-ups, and surgery. Furthermore, the knowledge of an affliction of one's heart seems especially frightening due to the common ambiguous and symbolic references to "the heart" in everyday language (Glaser, Harrison, & Lynn, 1964; Toker, 1971). An active psychoeducational preparation for heart surgery is of special importance since states of marked apprehension and depression may complicate cardiac surgery in childhood and adolescence (Barnes, Kenny, Call, & Reinhart, 1972).

An increasing number of children with *chronic renal disease* are treated with hemodialysis and kidney transplantation. Several unique features pertain to these procedures (Abram, 1970; Bernstein, 1971). The life-perpetuating kidney machine often create frightening fantasies in the child, such as fears of bleeding to death or of the machine assuming control of him. The use of immunosuppressive drugs cause Cushingoid appearance and interfere with the children's growth, already stunted by preexisting uremia. Consequently, these young patients often feel isolated and apart. This may be particularly difficult for the teen-ager, seeking independence from his family and a sense of identity among his peers. After kidney transplantation, many children find their parents tending to overprotect them and to use threats implying possible failure of the new kidney as a means of controlling their activities. The occurrence of "kidney rejection anxiety" at times of minor physical symptoms has been observed in children as long as six years after a successful transplantation. In cases of actual kidney rejection, requiring a return to hemodialysis, the young patient, like the adult, usually responds with a depressed, withdrawn state. Children in particular then tend to blame themselves for "destroying" the kidney given to them as a special gift, often by a family member. It should be noted, however, that follow-ups on children who have undergone renal transplantation have found many of them showing growth spurts as long as five years after surgery and a good adjustment as young adults (Lilly et al., 1971).

Children with *ulcerative colitis* and similar conditions often have unrealistic fears of certain food items harming them. Their frequent inability to control defecations cause much embarrassment. The common family preoccupation with the ill child's diet and with his stools requires energetic pediatric counseling. These children and their families often have to be prepared for a temporary or permanent ileostomy when other treatment methods fail. Such a procedure entails many realistic problems which are particularly stressful to an adolescent as he is beginning to establish intimate heterosexual friendships (McDermott & Finch, 1967). The counseling assistance of an older person with a successful ileostomy can be useful in supporting the young patient's self-image and confidence.

The recent interest in children and teenagers of *short stature*, often complicated by delayed sexual maturation (Rothchild & Owens, 1972), has shown that a major problem of the undersized child is related to his environment's tendency to baby him "as a dwarf" instead of treating him according to his chronological age. His sense of uniqueness may cause him to withdraw, leading to an inhibition of his cognitive and emotional development (Money & Pollitt, 1966). Some short youngsters cope by an excessive denial of their condition and become either good natured jokers with few aggressive strivings or spunky and overly assertive individuals.

The format of this paper does not permit further illustrations of specific emotional stress factors associated with many chronic handicaps and disorders in childhood, such as mental retardation (Mandelbaum, 1967), brain dysfunction and cerebral palsy (Birch, 1964; Gardner, 1968; Chess, Korn, & Fernandez, 1971; Minde, Hachett, Killon, & Silver, 1972), congenital amputees (Gurney, 1968; Roskies; 1972), orthopedic conditions (Myers, Friedman, & Weiner, 1970), cleft palate (Tisza & Gumperty, 1962), and cryptorchism (Cytryn, Cytryn, & Rieger, 1967). Helpful reviews of the psychological implications of long-term sensory, motor, visceral, and metabolic conditions in young patients are given by Prugh (1963), Apley and MacKeith (1968), Vernon et al. (1965), Kessler (1966), and Green and

Haggerty (1968). The unique emotional burdens associated with fatal illness in childhood and adolescence have recently been reviewed by Friedman (1968) and Easson (1970).

Additional Psychologic Threats

The child with a serious, chronic disease has to cope with threats of exacerbations, lasting physical impairment, and, at times, a shortened life expectancy. Other common concerns of his and his family relate to mounting medical expenses and the interference of his illness with schooling, leisure activities, vocational training, job opportunities, and later adult role as a spouse and a parent. In learning to live with a disability that demands continuous medical attention, often away from home, the growing child is expected to assume responsibility for his own care and accept certain limitations in his activities.

The final outcome of the child's attempts at mastering the continuous stress associated with his disability cannot be assessed until young adulthood. Each progressive step in his emotional, intellectual, and social development changes the psychologic impact of the illness on his personality and on his family and usually equips him with better means to cope (Mattsson & Gross, 1966b; Minde et al., 1972). Changes in the disease process and in familial circumstances will also affect the adaptational process.

COPING BEHAVIOR AND ADAPTATION IN CHILDREN

Several authors have used the conceptual framework of coping behavior to describe the responses of children and parents to such severe stress situations as serious illness, separation, and the threat of death (Murphy, 1962; Friedman, Chodoff, Mason, & Hamburg, 1963; Chodoff, Friedman, & Hamburg, 1964; Mattsson & Gross, 1966; Mattsson, Gross, & Hall, 1971). This term denotes all the adaptational techniques used by an individual to master a major psychologic threat and its attendant negative feelings in order to allow him to achieve personal and social goals. Coping behavior, then, includes the use of cognitive functions (perception, memory, speech, judgment, reality testing), motor activity, emotional expression, and psychologic defenses. (Defenses represent unconscious processes aiming at reappraisals and distortions of a threatening reality to make it more bearable (Murphy, 1962; Lazarus, 1966).) Successful coping behavior results in adaptation, which implies that the person is functioning effectively.

Many studies on long-term childhood disorders report a surprisingly adequate psychosocial adaptation of children followed to young adulthood (Langford, 1961; Prugh, 1963; Apley & MacKeith, 1968). These well-adapted patients have for years functioned effectively at home, in school, and with their peers, and with few limitations other than those realistically imposed by their disease and its sequelae. Their dependence on their family has been age-appropriate and realistic, and they have little need for secondary gains offered by the illness. From age 6 to 7, these children's use of such cognitive functions as memory, speech, and reality testing provided them with a beginning understanding of the nature of their illness. This allowed them to accept limitations, assume responsibility for their care, and assist in the medical management. This appropriate appearance of a sense of self-protection served the vital function of self-preservation and precluded the development of helpless, inactive dependence on their environment (Frankl, 1963). While slowly accepting his physical limitations, the well-adjusted child finds satisfaction in a variety of compensatory motor activities and intellectual pursuits, in which the parents' encouragement and guidance assumes great importance.

In addition to cognitive flexibility and compensatory physical activities, the appropriate release and control of emotions is an essential coping technique. The expression of anxious, sad, impatient, and angry feelings at times of exacerbations, and of confidence and guarded optimism during periods of clinical quiescence is characteristic of well-adapted children with a chronic illness.

In terms of psychologic defenses, most of these patients use denial as well as isolation in coping with their emotional distress caused by pain, malaise, and interrupted plans. They also show an adaptive use of denial of the uncertain future, which enables them to maintain hope for recovery at times of crisis, for more effective medical care, and for a relatively normal, productive adult life. Identification with other young and adult patients afflicted with a chronic handicap is a helpful defense for many children. Learning about and associating with others who are successful in dealing with similar problems can effectively support the development of a positive self-image as a socially competent and productive individual. Many of the well-adapted young patients display a certain pride and confidence in themselves, as they become successful in mastering the ongoing stress associated with their illness.

The nature of the specific illness appears less influential for a child's successful adaptation than such factors as his developmental level and available coping techniques, the quality of the parent-child relationship, and the family's acceptance of the handicapped member (Prugh, 1963; Apley & MacKeith, 1968; Freeman, 1968). Regarding the latter point, the parents' ability to master their initial reaction of fear and guilt, and their tendency to overprotect the child has received much emphasis (Solnit & Stark, 1961; Tisza, 1962; Prugh, 1963; Mattsson & Gross, 1966a; Green, 1967; Findlay, Smith, Graves, & Linton, 1969).

Children and adolescents with prolonged poor adjustment to their chronic disorder tend to show one of the three following behavioral patterns

(Prugh, 1963; Agle, 1964; Mattsson & Gross, 1966a). One group is characterized by the patients' fearfulness, inactivity, lack of outside interests, and a marked dependency on their families, especially their mothers. These youngsters present the psychiatric picture of early passive dependent states and their mothers are usually described as constantly worried and overprotective of them.

The second group contains the overly independent, often daring young patients, who may engage in prohibited and risk-taking activities. Such youngsters make a strong use of denial of realistic dangers and fears. At times their reality sense is impaired and they seem to seek out certain feared situations, challenging the risk of trauma. Since early childhood, many of these rebellious patients have been raised by oversolicitous and guilt-ridden mothers. Usually at puberty, they rebel against the maternal interference and turn into overly active, defiant adolescents.

A third, less common pattern of maladjustment is seen in older children and adolescents with congenital deformities and handicaps. They appear as shy and lonely people harboring resentful and hostile attitudes towards normal persons, whom they see as owing them payment for their life-long sufferings (Freud, 1957). Usually these patients were raised in a family that emphasized their defectiveness and tended to isolate or "hide" them in an embarrassed fashion. They came to identify with their family's view of them and developed a self-image of a defective outsider.

These illustrations of prolonged maladaptation to a chronic illness differ from more temporary situations, where the disease and its management become the vehicle for conflicts between the patient and his parents, siblings, friends, or school. Overt or covert refusal to cooperate in the medical regimen can be used as an effective weapon by a resentful young patient. Practically all children with a chronic disability will occasionally try to take advantage of their disease in order to avoid unpleasant situations, as for instance a disciplinary action or a school test.

EMOTIONAL STRESS AND COPING BEHAVIOR OF PARENTS

When a serious, long-term illness afflicts a child, the initial reaction of his parents usually includes acute fear and anxiety related to the possible fatal outcome of the disease. A closely associated stage is that of parental disbelief in the diagnosis, particularly if the obvious signs of illness have subsided (Tisza, 1962). The parents might then complain about being poorly informed by the physician and occasionally "shop around" for additional medical opinion, which will disprove the initial diagnosis. Beyond those denying, often uncooperative attitudes of the parents, feelings of mourning the "loss" of their desired normal child and feelings of self-blame in regard to their ailing child usually begin to emerge (Solnit & Stark,

1961; Glaser, Harrison, & Lynn, 1964). When the parents become aware of and can verbalize these feelings, they are able to accept the reality of the serious disability and its impact on the whole family.

A crucial factor in determining the parents' acceptance is their ability to master resentful and self-accusatory feelings over having transmitted or in some way "caused" their child's disorder (Solnit & Stark, 1961; Tisza, 1962; Mattsson & Gross, 1966a; Green, 1967; Findlay et al., 1969). Those parents who remain highly anxious and guilt-laden about their ill child tend to cope with their emotional distress by overprotecting and pampering him, and by limiting his activities with other children. Such prolonged parental overconcern, usually more prominent among mothers, can often be related to one of the following predisposing factors (Green & Solnit, 1964; Mattsson & Gross, 1966b): the child suffered a life-threatening condition at birth or as an infant, from which the family did not believe he would recover; the child is afflicted with a hereditary disorder present among relatives; the child's illness reactivates emotional conflicts in the parents stemming from the past death of a close relative; or the child was unwanted, causing a mixture of loving and rejecting feelings, particularly in the mother.

Any child being raised by oversolicitous, controlling, and fearful parents senses the parental expectation of his vulnerability and likely premature death (Green & Solnit, 1964). He may either accept this tacit view and assume passive-dependent characteristics, or he may rebel against the parents' concerns and become a daring, careless youngster, who seems to challenge their notions of his fragile condition.

The factors mentioned here as common determinants of prolonged parental overconcern also may lead to parental rejection or neglect of a disabled child and to extreme parental denial of the severity of the illness. These latter types of reaction are infrequent compared to the former one of overprotection. Again, strong unresolved feelings of guilt for their child's illness are often present in such detached and uncooperative parents (Mattsson & Gross, 1966a; Apley & MacKeith, 1968). They may talk angrily about all the inconvenience their child's ailment causes the family, and they often blame crises and complications on the child or the medical staff. In addition, they frequently "forget" instructions about the home care and are inconsistent in guiding their child. Such a child, when sensing the parental rejection, will often respond with both despondent and defiant attitudes, which greatly jeopardize his clinical condition.

Parents who have successfully adapted to the challenge of raising a chronically ill child will enforce only necessary and realistic restrictions on him, encourage self-care and regular school attendance, and promote reasonable physical activities with his peers. These well-adapted parents use some common psychologic defenses in coping with the constant strain caused by their child's illness (Mattsson & Agle, 1972). For example, they tend to isolate and deny their anxious and helpless emotions, especially during a medical crisis, which helps them to remain calm and assist effectively in the medical care. When the crisis is over, many parents experience a rebound phenomenon of feeling depressed and irritable, indicating that certain painful affects have been denied consciousness until that time when it is safer to experience them.

It is common among parents of handicapped children to show attitudes of critical superiority towards health specialists, particularly towards house officers. Some of this criticism may be valid, but one also senses that the parents are trying to ward off, by denial, their long-standing helpless feelings in this manner. They may also displace and project helpless and angry feelings about their child's condition onto various medical professionals and blame them for delays or mistakes in treating their child. Closely related to denial is rationalization, that is, the defensive use of rational explanations, valid or invalid, in an attempt to conceal some painful emotions from oneself. One commonly hears from parents of chronically ill children that the disorder has enriched the whole family, both emotionally and spiritually, and has developed their sense of compassion and tolerance. While indeed there may be some truth in such statements, these attitudes assist the parents—often the healthy siblings too—in hiding from themselves sad and resentful affects related to their unique burden.

All effectively coping parents, along with their sick children, use intellectual processes to master distressing emotions caused by the illness; that is, they rely on the coping technique of "control through thinking" (Bibring, Dwyer, Huntington, & Valenstein, 1961). The parents often make it a point to learn all they can about the medical, physiological, and even the psychological aspects of the disease. Thus, they lessen their anxiety by familiarizing themselves with the likely future course of development of the child.

The association and identification with other parents of seriously ill children is helpful to many parents. Informally and in group discussions, at times conducted by a health specialist, they can share many of their distressing hardships and learn to adopt more realistic and relaxed child caring attitudes and also pass on their positive experiences to less knowledgeable parents (Mandelbaum, 1967; Mattsson & Agle, 1972).

CONCLUSION

The successful psychological management of a child with a long-term physical illness and his family depends on two interrelated factors (Tisza, 1962; Prugh, 1963; Mattsson & Gross, 1966a; Green, 1967; Apley & MacKeith, 1968; Solnit, 1968): 1) the continuous "personalized" support and counselling by the physician, who should be alert to all the incompatible feelings with which both the patient and his parents are coping; these affects are normal reactions, which often will subside if given time and verbal expression; and 2) the parents' acceptance of the disease with its uncertain course and impact on the family, which implies that they have gradually mastered their conflicting emotions aroused by their child's ailment.

The parents as well as their child require repeated, truthful, and comprehensible information about the illness, its etiology, and therapeutic concepts. Whenever possible, they should be prepared for procedures and likely changes in clinical manifestations. Such preparation helps to mobilize their intellectual functions and psychologic defenses to cope with the anticipated stress. The physician should make sure that his explanations and plans are understood by the parents and the young patient, and well coordinated with the collaborative efforts of his medical, nursing, and social service colleagues. The medical team and the parents can greatly assist the ill child by encouraging him to ask questions and to verbalize distressing feelings.

The parents need instruction to develop in their child an increasing responsibility for self-care and protection. The goal of raising the handicapped child as normally as possible may be achieved by promoting reasonable activities with other children and regular schooling, modified by individual needs. Overprotection and undue restrictions, both at home and in school, should be discouraged. The father's active involvement in the child-rearing can be fostered by his assuming major responsibility for helping his ill youngster to succeed in compensatory activities and interests. In terms of the healthy siblings, the physician should assess whether they are receiving needed parental love and attention as well as acceptance of their frequent feelings of anxiety, resentment, and guilt towards their ailing brother or sister.

The physician should tactfully call attention to parental attitudes of overindulgence, lenient discipline, or neglect which can endanger the child's emotional growth. He may suggest a psychiatric consultation when he notices many unresolved conflicts in the parents responsible for prolonged overprotective, inconsistent, or rejecting handling of the child. Psychiatric intervention can also be of value for some young patients with marked difficulties in adapting to their long-term illness, such as children showing defiant, risk-taking behavior, a fearful, passive dependence, or hostile, embittered attitudes towards their environment and life situation.

REFERENCES

Abram, H. S. Survival by machine: The psychological stress of chronic hemodialysis. *Psychiatric Medicine*, 1970, *1*, 37.
Agle, D. P. Psychiatric studies of patients with hemophilia and related states. *Archives of Internal Medicine*, 1964, *114*, 76.

Apley, J., & MacKeith, R. *The child and his symptoms*, pp. 209–215, 216–240. Philadelphia: F. A. Davis Co., 1968.

Barnes, C. M., Kenny, F. M., Call, T., & Reinhart, J. B. Measurement in management of anxiety in children for open heart surgery. *Pediatrics*, 1972, *49*, 250.

Bernstein, D. M. After transplantation—The child's emotional reactions. *American Journal of Psychiatry*, 1971, *127*, 1189.

Bibring, G. L., Dwyer, T. F., Huntington, D. S., & Valenstein, A. F. A study of the psychological processes in pregnancy and of the earliest mother-child relationship. Appendix B: Glossary of defenses. *Psychoanalytic Study of the Child*, 1961, *16*, 62.

Birch, H. G. *Brain-damage in children. The biological and social aspects*. Baltimore: The Williams & Wilkins Co., 1964.

Carey, W. B., & Sibinga, M. S. Avoiding pediatric pathogenesis in the management of acute minor illness. *Pediatrics*, 1972, *49*, 553.

Chess, S., Korn, S. J., & Fernandez, P. B. Psychiatric disorders of children with congenital rubella. New York: Brunner-Mazel, 1971.

Chodoff, P., Friedman, S. B., & Hamburg, D. A. Stress, defenses, and coping behavior: Observations in parents of children with malignant disease. *American Journal of Psychiatry*, 1964, *120*, 743.

Cytryn, L., Cytryn, E., & Rieger, R. E. Psychological implications of cryptorchism. *Journal of the American Academy of Child Psychiatry*, 1967, *6*, 131.

Dubo, S., McLean, J., Ching, A., Wright, H., Kauffman, P., & Sheldon, J. A study of relationships between family situation, bronchial asthma, and personal adjustment in children. *Journal of Pediatrics*, 1961, *59*, 402.

Easson, W. M. *The dying child. The management of the child or adolescent who is dying*. Springfield, Ill.: Charles C Thomas Publisher, 1970.

Findlay, I. I., Smith, P., Graves, P. J., & Linton, M. L. Chronic disease in childhood: A study of family reactions. *British Journal of Medicine*, 1969, *3*, 66.

Frankl, L. Self-preservation and the development of accident proneness in children and adolescents. *Psychoanalytic Study of the Child*, 1963, *18*, 464.

Freeman, R. D. Emotional reactions of handicapped children. In S. Chess and A. Thomas (Eds.), *Annual progress in child psychiatry and child development*, pp. 379–395. New York: Brunner-Mazel, 1968.

Freud, A. The role of bodily illness in the mental life of children. *Psychoanalytic Study of the Child*, 1952, *7*, 69.

Freud, S. Some character types met with in psychoanalytic work. I. The "exceptions" (Standard ed., Vol. 14), pp. 311–315. London: Hogarth Press, 1957. (Originally published in 1916.)

Friedman, S. B. Management of fatal illness in children. In M. Green & R. J. Haggerty (Eds.), *Ambulatory pediatrics*, pp. 753–759. Philadelphia: W. B. Saunders Co., 1968.

Friedman, S. B., Chodoff, P., Mason, J. W., & Hamburg, D. A. Behavioral observations on parents anticipating the death of a child. *Pediatrics*, 1963, *32*, 610.

Gardner, R. A. Psychogenic problems of brain-injured children and their parents. *Journal of the American Academy of Child Psychiatry*, 1968, *7*, 471.

Glaser, H. H., Harrison, G. S., & Lynn, D. B. Emotional implications of congenital heart disease in children. *Pediatrics*, 1964, *33*, 367.

Green, M. Care of the child with a long-term life-threatening illness: Some principles of management. *Pediatrics*, 1967, *39*, 441.

Green, M., & Haggerty, R. J. The management of long-term illness. Part IV. In M. Green & R. J. Haggerty (Eds.), *Ambulatory pediatrics*, pp. 441–468. Philadelphia: W. B. Saunders Co., 1968.

Green, M., & Solnit, A. J. Reactions to the threatened loss of a child: A vulnerable child syndrome. *Pediatrics*, 1964, *34*, 58.

Gurney, W. Congenital amputee. In M. Green & R. J. Haggerty (Eds.), *Ambulatory pediatrics*, pp. 534–540. Philadelphia: W. B. Saunders Co., 1968.

Jessner, L. Some observations on children hospitalized during latency. In L. Jessner & E. Pavenstedt (Eds.), *Dynamic psychopathology in childhood*, pp. 257–268. New York: Grune & Stratton, 1959.

Kessler, J. W. *Psychopathology of childhood*, pp. 332–367. Englewood Cliffs, N.J.: Prentice-Hall, 1966.

Langford, W. S. The child in the pediatric hospital: Adaptation to illness and hospitalization. *American Journal of Orthopsychiatry*, 1961, *31*, 667.

Lazarus, R. S. *Psychological stress and the coping process*, pp. 258–266. New York: McGraw-Hill Book Co., 1966.

Lilly, J. R., Giles, G., Hurvitz, R., Schroter, G., et al. Renal homotransplantation in pediatric patients. *Pediatrics*, 1971, *47*, 548.

McCollum, A. T., & Gibson, L. E. Family adaptation to the child with cystic fibrosis. *Journal of Pediatrics*, 1970, *77*, 571.

McDermott, J. F., & Finch, S. M. Ulcerative colitis in children. Reassessment of a dilemma. *Journal of the American Academy of Child Psychiatry*, 1967, *6*, 512.

Mandelbaum, A. The group process in helping parents of retarded children. *Children*, 1967, *14*, 227.

Mason, E. A. The hospitalized child—His emotional needs. *New England Journal of Medicine*, 1965, *272*, 406.

Mattsson, A., & Agle, D. P. Group therapy with parents of hemophiliacs: Therapeutic process and observations of parental adaptation to chronic illness in children. *Journal of the American Academy of Child Psychiatry*, 1972, *11*, 558.

Mattsson, A., & Gross, S. Social and behavioral studies on hemophilic children and their families. *Journal of Pediatrics*, 1966a, *68*, 952.

Mattsson, A., & Gross, S. Adaptational and defensive behavior in young hemophiliacs and their parents. *American Journal of Psychiatry*, 1966b, *122*, 1349.

Mattsson, A., Gross, S., & Hall, T. W. Psychoendocrine study of adaptation in young hemophiliacs. *Psychosomatic Medicine*, 1971, *33*, 215.

Mattsson, A., & Weisberg, I. Behavioral reactions to minor illness in preschool children. *Pediatrics*, 1970, *46*, 604.

Minde, K. K., Hachett, J. D., Killon, D., & Silver, S. How they grow up: 41 physically handicapped children and their families. *American Journal of Psychiatry*, 1972, *128*, 1554.

Money, J., & Pollitt, E. Studies in the psychology of dwarfism. II. Personality maturation and response to growth hormone treatment in hypopituitary dwarfs. *Journal of Pediatrics*, 1966, *68*, 381.

Murphy, L. B. The widening world of childhood. New York: Basic Books, 1962.

Myers, B. A., Friedman, S. B., & Weiner, I. B. Coping with a chronic disability: Psychosocial observations of girls with scoliosis treated with the Milwaukee brace. *American Journal of Diseases of Children*, 1970, *120*, 175.

Pless, I. B. Epidemiology of chronic disease. In M. Green & R. J. Haggerty (Eds.), *Ambulatory pediatrics*, pp. 760–768. Philadelphia: W. B. Saunders Co., 1968.

Prugh, D. G. Toward an understanding of psychosomatic concepts in relation to illness in children. In A. J. Solnit & S. A. Provence (Eds.), *Modern perspectives in child development*, pp. 246–367. New York: International Universities Press, 1963.

Purcell, K., Brody, K., Chai, H., Muser, J., Molk, L., Gordon, N., & Means, J.

194   Mattson

The effect on asthma in children of experimental separation from the family. *Psychosomatic Medicine*, 1969, *31*, 144.

Purcell, K., & Weiss, J. H. Asthma. In C. G. Costello (Ed.), *Symptoms of psychopathology*, pp. 597–623. New York: John Wiley & Sons, 1970.

Robertson, J. *Young children in hospitals*. New York: Basic Books, 1958.

Roskies, E. *Abnormality and normality: The mothering of thalidomide children.* Ithaca, N.Y.: Cornell University Press, 1972.

Rothchild, E., & Owens, R. P. Adolescent girls who lack functioning ovaries. *Journal of the American Academy of Child Psychiatry*, 1972, *11*, 88.

Rutter, M., Tizard, J., & Whitmore, K. *Handicapped children. A total population prevalence study of education, physical, and behavioral disorders.* London: Longmans, 1968.

Shrand, H. Behavior changes in sick children nursed at home. *Pediatrics*, 1965, *36*, 604.

Solnit, A. J. Psychotherapeutic role of the pediatrician. In M. Green & R. J. Haggerty (Eds.), *Ambulatory pediatrics*, pp. 159–167. Philadelphia: W. B. Saunders Co., 1968.

Solnit, A. J., & Stark, M. H. Mourning and the birth of a defective child. *Psychoanalytic Study of the Child*, 1961, *16*, 523.

Stewart, W. H. The unmet needs of children. *Pediatrics*, 1967, *39*, 157.

Swift, C. R., & Seidman, F. L. Adjustment problems of juvenile diabetes. *Journal of the American Academy of Child Psychiatry*, 1964, *3*, 500.

Tietz, W., & Vidmar, T. The impact of coping styles on the control of juvenile diabetes. *Psychiatric Medicine*, 1972, *3*, 67.

Tisza, V. B. Management of parents of the chronically ill child. *American Journal of Orthopsychiatry*, 1962, *32*, 53.

Tisza, V. B., & Gumperty, E. The parents' reactions to the birth and early care of children with cleft palate. *Pediatrics*, 1062, *30*, 86.

Toker, E. Psychiatric aspects of cardiac surgery in a child. *Journal of the American Academy of Child Psychiatry*, 1971, *10*, 156.

Vernon, D., Foley, J., Sipowicz, R., & Schulman, J. *The psychological responses of children to hospitalization and illness. A review of the literature.* Springfield, Ill.: Charles C Thomas Publisher, 1965.

THE ADAPTATION OF PARENTS TO THE BIRTH OF AN INFANT WITH A CONGENITAL MALFORMATION: A Hypothetical Model

Dennis Drotar, Ann Baskiewicz,
Nancy Irvin, John Kennell, and Marshall Klaus[1]

The birth of an infant with a congenital malformation presents complex challenges to the pediatrician who will care for the affected child and his family (Hare, Laurence, Paynes, & Rawnsley, 1966; Johns, 1971; National Association for Mental Health Working Party, 1971; Fletcher, 1974). Despite the relatively large number of infants with congenital anomalies (Villumsen, 1971), our understanding of how parents develop an attachment to a malformed child remains incomplete. Although previous investigations are in agreement that the child's birth often precipitates major family stress (Rose, 1961; Hare et al., 1966; Johns, 1971; National Association for Mental Health Working Party, 1971; Villumsen, 1971; Roskies, 1972; Fletcher, 1974), there have been relatively few descriptions of the process of family adaptation (Hare et al., 1966; Johns, 1971; Roskies, 1972) during the infant's first year of life. A major advance was Solnit and Stark's discussion of the need for parents to mourn the loss of their expected, normal child (Solnit & Stark, 1961). Other observers (Waterman, 1948; Zuk, 1959; Michaels & Shuoman, 1962) have noted the pathological aspects of family reactions including the chronic sorrow which envelops the family with a defective child (Olshansky, 1962). There has been less emphasis on the more adaptive aspects of parental attachment to children with malformations.

This report, which is based on an analysis of interviews with parents of 20 children with congenital malformations, describes a hypothesized sequence of parental reactions to the infant's birth and focuses on the process of parental attachment. Knowledge of these stages of parental reactions provides a clinically useful framework for pediatric intervention with parents.

Reprinted from *Pediatrics* 56(5), pp. 710–717, © 1975, American Academy of Pediatrics, with permission.

Supported in part by the Grant Foundation and Educational Foundation of America and Public Health Service grant MC-R-390337.

[1]All from the Department of Pediatrics, Case Western Reserve University School of Medicine, Cleveland, OH.

METHOD

Subjects

The parents (20 mothers and 5 fathers) of 20 children with congenital malformations who had been hospitalized at Rainbow Babies and Childrens Hospital during a two-month period were interviewed regarding their reactions to the births. The children represented a range of common malformations including Down's syndrome, congenital heart disease, microcephaly, cleft palate, and others as shown in Table 1. The mean age of the mothers was 26 years. The mean occupational level of the sample was 2.6 (semiprofessional administrative personnel) and educational level was 3.2 (partial college training) according to Hollingshead and Redlich (1958).

Data Analysis

The interview information was obtained by a series of open-ended questions regarding parents' emotional reactions and perception of the child's malformation as shown in Table 2. The interviews were audio-taped, took approximately 1½ hours, and the time of the interviews ranged from within a few days of the birth to as long as five years later with the exception of one interview at 13 years. Sixty-five percent of the interviews were in the first year. We recorded the reactions of parents who had just learned about the anomaly as well as reports of memories of the early crisis situation.

Analysis of each interview involved transcription, followed by an analysis of statements made in the interviews. Those with common characteristics were grouped together and then placed into broad qualitative categories or stages by two of the authors who did not conduct the initial interviews or have information concerning the child's problem.

RESULTS

Despite the great variation among the children's malformations and parental backgrounds, a surprising number of common themes emerged from the parents' discussion of their reactions. In general, they vividly recalled the events surrounding the birth and described both their reactions and the reactions of others around them in great detail. Many of the parents seemed to struggle with common issues and went through identifiable emotional reactions. Figure 1 represents a generalization of the complex reactions of the parents. Although there was a variation in the amount of time that each dealt with the issues of a specific stage, the following sequence reflected the course of most parents' reactions to their congenitally malformed infant.

Table 1. Clinical data

Case no.	Anomaly	Sex	Visible anomalies	Nonvisible anomalies	Infant's age at parental interview	Other congenital anomalies in family
1	Extrophy of bladder	M	+	–	2 wk	No
2	Extrophy of bladder	M	+	–	6 mo	Yes
3	Down's syndrome	F	+	+	7 mo	No
4	Down's syndrome	M	+	+	18 mo	No
5	Trisomy 13–15 bilateral cleft lip and palate	F	+	+	7 days	Yes
6	Coffin syndrome—motor and mental retardation	F	+	+	23 mo	No
7	Cleft palate	F	–	+	2 mo	No
8	Cleft lip	F	+	–	2 wk	No
9	Bilateral cleft lip and palate; horseshoe kidney	M	+	+		Yes
10	Severe congenital lymphedema	M	+	+	11 mo	Yes
11	Microcephaly with mental retardation	M	+	+	6 mo	No
12	Multiple congenital malformations	M	+	+	2 wk	No
13	Absent lower right forearm	F	+	–	2 wk	Yes
14	Ichthyosis	F	+	–	3 yr	No
15	Congenital myopathy with abnormal facies	M	+	+	5 yr	No
16	Imperforated anus; vaginal fistula; absent left radius	F	+	+	2 mo	Yes
17	Multiple vertebral anomalies; congenital heart disease	F	+	+	5 yr	No
18	Frontal encephalocele; cleft lip and palate	F	+	+	13 yr	Yes
19	Bilateral choanal atresia; coloboma of right eye	F	–	+	1 wk	Yes
20	Mental retardation; unknown etiology	M	–	+	3 yr	No

Table 2.   Congenital anomaly questionnaire format

I.   Parental perception of the child's deformity
1.   When did you first suspect your baby had a problem?
2.   How did you find out?
3.   What were you told?
4.   When?
5.   How did you feel?

II.   Parental feelings
1.   What has happened since then up to the present with the baby?
2.   With the both of you?

III.   Assessment of parental attachment
1.   Does it seem like the baby is yours? When?
2.   Do you feel close to the baby?
3.   When did you start to feel close to the baby?
4.   Do you consider your baby cuddly?
5.   How did you go about naming the baby?

IV.   Effects of the anomaly
1.   Could you go back to the time of the baby's birth and say how each of you had adapted to the situation?
2.   Have you shared your feelings together?
3.   How much have you cried?
4.   Do you find yourself very blue? Very angry? Irritable?
5.   Have you found yourself doing unusual things? Having unusual thoughts?
6.   Has there been a change in your health?
7.   Your outlook for the future?
8.   Your eating? Sleeping? Dreaming? Mood?
9.   What changes have you noticed in each other, in your friends, and in your relatives?
10. Could you compare your family life since the baby was born with the way it was before?

V.   Parental attitudes toward handling of the situation
1.   To review, could you tell me again what stages you remember going through since the baby was born?
2.   What helped?
3.   What didn't help?
4.   What suggestions would you have for other families in the same situation?
5.   What could doctors do that would be helpful?

First Stage: Shock

Most parents' initial response to the news of their child's anomaly was overwhelming shock. All but two of the parents reported reactions and sensations indicating an abrupt disruption of their usual feeling states. Many parents confided that this early period was a time of irrational behavior, characterized by much crying and feelings of helplessness. One mother said, "It was a big blow. It just shattered me" (case 6).

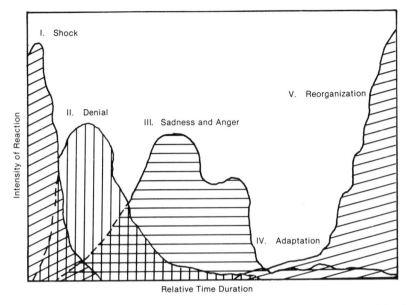

Figure 1. Hypothetical model of a normal sequence of parental reactions to the birth of a malformed infant.

Six mothers emphasized the fact that they were totally unprepared for the news of the child's anomaly. All but one mother reported they had naturally expected a normal child.

Second Stage: Denial

Once parents had recognized their feelings of shock, many tried either to escape the information of their child's anomaly or to cushion the tremendous blow. Each reported a wish to be free from the situation or to deny its impact. One father graphically described his disbelief: "I found myself repeating 'it's not real' over and over again." Other parents mentioned that the news of the baby's birth just didn't make sense. One man (case 5) admitted, "I just couldn't believe it was happening to me. I thought it was unreal and I would soon wake up."

Although every parent reported his disbelief of his child's malformation, the intensity of the parents' denial varied considerably, depending on the visibility of the malformation.

Third Stage: Sadness, Anger, and Anxiety

Accompanying and following the stage of disbelief were intense feelings of sadness and anger. The most common emotional reaction was sadness. Twelve parents described their sadness and noted that they had cried a good deal. One mother reported, "I felt terrible. I couldn't stop crying. Even after a long while I still cried about it."

Seven families were disrupted by angry feelings. For example, one mother reported that she was quite angry upon learning her infant had Down's syndrome. "I never hated the baby, I hated what she was. I didn't care if she died" (case 3). One father said, "I just wanted to kick someone" (case 14). Another mother (case 11) noted that she "hated him (the baby) or hated myself. I was responsible. I still can't lose that feeling completely." Many directed their anger toward themselves, toward the baby, or outwardly toward hospital staff and other people.

Eleven parents described intense feelings of anxiety as being a part of their initial reactions to their babies. Many mothers feared for their babies' lives despite in most instances strong reassurance. Five parents spontaneously verbalized fears that the babies might die. This fear caused a number of parents to feel reluctant to become attached to or interact with the babies. Mothers felt isolated and estranged from their children. One mother (case 17) said that she initially perceived her child as "non-human." "Holding him with that tube distressed me. Initially I held him only because it was the maternal thing to do." Another explained, "It was just as if it were someone else's baby. I couldn't hold him" (case 1).

Hesitance regarding their attachment to the babies was seen in almost all of the mothers. Their fear that the babies would die seemed to be an issue in their hesitancy regarding interactions. As one mother put it, "I didn't feel close to the baby at first. I was afraid I was going to lose her" (case 7). Others mentioned that sadness and disappointment regarding the abnormality seemed to affect their relationship with the malformed infants.

Fourth Stage: Adaptation

Ten of the parents reported a gradual lessening of the anxiety and intense emotional reactions. Along with a lessening of feelings of emotional upset, they reported increased comfort with their situation and confidence in their ability to start caring for the babies. According to their own descriptions, parents varied in the length of time required to reach the period of adaptation. Sometimes many months elapsed before their intense emotional reactions subsided. Even at best, this adaptation continued to be incomplete, for one parent reported that "tears come even yet, years after the baby's birth" (case 14).

Characteristics of Adaptation and Attachment

The parents' adaptation appeared to be a gradual process which involved their coping with a number of complex issues including their anxieties and sadness related to the infants. Eight mothers described their babies as vulnerable and expressed concern about hurting them. Mothers remained very conscious of putting the babies through too much pain and were especially vigilant concerning their physical condition. Some parents believed that their attachment to the children had started when they first had contact with the infants in the hospital. For example, one mother (case 14) reported, "When they gave her to me and put her in my arms, then she was mine." A majority of the parents who had children with a visible malformation reported seeing the infants for the first time and revealed that the children were much better than they had expected. One parent reported, "We had been conjuring up all kinds of things—that there could be something wrong with every organ. But then what I saw was a relatively normal baby." (The malformation in this instance was repairable; case 8.)

Four mothers made comments concerning their belief that taking care of their children was now "just like taking care of a normal child." Five mothers reported that they had especially unique, close attachments to their babies. The children were also considered "very special." In this regard, parents were reluctant to describe overtly rejecting attitudes toward their child, although one mother did report that she'd rather have her child "die than be a vegetable later on" (case 5).

Fifth Stage: Reorganization

The period of reorganization was a complex time in which parents described a more rewarding level of interaction with their infants. Parents also dealt with such issues as their responsibility for their children's problems. Four mothers spontaneously reported that they had to assure themselves that the babies' problems were "nothing I had done." On the other hand, three parents seemed content with the recognition that their child's birth "just happened." Other parents continued to search for possible causes, scrutinizing diets and other aspects of their prenatal care to find a cause for the malformations.

A positive long-term acceptance of the child also involved the parents' mutual support of one another throughout the time after the birth. Parents reported that they felt alone and isolated during the period following the baby's birth and found it difficult to face family and friends with the news of the baby's malformation. Seven couples reported that they relied heavily on one another during this period. One couple said, "We worried more about each other than the baby. We needed each other more during this time" (case 14). One woman spoke positively of her husband's support. "He's the only way I'm holding up still. We couldn't have gotten through this without each other." Six couples reported that the experience of the birth seemed to draw them closer together. However, in other instances the crisis of the birth separated parents, particularly those who blamed one another for the baby's birth (case 11). In another instance, one mother remembered that her husband did not provide emotional support for her, but rather turned on her, saying, "You always had to have everything just so. Now you don't have everything just so and you can't change it" (case 3).

DISCUSSION

The results of the present study suggest that parental reactions to the birth of a child with a congenital malformation may follow a predictable course. For most parents, initial shock, disbelief, and a period of intense emotional upset (including sadness, anger, and anxiety) were followed by a period of gradual adaptation, which was marked by a lessening of intense anxiety and emotional reaction. Adaptation was characterized by an increase in the parents' ability to care for their babies and in their satisfaction with their children. The stages of parental reactions reported here are consistent with previous observations of parental reactions to children with malformations (Hare et al., 1966; Johns, 1971; Roskies, 1972) and to other crisis situations, such as a terminally ill child (Friedman, Chodoff, Mason, & Hamburg, 1963). The shock, disbelief, and denial (Geleerd, 1965) reported by many parents seemed to be an understandable attempt to escape the traumatic news of the baby's malformation, which was so discrepant from usual parental expectations for their newborn that it was impossible to register except gradually.

The intense emotional turmoil described by parents who have given birth to a child with a congenital malformation corresponds to a period of crisis (Bloom, 1963; Caplan, Mason, & Kaplan, 1965; Rappoport, 1975) which is an "upset in a state of equilibrium caused by a hazardous event which creates a threat, a loss, or a challenge for the individual." A crisis includes a period of impact, a rise in tension associated with stress, and finally a return to equilibrium. During such crisis periods, a person is at least temporarily unable to respond with his usual problem solving activities to solve the crisis. Roskies (1972) noted a similar "birth crisis" in her observations of mothers who had given birth to children with birth defects caused by thalidomide.

Solnit and Stark (1961) have likened the crisis of the birth of a child with a malformation to the emotional crisis following the death of a child in that the mother must mourn the loss of her expected, normal infant. In addition, she must become attached to her actual living, damaged child. The present study also suggested that the sequence of parental reactions to the birth of a baby with a malformation differs from that which takes place following the death of a child. The mourning or grief work does not take place in the usual manner because of the issues raised by continuation of the child's life and the demands of the child's physical care which preoccupied most parents. The mothers' initiation of their relationship with their children was a major development in the reduction of the anxiety that followed the child's birth. As with normal children (Zuk, 1959), many parents' initial experience with their infants seemed to release positive feelings which aided the mother-child relationship following the stresses associated with the news of the child's anomaly. These observations are consistent with previous investigations of the importance of early physical contact between mother and child in the development of a positive mother-child relationship (Klaus, Kennell, Plumb, & Zuehlke, 1970).

It was significant to note that many mothers emphasized the baby's normality and strengths in reaching an adaptation to the child and in developing satisfaction with their child. The parents' emphasis on the normal aspects of their babies' development appeared to reflect the parents' positive adaptation rather than a simple denial of the disability. The parents' increasing attachment to their children led them to identify similarities between themselves and their babies. Roskies (1972) also noted that mothers of thalidomide children emphasized the normal aspects of their child's development in successfully coping with their physical limitations. Furthermore, recent studies (Berkson, 1974; Rosenblum, 1974) have documented animal mothers' compensatory responses to defective infants.

For many parents in the present study, the mother-child relationship remained fraught with anxieties which caused some mothers to establish what they described as "closer than normal" relationships with their children. The parents' ambivalent response to their children has been considered a possible explanation for the overly close relationship which often develops between a malformed child and his mother (Lax, 1972). Complexities of the ongoing physical care of children with congenital malformations are realistically much greater than those involved with normal children. In addition, the uncertain developmental prognosis for many of the children also added to parental concern about doing "the right thing." Furthermore, the recurrent hospitalizations required for the care of many children with malformations intensified parental anxieties, which had been initially created by the baby's birth and might start the process of reactions over again.

Other aspects of parental adaptation to the birth of a child with a malformation are characteristic of human adaptation to other crisis situations, particularly those which involve loss or threat. For example, the parents' search for an explanation for the anomaly was consistent with the observations of Friedman et al. that the parents of children with a fatal illness struggle to identify reasons to explain why their child was affected (Friedman et al., 1963). Parkes (1973) noted that an adult's adaptation to the death of a spouse often involved an attempt to make sense out of the event by trying to make it fit with one's conceptions of why things happen. In the present study, the parents' attempts to identify the reasons their children were born with malformations also involved deeply personalized struggles to attain philosophical or religious meaning out of their experiences.

The present results suggest that the maintenance of satisfactory relationships between the parents is often a crucial aspect of positive adaptation. The crisis of the baby's birth has the potential for bringing parents closer together through the mutual support and communications required in the complex adaptation to the child's birth. On the other hand, in some instances the baby's birth estranged parents from one another. The ongoing demands imposed by the baby's care increased the isolation between parents, particularly if they did not share responsibility for the child's care. Parents who each had a different time duration at each stage were termed asynchronous. They usually did not share these differing feelings with each other and seemed to have particular difficulty in their relationship with each other. Asynchronous parental reactions often resulted in a temporary emotional separation of the parents, and may be a significant factor in the incidence of parental separations following major family crises.

Despite the important similarities in parental reactions to the various malformations, there were differences in how parents negotiated the various stages of reaction. Some parents did not report initial reactions of shock and emotional upset, tending to intellectualize the baby's problem and focus on the facts related to the baby's condition rather than their own feelings. Other parents were not able to successfully cope with their very strong emotional reactions to the birth and, as a result, did not achieve an adequate adaptation; they seemed to be in a state of sorrow which lasted long after the birth (Olshansky, 1962).

However, the methodological problems inherent in the design of this pilot study made it difficult to determine the length of particular stages of parental reactions. A longitudinal investigation which allows one to separate concurrent from retrospective data is needed to determine more adequately the length and nature of the stages of parental response to the birth of a congenitally malformed child.

The present results have many implications for pediatric management. The fact that parental reactions may involve predictable stages allows the pediatrician to anticipate parental reactions and to adopt an approach to a situation which can arouse great discomfort in those who must manage the child. Further, since the parents' initial shock and disbelief limit the amount of information that they can absorb in regarding their child's condition, information regarding the child's handicap may have to be communicated very clearly and repeated many times (Giannini & Goodman, 1963; Goodman, 1964; Golden & Davis, 1974). It is particularly important to note that parental anger is a natural reaction and is often displaced onto the nurses and physicians attending the malformed infant. With the knowledge that parents' anger, sadness, and anxiety are predictable, but not pathological, emotional reactions should aid the physician in his attempts to provide supportive, calm communications which build trust for future productive interactions with the family. Parents' anxieties and loneliness during the baby's hospitalization may be alleviated by the support and availability of their physicians and nurses.

Prominent in the interviews were the marked loneliness and anxieties reported by many of the parents during the period immediately following their infant's birth. Mothers often had intense concerns about their infant's appearance, and fantasies that their children had died. However, the infants generally appeared much less affected and more normal than the parents' impressions of their condition. For this reason, in most instances we suggest that the newborn be brought to the parents as soon as possible after delivery and the child's problem discussed with the family in a way that emphasized the infant's normal attributes. Although there may be exceptional circumstances when parents might not be completely ready to initiate attachment to a child with malformations, encouragement of the parents' physical contact with their children serves to minimize the parents' estrangement from their child and awesome sense of the baby's abnormality. The long-term care of children with congenital malformations may be improved considerably by the pediatrician's interventions. The pediatrician's availability to the family not only following the crisis of the child's birth, but throughout the child's development as well, places him in a unique position to aid the family's adaptation to the child's malformation. Many of the emotional problems and family difficulties associated with the birth of infants with malformations (Walker, Thomas, & Russell, 1971; Bentovim, 1972; Mannoni, 1972) may not be inevitable consequences of parental reactions but may be prevented by constructive interventions (Caplan, 1961; Rose, 1961). However, interventions soon after the infant's birth are often difficult, particularly for young house officers who may feel helpless and anxious in their interviews with parents of malformed infants. We have found it useful to follow Barbero's (1973) suggestion (oral communication) to have house officers participate in such interviews with senior staff physicians who are effective models for interventions with families.

The complexities of the parents' emotional reactions provide strong support for the impression that without supportive pediatric intervention, the rearing of a child with a malformation is truly not "a fair test of motherliness of a woman or fatherliness in a man" (Fraiberg, 1971).

It is our hypothesis that pediatric advice, support, and parent counseling during the baby's first year of life will be a crucial aid in maximizing the development of the child with a congenital malformation and his family. Future studies are planned to test whether family counseling, based on a crisis intervention model, will result in significant improvement in the family's adjustment to the child's birth and the ongoing care of a child with a congenital malformation.

206   Drotar et al.

REFERENCES

Barbero, G. *Oral communication.* May, 1973.
Bentovim, A. Emotional disturbances of handicapped pre-school children and their families—Attitudes to the child. *British Journal of Medicine,* 1972, *2,* 579.
Berkson, G. Social responses of animals to infants with defects. In M. Lewis & L. A. Rosenblum (Eds.), *The effect of the infant on its caregiver,* p. 233. New York: John Wiley & Sons, 1974.
Bloom, B. Definitional aspects of the crisis concept. *Journal of Consulting Psychology,* 1963, *27,* 42.
Caplan, G. An approach to community mental health. New York: Grune & Stratton, 1961.
Caplan, G., Mason, E., & Kaplan, D. Four studies of crisis in parents of prematures. *Community Mental Health Journal,* 1965, *1,* 149.
Cushna, B., & Crocker, A. Three years is still too late. In H. Ohberg (Ed.), *Focus on exceptionality, readings in special education.* New York: Simon & Schuster, 1973.
Fletcher, J. Attitudes toward defective newborns. *Hastings Center Studies,* 1974, *2,* 21.
Fraiberg, S. Intervention in infancy: A program for blind infants. *Journal of the American Academy of Child Psychiatry,* 1971, *10,* 381.
Friedman, S. B., Chodoff, P., Mason, J. W., & Hamburg, D. A. Behavioral observations on parents anticipating the death of a child. *Pediatrics,* 1963, *32,* 610.
Geleerd, E. R. Two kinds of denial: Neurotic denial and denial in the service of the need to survive. In M. Schur (Ed.), *Drives, affects, and behavior* (Vol. 2), p. 118. New York: International Universities Press, 1965.
Giannini, M. J., & Goodman, L. Counseling families during the crisis reaction to mongolism. *American Journal of Mental Deficiency,* 1963, *67,* 743.
Golden, D. A., & Davis, J. G. Counseling parents after the birth of an infant with Down's syndrome. *Children Today,* 1974, *3,* 7.
Goodman, L. Continuing treatment of parents with congenitally defective infants. *Social Work,* 1964, *9,* 93.
Hare, E. H., Laurence, K. M., Paynes, H., & Rawnsley, K. 1966. Spina bifida cystica and family stress. *British Journal of Medicine,* 1966, *2,* 757.
Hollingshead, A. B., & Redlich, F. C. *Social class and mental illness.* New York: John Wiley & Sons, 1957.
Johns, N. Family reactions to the birth of a child with a congenital abnormality. *Medical Journal of Australia,* 1971, *7,* 277.
Klaus, M., Kennell, J., Plumb, N., & Zuehlke, S. Human maternal behavior at the first contact with her young. *Pediatrics,* 1970, *46,* 182.
Lax, R. Some aspects of the interaction between mother and impaired child: A mother's narcissistic trauma. *International Journal of Psychoanalysis,* 1972, *53,* 339.
Mannoni, M. *The backward child and his mother.* New York: Random House, 1972.
Michaels, J., & Shuoman, H. Observations on the psychodynamics of parents of retarded children. *American Journal of Mental Deficiency,* 1962, *66,* 568.
National Association for Mental Health Working Party. The birth of an abnormal child: Telling the parents. *Lancet,* 1971, *2,* 1075.
Olshansky, S. Chronic sorrow: A response to having a mentally defective child. *Social Casework,* 1962, *43,* 190.

Parkes, C. M. *Bereavement: Studies of grief in adult life*. New York: International Universities Press, 1973.

Rappoport, L. The state of crisis: Some theoretical considerations. In H. J. Parad (Ed.), *Crisis intervention*, p. 22. New York: Family Service Association, 1975.

Robson, K., & Moss, H. Patterns and determinants of maternal attachment. *Journal of Pediatrics*, 1970, *77*, 976.

Rose, J. A. The prevention of mothering breakdown associated with physical abnormalities of the infant. In G. Caplan (Ed.), *Prevention of mental disorders in children*. New York: Basic Books, 1961.

Rosenblum, L. A., & Youngstein, K. P. Developmental changes in compensatory dyadic response in mother and infant monkeys. In M. Lewis & L. A. Rosenblum (Eds.), *The effect of the infant on its caregiver*, p. 141. New York: John Wiley & Sons, 1974.

Roskies, E. *Abnormality and normality: The mothering of thalidomide children*. New York: Cornell University Press, 1972.

Solnit, A. J., & Stark, M. H. Mourning and the birth of a defective child. *Psychological Studies of Children*, 1961, *16*, 523.

Villumsen, A. L. Environmental factors in congenital abnormality. *Obstetrical and Gynecological Surgery*, 1971, *26*, 635.

Walker, J. H., Thomas, M., & Russell, J. T. Spina bifida and the parents. *Developmental Medicine and Child Neurology*, 1971, *13*, 462.

Waterman, J. H. Psychogenic factors in parental acceptance of feeble-minded children. *Diseases of the Nervous System*, 1948, *9*, 184.

Zuk, G. H. Religious factor and the role of guilt in parental acceptance of the retarded child. *American Journal of Mental Deficiency*, 1959, *64*, 145.

LONG TERM AND FATAL ILLNESS AND THE FAMILY

Norman B. Gordon[1] *and Bernard Kutner*[2]

In recent years the problems created by interaction between the ill individual and members of his family have received considerable attention. An important part of this problem relates to familial aspects of fatal and long-term illness in children. Interest in childhood illness has been stimulated by both scientific and public interest in poliomyelitis, muscular dystrophy, mental retardation, cerebral palsy, leukemia, cystic fibrosis, Tay-Sachs disease and other illnesses. Despite these interests relatively little attention has been devoted to the impact of serious childhood diseases on the life of the family unit as a whole.

It is the purpose of this paper to examine some of the familial consequences of serious childhood illness, to review existing literature on this subject, and to examine some aspects of the problem concerning social and medical science.

PSYCHOLOGICAL AND SOCIAL CONSEQUENCES OF CHILDHOOD ILLNESS

The family crisis created by the discovery and ensuing need to manage a seriously ill child may initiate a series of complex reactions, depending upon the nature of the illness. One or more of the following may occur:

1. There may be an initial traumatic reaction when the diagnosis is revealed to the parents.
2. The parents' self attitudes as well as their relationships with other members of their families, friends and neighbors, may be seriously altered.
3. There may be a difficult adjustment to the medical needs of the sick child.
4. A variety of relationships with physicians and other medical personnel in clinics and hospitals must be established.

Reprinted from *Journal of Health and Human Behavior 6*, pp. 190–196, © 1965, The American Sociological Association.

This article is the product of Unit for Research in Aging, Albert Einstein College of Medicine, supported by Grant HD-00674, National Institutes of Health, U.S. Public Health Service.

[1]From Graduate School of Education, Yeshiva University.

[2]From Department of Preventive and Environmental Medicine, Albert Einstein College of Medicine, Yeshiva University.

5. A long term readjustment in way of life depending upon the nature of the illness and the economic, biological and social consequences following in its wake may be required.

6. Latent emotional problems may be brought to the surface by the demands of the situation.

The afflicted family usually evolves a set of behaviors and attitudes to attempt to cope with the circumstances. Even though there are individual differences in ability to absorb the facts and to deal with their ramifications the kind of problems presented to parents go far beyond customary experience. Their responses may be adaptive or maladaptive involving all levels of both psychological and social reactivity. What is known of such familial reactions? What is known of the potential and actual roles played by physicians?

THE INITIAL REACTION

The initial parental reaction to the discovery of a serious childhood illness may trigger an emotional trauma as well as a host of judgments, decisions and activities. The physician rendering the diagnosis may play a key role in managing the emotional reaction, reducing confusion and anxiety and in helping parents approach the ensuing problems realistically. Yet Korkes (1955), in a thorough-going study of the impact of children's mental illness and behavior disorders on families, found that only 17 per cent of her sample arrived at convictions about the cause of their children's illness through professional advice. Bruch (1949) in a study of diabetic children pointed to a conflict between the physician's need to instruct parents concerning the seriousness of the illness and his desire to avoid fright and unnecessary anxiety. Bozeman, Orbach, and Sutherland (1955) have dealt with the impact on the mother of the occurrence of leukemia in her child. They refer to the period immediately following the diagnosis as a time of "intense parental anxiety manifested by hostility towards doctors." Thus ". . . failure to comprehend information given, acute feelings of personal responsibility for the illness, disruption of functioning, and separation fears" are some of the earmarks of the characteristic response. They go on to point out that "The physician's responsibility therefore cannot stop with the treatment of the child. It must also include an effort to alleviate the poignant and pathetic reaction of the parents. The physician who manages the child's care during diagnostic procedures and the first doctors with whom a mother has contact in the treatment institution, play the most important role in doing this."

In an attitude study of parents with mentally retarded children, Koch, Graliker, Sands, and Parmelee (1959) found that parents tended to be critical of what and how they were told about the diagnosis and prognosis of the child. Almost 50 per cent of over 100 families were critical of the medical care they received in this respect. Complaints ranged from lack of interest and bluntness by the physicians, to claims of unfairness in predicting the future and a tendency to rush hospitalization. In another study, Graliker, Parmelee, and Koch (1959) examined the initial reactions and concerns of the parents to the diagnosis of mental retardation. Nearly a third of the parents of 67 children rejected the diagnosis. The major parental concerns expressed were the actual cause of the retardation and feelings of their own rejection of the child. The authors concluded that the initial contact with the parents at time of diagnosis must concentrate on the nature of the illness, its causes and probable effects. Future care and counseling concerning course of action should take place during subsequent contacts.

In sum, the usual initial responses of parents when they learn of a serious or fatal diagnosis in their child may include: 1) shock 2) anxiety and confusion 3) denial 4) rejection of the child and 5) criticism of the diagnosing physicians.

PHYSICIAN'S ROLE IN DIAGNOSIS AND BEYOND

Although the physician who discovers a long term or fatal childhood illness may regard his function as the conclusive establishment of the diagnosis, parents in most cases demand much more. Frequently, they require advice regarding the need for further confirmation of the diagnosis, whether and when hospitalization may be necessary, management of the afflicted child's daily needs, family planning and a host of other problems. Existing reports of parents' views of the physician's role in such situations reveal considerable variation in the perceived practices of the diagnosing and consulting physician.

Waskowitz (1959) refers to the fact that only 25 per cent of parents he interviewed reported that their contacts with professional personnel such as physicians and clinic personnel were satisfactory either in devoting sufficient time and interest to their problems, or dealing with them in an understanding manner. The shock of diagnosis, which came as a sentence of death, was followed by feelings of aloneness, being set apart and by confusion. While institutional care for their children was frequently recommended only 1 in 20 followed this advice. Parents' complaints concerning the medical care they received included concern over crudeness, bluntness, lack of concern, evasion of issues by the physician and the use of complicated terminology.

Truitt (1954) stated that physicians are not agreed that there is any best time when parents should be informed of the diagnosis of muscular dystrophy. Some believe that parents should be informed as soon as possible, others hold that parents may well have as many months as possible without the burden of such knowledge. He reports that many parents do not believe the diagnosis, some pin hopes on medical miracles, others simply bemoan their fate. He feels that it is extremely important to give parents time to be listened to and to allow them to ventilate their fears and lack of knowledge in order to fully understand what is happening.

Richmond and Waisman (1955) in a study of children with malignant diseases, point to the psychological effect of diagnosis as the "most deep-seated of all anxieties, that of separation of a loved one." This has deeper meaning than most separation anxieties, which parents and children face, because of the finality of separation which comes with death. The psychological depth of this reaction indicates the importance of the physician's precision in diagnosis. Publicity and cancer education have made people increasingly aware of, and sometimes anxious, concerning the possibility of this diagnosis. "Thus, promptness and skill in diagnosis of the physical disorder may have far-reaching effects psychologically in management."

Davis (1956) points to the important role of the physician in defining "time perspective" for parents. The physician must "communicate to the parents that the uncertainty (in diagnosis and prognosis) stems from the nature of the disease and not from therapeutic incompetence or unwillingness to speak the truth." Since the physician is not always believed, his failure to convince may lead to medical "shopping." Henley and Albam (1955) speak of resentment towards the physician for not diagnosing muscular dystrophy early enough, and a long period of unwillingness on the part of the parents to accept the diagnosis. Bernstein and Malter (1957) in a survey of muscular dystrophy found that difficulties in diagnosis and pessimistic prognoses make parents initially depressed. Parents expressed guilt feelings about the hereditary possibilities of the disease and felt that they were to blame. Greene (1957) reports that a common parent reaction in muscular dystrophy is the "spoiled child syndrome": trying to do everything to make the child happy presumably as a reaction formation to their guilt for the child's disease. Frick (1952) noted that in cardiovascular illness, parents also blame themselves and want to shield the child from further possible harm, undermining the child's confidence. Medical management of the illness and surgical care are made more difficult.

Another indication of the complex reactions created in parents may be found in Kozier (1957) commenting on casework with parents, that parents are often tense about their own parenthood, and are anxious for status and achievement. The discovery of a severe brain defect usually results in intense emotional difficulties in planning for the care of their sick child.

Kanoff, Kutner, and Gordon (1962), in a recent study of 25 families having children with Tay-Sachs disease[3] confirm most of the above find-

[3]An illness leading to fatality in the second or third year caused by an hereditary fault in fatty metabolism and is usually diagnosed during the first year. Symptoms are regression in motor behavior.

ings. A major focus of each of the interviews with the parents was concerned with the initial discovery of the illness, the "diagnostic scene" and the events that ensued. The majority of the parents reported some degree of dissatisfaction with the physician making the diagnosis. While the details of these encounters are an important matter in their own right, they are significant here, since they play an important role in the decisions and actions parents subsequently took. Where the encounter with the diagnosing physician was unsatisfying, either from an informational or emotional point of view (in terms of the parents' ability to incorporate the facts into the frame of reference of their own observations and knowledge), they resorted to a number of inappropriate steps or sought solutions against medical advice. In some instances parents were given the advice to hospitalize the child at once and/or to have no further children. These recommendations were very difficult to cope with since they ran counter to the needs and aspirations of parents with young children, and to the frequently healthy and well-developed appearance of their infants. Exceedingly skillful psychologic care is needed if parents are to face facts appropriately. The injunction to "hospitalize immediately" may make sense to those who have been concerned with the hospital care of such children and are anxious to protect parents from futile hopes. Yet the advice may make little sense to nurture-oriented parents. The perceived coldness of the information is greeted by the parents as issuing from a disinterested physician, and may contribute to their taking steps to obtain cures or to disprove the diagnosis.

Similarly the injunction—"have no more children," when parents may have strong child-rearing motives (and may not have been convincingly informed of the genetic facts) may lead to deprivation, doubting and even parental conflict. Parents may wish to risk further pregnancies, they may need advice concerning adoption, and they may need help in merely accepting the known facts.

The most significant finding in the above study is that families managed in some manner to re-orient their lives to encompass the new and serious events despite a high psychological and social cost.

A precise understanding of the cause of serious illness, opportunities to accurately assess related facts, assistance in managing emotional crises, and planning for the future are among the essential ingredients of satisfactory familial adjustment. Continuing guilt, shame and anxiety may then be treated as routine conditions. The physician is expected to take the role of humane counselor, advisor and expert professional resource to parents beyond the diagnosis. It would appear that the constellation of events which follow the diagnosis faces the physician with a crucial task, the successful handling of the long term effects upon the parents.

A serious long term or fatal illness in a child provokes a set of crises during which parents are led to question matters often never given a second thought. Parental knowledge and understanding of the disease, its etiology, course and implications appear related to their actions in dealing with it. A severe burden is placed on parents to secure and comprehend sufficient and acceptable information despite the emotional overlay created by knowledge of the disease. Along with the task of understanding the medical facts, parents must be prepared to make a number of short and long term decisions— whether to continue normal care or to secure special services, how to inform other children, family and friends, and how to plan future family life. At the same time uncertainty and doubt arise about the cause of the illness, their role in its origins and the actions they might take to alter its course. In the studies cited, ignorance concerning the illness varies in inverse proportion to parents' reports of satisfactory relationships with physicians and medical personnel, as well as with their ability to adjust to the demands of their child's illness and its implications. Other questions remain. What factors contribute to the parents' ability or failure to function normally and to make logical decisions in regard to the sick child? What is the impact of the illness on parents' self-image and their ability to adequately cope with the more subtle aftermaths while they re-orient their lives?

LONG TERM ALTERATIONS IN PARENTS' CONCEPTIONS

One of the most significant studies of parental reactions to serious childhood illness is that of Korkes (1955). She views parents in a stress situation "wherein the power to control the difficulty is not in their hands." This stress produces almost immediate changes of self-perception and initiates more enduring alterations in long-term goals and aspirations. She describes certain socio-psychological changes involving:

1. A feeling of exclusion from the "normal community."
2. A loss of rewards of "free communication."
3. A loss of rewards of anticipated pleasure of child rearing.
4. A period of prolonged stress from which escape is impossible.

Among the consequences may be one or more of the following: changes in the perception of the sick child from positive to negative valence, in their own roles as parents (i.e., some parents "abandon" the child to an institution), and in their relationships to the larger family group and to others (i.e., greater social isolation). Major variables in these changes are the nature and duration of the illness, parents' perception of their causal role in the illness and their role in controlling it. Objectively, illnesses may be divided by degrees of parental "culpability" ranging from least "culpable" (hereditary "errors", birth injuries and chance traumatic accidents) to most "culpable" (emotional or behavioral disorders, injuries from parental punishment, etc.).

Regardless of the true nature of the objective causal factors, parents may not perceive the facts accurately and may experience guilt feelings or blame themselves or each other for some actual or imagined behavior assumed to have contributed to the child's condition. Even in the case of hereditary diseases some parents may perceive the illness as resulting from their own inappropriate behavior or that of their spouse. In less understood illnesses such as juvenile diabetes or cerebral palsy, parents may look inwardly in the search for causes in each other's behavior. The distortion may be of reverse order: denying involvement in the development of a behavior disorder rooted in a disturbed household.

When an illness is discovered about which there is little public information, or about which there is attached a stigma (hereditary or mental illness) or a doubt over the etiology, major problems may arise between husband and wife. Where little information is available or made available to parents, they may either blame themselves or each other for some hereditary imperfection presumed to be the causal factor. At a time when each needs the other for maximum support faulty comprehension may block an important avenue of communication and lead to emotional or marital disturbance.

Murstein (1960) stressed the importance of cognition of the way parents perceive the consequences of childhood illness. The changes in perception of role as well as relationships with others are functions of the way parents come to understand the illness of their child. Korkes (1955) indicated that seven out of ten parents in her sample arrived at the etiology of the illness by themselves. Furthermore, over half of the families reported difficulty in communication between husband and wife largely because of lack of understanding of the nature of the illness. Parents of the Tay-Sachs children in Kanoff et al. (1962) reported an initial unwillingness to communicate with each other until the facts of etiology became clarified.

Farber (1959), Bakwin (1956), Kanner and Eisenberg (1957), and Cobb (1956) have all pointed to the critical changes that take place as the parents' self-images are altered through the impact of their children's illnesses.

Brown, Mally, and Kane (1960) report on 28 hemophilic children in which the mothers' awareness of the fact that they were the hereditary carriers of the illness resulted in extreme guilt reactions. In some cases mothers appeared to deny the existence of the disease. The rearing of these children was perceived by the mothers as a continuous struggle between life and death, in which the mother's role gradually evolved as the "protector of the child." On the other hand, fathers demonstrated extreme fear at interaction with their children lest some accident result in serious bleeding. The mother's behavior became characterized by extreme guilt and the father's by ambivalence toward the child due to his anxiety and the resultant thwarting of his parenthood ambitions.

SUGGESTED APPROACHES TO
THE PROBLEM OF PARENT COUNSELING

An approach to dealing with the manifold familial problems that arise in connection with serious childhood illness has been suggested by Korsch, Fraad, and Barnett (1954) and Korsch and Barnett (1961). The former study reports on the successful use of pediatric discussions with parent groups whose children were under treatment for nephrosis. The major benefit of this procedure was that it provided an important outlet for the expression of parents' concerns about their child, and their doubts about how to manage him. It provided an opportunity for parents to discuss a host of related problems pertaining to the illness. This enabled parents and medical staff to attend to a wide range of social and psychological problems as well as to provide parents with an opportunity to raise practical problems of child care. An added benefit of this procedure was the opportunity offered to provide training for residents and nurses in the broad field of family management attendant upon the serious illness of a child.

The latter study (Korsch & Barnett, 1961) likewise deals with families whose children are afflicted with nephrosis and points to the fact that the physician is in a position to "make a significant continuing contribution to the welfare and comfort of patient and family." Furthermore it is pointed out that the families "need the physician's support and reassurance in dealing with their own anxieties and mixed feelings, so that they can be as supportive and reassuring as possible in their relationship to the sick child whose attitudes about his illness, his treatment, and himself as a person will largely reflect the attitudes of his parents."

These two studies underline the conclusions derived from the work previously cited. Serious childhood illness creates broad psycho-social problems. Parents and physicians deal with them in ways that vary greatly and do not always yield the desired ends. Before proposing any formula for action, however, much systematic information is needed to serve as the basis for a convincing approach to this problem.

RESEARCH IMPLICATIONS

The reactions of parents when a serious childhood illness occurs in a family appear to hinge on the inter-relationship between information, emotional reaction and decision-making in a crisis situation. Several stages have been identified as focal points of the consequences of this interaction. The entire situation is complicated by the nature of the particular independent variables involved—i.e., the precise nature of the illness, age at onset, the presence of other children, etc. The following is an attempt to organize the findings into logically identifiable problem areas in which the major focus is on sets of circumstances that are characteristic consequences of serious childhood illness.

1. *Pre-diagnostic factors* Children may have distinct signs of abnormality for some time before parents take any overt action to discover their cause or seek professional advice. Parents vary considerably in the way in which they react to symptoms of abnormality in their children even when others call them to their attention. Many deny such symptoms for varying periods of time, and are overtly fearful of medical or psychologic confirmation of their fears. This behavior may have important consequences on the eventual impact of the diagnosis. An important research issue is a determination of the factors associated with early or delayed recognition of symptoms and the degree of temporal delay in seeking definitive advice.

2. *The diagnostic scene* The set of circumstances that occur at the diagnosis presents a complex situation for both the diagnosing physician and the parents. At least two major factors emerge as research problems:

   a. The effects upon parents of the manner in which the physician informs parents about the disease and its medical ramifications; and the actions he recommends parents take to deal with its consequences, and

   b. the manner in which the social and psychological impact of the diagnosis affects parents over time.

   Parents' abilities to comprehend the facts concerning the disease and to make intelligent decisions are influenced by their emotional reactions and anxiety about how they will be received by others as parents of a handicapped child. Emotional shock, aroused fears and anxieties, and the cognitional disruption caused by the knowledge that a child is seriously or fatally ill, make difficult the acceptance of a diagnosis and planning for the future. Long term study of parent behavior at systematic time intervals from the "diagnostic scene" are needed in order to evaluate the communication patterns of physician and parents which are most and least effective in determining successful decision-making and later adjustment.

3. *Hospitalization* In the case of both serious mental and physical illnesses, the advice most frequently given by physicians is the hospitalization of the sick child. This involves the severest kinds of conflicts for parents and it is frequently viewed as a separation akin to that of death or abandonment. What may appear as an obvious and inevitable solution, in objective terms, requires a profound change in attitudes in parents. Since hospitalization as a parental decision has many ramifications, studies of the decision-making process and of the factors associated with early, late or no hospitalization would be enlightening.

4. *Long-term readjustment problems*   The effect of a serious illness in a child on family planning is a variable function of parental age, birth order of the sick child and the specific nature of the particular illness (i.e., whether it is hereditary or not, or whether it involves the parents in serious economic, psychological or child-management difficulties). The future of a family is a major problem for parents as it may bring to the surface latent distortions in self-image and difficulties in family integration, as major marital aims and ambitions are thwarted in one degree or another. Along with plans for such matters as further child bearing, the long term problems of re-adjustment may involve an entire shift in the frame of reference of the parents and their social and interpersonal relationships. Such re-adjustments include such miscellaneous problems as:

a. adjustment to death, separation or atypicality in a child.
b. the overt insinuation of latent emotional problems brought to the surface by the illness-produced crisis.
c. altered relationships with other family members, friends and neighbors.
d. long-range economic re-adjustment necessitated by medical costs, and the added burden of physical care of the child.
e. general re-evaluation of spiritual and religious attitudes. A systematic investigation of this problem area would be an important contribution to an understanding of parent behavior in response to crisis situations.

CONCLUSION

An outline of a problem area defined as the impact of serious or fatal childhood illness on the family has been presented. Many facts are known about the psycho-social impact of such fundamental disruptions in the normal family life cycle, but full understanding of the problems and the available means for aiding afflicted individuals to cope with the consequences are imperfect. The emotional pain, social stigmata, cognitional disruption and economic consequences attending such events are matters often left almost entirely to the individuals concerned. The entire set of circumstances suggests the need for a line of both practical and theoretical research to examine such aspects of the problem as family decision-making and stress, physician-family relationships in serious illness as well as the long-term impact of serious health events on child-rearing practices and family well being. It is hoped that behavioral scientists will pay increased attention to this fruitful research area.

REFERENCES

Bakwin, H. Informing the parents of the mentally retarded child. *Journal of Pediatrics*, 1956, *49*, 486–498.

Bernstein, H., & Malter, S. *A social survey of muscular dystrophy*. New York: Professional Educational Services, Scientific Department, Muscular Dystrophy Associations of America, 1957.

Bozeman, M. F., Orbach, C. E., & Sutherland, A. M. Psychological impact of cancer and its treatment. III. The adaptation of mothers to the threatened loss of their children through leukemia, Part I. *Cancer*, 1955, *8*, 1–19.

Brown, W. J., Mally, M., & Kane, R. P. Psycho-social aspects of hemophilia: A study of twenty-eight hemophilic children and their families. *American Journal of Orthopsychiatry*, 1960, *30*(2), 730–740.

Bruch, H. Physiologic and psychologic interrelationships in diabetes in children. *Psychosomatic Medicine*, 1949, *11*(4), 200–211.

Cobb, B. Psychological impact of long illness and death of a child on the family circle. *Journal of Pediatrics*, 1956, *49*, 746–751.

Davis, F. Definitions of time and recovery in paralytic polio convalescence. *American Journal of Sociology*, 1956, *62*, 582–587.

Farber, B. Effects of a severely mentally retarded child on family integration. *Monographs of the Society for Research in Child Development*, 1959, *24*(2).

Frick, A. Emotional significance of cardiovascular disease in children. In *Children with congenital heart disease*, pp. 1718–1721. New York: Bureau for Handicapped Children, New York City Department of Health and New York Heart Association, 1952.

Graliker, B. V., Parmelee, A. H., Sr., & Koch, R. Attitude study of parents of mentally retarded children. II. Initial reactions and concerns of parents to a diagnosis of mental retardation. *Pediatrics*, 1959, *24*(5), 1.

Greene, J. L. *Emotional factors in children with muscular dystrophy*. New York: Muscular Dystrophy Associations of America, 1957.

Henley, T. F., & Albam, B. A psychiatric study of muscular dystrophy, the role of the social worker. *American Journal of Physical Medicine*, 1955, *34*(1), 258–264.

Kanner, L., & Eisenberg, L. Childhood problems in relation to the family. Summary of a seminar. *Journal of Pediatrics*, 1957, *20*(1), 155–164.

Kanoff, A., Kutner, B., & Gordon, N. B. The impact of Tay-Sachs disease on the family. *Pediatrics*, 1962, *29*, 37–45.

Koch, R., Graliker, B. V., Sands, R., & Parmelee, A. H., Sr. Attitude study of parents with mentally retarded children; evaluation of parental satisfaction with the medical care of a retarded child. *Pediatrics*, 1959, *23*, 582–584.

Korkes, L. *The impact of mentally ill children upon their families*. Trenton, N.J.: State Department of Institutions and Agencies, 1955.

Korsch, B., & Barnett, H. L. The physician, the family and the child with nephrosis. *Journal of Pediatrics*, 1961, *58*, 707–715.

Korsch, B., Fraad, L., and Barnett, H. L. Pediatric discussions with parent groups. *Journal of Pediatrics*, 1954, *44*(6), 703–717.

Kozier, A. Casework with parents of children with severe brain defects. *Social Casework*, 1957, *38*(4), 183–189.

Murstein, B. The effect of long term illness of children on the emotional adjustment of parents. *Child Development*, 1960, *31*, 157–171.

Richmond, J. B., & Waisman, H. A. Psychologic aspects of children with malignant diseases. *American Journal of Diseases of Children*, 1955, *89*, 42–47.

Truitt, C. J. *Personal and social adjustment of children with muscular dystrophy.* Paper in symposium on Clinical Management of Patients. 3rd Medical Conference, Muscular Dystrophy Associations of America, New York, October 8–9, 1954.

Waskowitz, C. H. The parents of retarded children speak for themselves. *Journal of Pediatrics*, 1959, *54*, 319–329.

PERSONAL STATEMENT · · · · · ·
Karen

Medical History: Karen

Age	Medical Problem
4 weeks (4½ pounds)	Open heart surgery
10 months	Cerebral palsy diagnosed
2½ years	Brace on leg to allow for walking
6 years	Heel cord surgery
7 years	Open heart surgery
10 years	Muscle transplant—arm

I am the mother of this child. While it is she who must bear the trauma, the pain, and the limitations, it is I who suffers with her and sometimes, truthfully, because of her.

After writing the brief medical history, I thought I would try to compute the hours spent in and traveling to and from hospitals. I found it impossible—the hours are uncountable. Which is worse, I think—life-or-death surgery with comparatively little follow-up or routine orthopedic surgery, which requires trips to Boston (20 miles one way) three times a week for physical therapy? It has been almost a year since the last surgery and we are still making the trip twice a month. The exercises are never ending, the casts must be continually replaced, and trying to motivate acceptance of these responsibilities by Karen was, until recently, next to impossible.

She is mine forever, I sometimes think. I will never forget the doctor's response when I asked when all this would stop. His answer was to the point—"When her husband takes over." To him, she is not a person but an arm or a leg, depending on where the problems lay at the time.

I think back to her day of birth—thrilled with another girl. Karen was preemie weight but full term. Because she nursed well, she was allowed to come home with me. Symptoms began to appear within a few weeks, but nothing that didn't seem too unusual. A doctor who cared enough saw her once or twice a week to check and called me often when I didn't call him. Because he cared enough to keep a close watch, he was able to diagnose a congenital heart defect before it was too late—he saved her life. I had never dreamed of a problem of such magnitude.

The diagnosis was a septal defect in the heart. In other words, a hole in the heart that allowed oxygenated blood to mix with deoxygenated blood. Emergency surgery was needed to repair the defect. The doctors would not give us any odds on Karen's survival of the surgery, but she had no chance at all if surgery was not performed. Karen was, at the time, one of the smallest (although not the youngest) infants to survive this surgery. We thought our problems were over until we discovered (when she was 10½ months old) that Karen had cerebral palsy. It was years before I could say those last two words—cerebral palsy. I always said that she had damage to the motor area of the brain. Somehow that didn't seem so bad.

The cause will always remain unknown. It could be congenital, it could be due to a lack of oxygen before the corrective heart surgery, or it could have happened during the surgery at a time when techniques were not perfected for working on such a small child (she was hooked up to an adult size heart-lung machine, for example). The cause is unimportant. It is the effects that we must deal with.

At first the attention a family gets in these circumstances is unbelievable. You're special, everyone wants to help, and there is a certain amount of glory or martyrdom involved. "How do you manage?" they ask. They could **never** do it. Well, the answer to that is, you do it because you have to. There is no one else to do it for you. You only wonder how you managed after the latest crisis has passed. Then it's on to the next crisis—always another one to look forward to. It's almost as if this child will be mine forever—in the sense that I will always be responsible for her. While this may sound selfish, I can't imagine any parent wanting to keep their children with them for the rest of their lives. Cop out? Maybe it is, but I can't help it.

How do we feel about Karen? It was a long time before I could say that sometimes I hate her for all the problems she presents. A parent cannot easily voice this emotion regarding a child, especially a handicapped child—it's almost inhuman. Karen's sisters could say "hate" much easier—children's feelings are much closer to the surface than those of adults.

On the other hand, these same sisters who sometimes hate her will rise to her defense when they see that she is treated badly. She is not, however, an easy child to get along with. Although Karen functions well in school with a great deal of supportive help (resource room, counseling, etc.) she is socially immature and has no real friendships to rely on. It is we at home who care for her who must bear the brunt of her frustrations—acting out and generally behaving abominably.

Of course we love Karen, but it is often difficult to show openly. A child of Karen's temperament can drain your emotions. The more affection and attention you give, the more she wants. I often feel as though I am bled dry. She is all consuming.

Sometimes I feel pity. What will she be able to do? Because she appears almost normal, people expect normalcy from her. For that matter, so do we, for I am always afraid of selling her short. We demand that she perform tasks that are within her capabilities—even more. If I tie her shoes for her now, who will do it when I'm not here? She needs to know how to tie shoes with one hand. She must learn in spite of herself.

Often I feel compassion. How do you console a child who has no "real" friends? What playmates she does have are not above tormenting her in insidious ways. What do you say when she tells you that the kids at school call her "mental"? How does it feel knowing that if someone comes to call for you, it is only because no one else can come out to play? Telling her not to pay attention is almost ludicrous. These things hurt us both, but it is very difficult to build self-image in a child who is "different" and intelligent enough to know it.

I always feel guilty—not because I've somehow done this to her, but because she is so much better off than other victims of cerebral palsy. Cerebral palsy can be devastating to the point of total immobility and retardation. Karen is neither. Why then should I complain? I guess I can only say that this is our problem, and it is we who must deal with it.

At night I cry when I see her sleeping. She sleeps relaxed, the spasticity is gone, the CP seems to have disappeared for 12 hours or so. But in the morning, Karen still limps, her hand is still misshapen and she still has trouble with school work and social adjustment. I cry now.

What will Karen be when she grows up? My head knows that there's a place for her somewhere—my heart wonders if she'll find it.

RECOMMENDED READINGS FOR SECTION I

Anthony, E. J. The mutative impact on family life of serious mental and physical illness in a parent. *Canadian Psychiatric Association Journal*, 1969, *14*, 5.

Bane, M. J. *Here to stay*. New York: Basic Books, 1976.

Baum, M. Some dynamic factors affecting family adjustment to the handicapped child. *Exceptional Children*, 1962, *28*, 387-391.

Bronfenbrenner, U. Nobody home: The erosion of the American family. *Psychology Today*, 1977, May, 53-61.

Christopherson, V. The patient and family. *Rehabilitation Literature*, 1962, February, 34-41.

Cobb, A. B. *Medical and psychological aspects of disability*. Springfield, Ill.: Charles C Thomas Publisher, 1973.

Coelho, G., Hamburg, D., & Adams, J. (Eds.). *Coping and adaptation*. New York: Basic Books, 1974.

Gath, A. The impact of an abnormal child upon the parents. *British Journal of Psychiatry*, 1977, *130*, 405-410.

Glick, P. A demographer looks at American families. *Journal of Marriage and the Family*, 1975, February, 15-26.

Hall, J., & Weaver, B. (Eds.). *Nursing of families in crisis*. Philadelphia: J. B. Lippincott Co., 1974.

Handy, I. Psychological aspects of chronic disability. *Journal of the American Geriatrics Society*, 1969, *17*(1), 105-111.

Jordan, T. Physical disability in children and family adjustment. *Rehabilitation Literature*, 1963, *24*, 11.

Krupp, N. Adaptation to chronic illness. *Postgraduate Medicine*, 1976, *60*, 5.

Lewis, J. The family and physical illness. *Texas Medicine*, 1976, *72*, 43-49.

Lipowski, Z. J. Physical illness, the individual, and the coping process. *Psychiatry in Medicine*, 1970, April, 91-102.

Litman, T. The family and physical rehabilitation. *Journal of Chronic Diseases*, 1966, *19*, 211-217.

Marinelli, R., & Dell Orto, A. *The psychological and social impact of physical disability*. New York: Springer Publishing Co., 1977.

Mercer, R. Crisis: A baby is born with a defect. *Nursing*, 1977, November, 45-47.

Moos, R. (Ed.). *Coping with physical illness*. New York: Plenum Medical Book Co., 1977.

Mowrer, O. H. New hope and help for the disintegrating American family. *Journal of Family Counseling*, 1975, *3*(1), 17-23.

Nav, L. Why not family rehabilitation. *Journal of Rehabilitation*, 1973, May–June, 14–17.

Olsen, E. The impact of serious illness on the family system. *Postgraduate Medicine*, 1970, February, 169–174.

Parks, R. Parents reactions to the birth of a handicapped child. *Health and Social Work*, 1977, *2*(3), 52–66.

Pearse, M. The child with cancer: Impact on the family. *The Journal of School Health*, 1977, March, 174–178.

Poznanski, E. Emotional issues in raising handicapped children. *Rehabilitation Literature*, 1973, *34*, 11.

Rakel, R. *Principles of family medicine.* Philadelphia: W. B. Saunders Co., 1977.

Reinhardt, A., & Quinn, M. (Eds.). *Family-centered community nursing.* St. Louis: C. V. Mosby Co., 1973.

Reinhardt, A., & Quinn, M. (Eds.). *Current practice in family-centered community nursing.* St. Louis: C. V. Mosby Co., 1977.

Roessler, R., & Bolton, B. *Psychosocial adjustment to disability.* Baltimore: University Park Press, 1978.

Roghmann, K., Hecht, P., & Haggerty, R. Family coping with everyday illness: Self reports from a household survey. *Journal of Comparative Family Studies*, 1973, *4*, 49–62.

Sasano, E., Shepard, K., Bell, J., Davies, N., Hansen, C., & Sanford, T. The family in physical therapy. *Physical Therapy*, 1977, *57*, 153–159.

Schram, R. Marital satisfaction over the family life cycle: A critique and proposal. *Journal of Marriage and the Family*, 1979, *41*(1), 7–14.

Shorter, E. *The making of the modern family.* New York: Basic Books, 1975.

Skipper, J., Fink, S., & Hollenback, P. Physical disability among married women: Problems in the husband-wife relationship. *Journal of Rehabilitation*, 1968, September–October, 16–19.

Snyder, J., & Wilson, M. Elements of a psychological assessment. *American Journal of Nursing*, 1977, February, 235–239.

Sobol, E., & Ribischon, P. *Family nursing.* St. Louis: C. V. Mosby Co., 1975.

Strauss, A. *Chronic illness and the quality of life.* St. Louis: C. V. Mosby Co., 1975.

Stubbins, J. (Ed.). *Social and psychological aspects of disability.* Baltimore: University Park Press, 1977.

Thompson, B., & Clifford, K. The disabled person and family dynamics. *Accent on Living*, 1972, Summer, 18–24.

Travis, G. *Chronic illness in children.* Stanford, Cal.: Stanford University Press, 1976.

SECTION II

THE FAMILY REACTION TO SPECIFIC TRAUMAS

When working with patients, the health professional is not just dealing with disabled individuals but with the spouse or parents, the children, relatives, and sometimes friends. The disability will usually affect all family members, because the family represents a group relationship. Section I emphasizes the interrelationship between problems of disability and family concerns. Section II continues this theme, but highlights some of the differential effects certain disabilities or chronic illnesses have on family life.

Disabling or life-threatening conditions usually cause feelings of grief, anxiety, and helplessness in family members. Diseases progress in different ways; with some there are periods of remission and exacerbation, e.g., multiple sclerosis, and with others there is a rapid, progressive deterioration, e.g., many forms of cancer. Such changes in disease progression can cause family members to react emotionally in different ways than when an illness has stabilized in its course. Uncertainty, hesitancy to make long-range family plans, and the fears that accompany living with the unknown can all be shared by family members as they attempt to cope with disability impact on family life.

The personal statements of Daniel and Geraldine in this section identify the many family emotions that occur with specific diseases. Both accounts were written by the parents. One involves a child and the other, a young woman, married with a young son. Both of the stories allow the reader to enter the lives of these families and learn how each family has coped. The parents of Daniel have devoted much energy to preventing the crisis caused by the disease from becoming destructive to their own relationship. The illness actually has brought the family closer together. How all of this is accomplished is explained in their statement, and they offer suggestions to health professionals on what has helped them live with the reality of the serious illness.

The mother of Geraldine relates how she dealt with her daughter's illness, and illustrates the influence the daughter's husband had during the devastating course of the disease. He continually searched for a new cure but also provided his wife with a reason to live. It was not to be, and the story indicates that chronic sorrow lives with many family members.

All of the material in Section II provides further information for the helping professional on family dynamics during disability or illness trauma. The articles explain the family responses to traumatic head injury, progressive neurological diseases, and terminal illness. With the personal statements and text written by the authors, they further suggest the influences the family can have on the patients. Such influences represent perspectives for family intervention.

PERSONAL STATEMENT ......
Daniel

The profound emotional impact of what it meant
to be a parent of a sick child occurred when
Daniel was born. The first morning he was
taken to a special care unit since his head was
swollen. At this time we were faced with a crisis
that we would survive but that would be a
precursor of many more to follow.

Being in the hospital for the first few days
exposed us to the feelings of horror, uncertainty, helplessness, and confusion. We had a
baby who was ill and we could do nothing about
it. What made a difference was the hospital staff
who were able to support us and show us that
they cared and were concerned about our emotional well-being as well as the physical well-
being of our child.

At this point we began our journey into the
uncertainty of having a problem without a
definite diagnosis. After the circumcision,
Daniel bled; at 5½ months, black and blue
marks appeared. But what could be wrong?
Daniel was so healthy and active. The turning
point came after a series of tests when we
received a phone call from Children's Hospital.
We knew it was serious when the doctor would
not tell us over the phone what the diagnosis
was. The ride to the hospital was terrifying. Did
he have leukemia? Was it a fatal disease? The
words of the doctor will stay with us forever.
"Daniel has a very serious disease that is compatible with a normal life-style: He is a severe
hemophiliac." At this point the implications of
this were not known to us. We were unfamiliar
with hemophilia and were caught off guard.
Having two physicians in the family helped us
with the medical aspects of the disease but we
had to find out as much as possible on our own.
Reading the literature that first evening scared

229

us more than helped us. At this point we felt we
were alone. We did not know anyone who had a
hemophilic child.

The questions we asked were: Why did it
happen to us? How can we go on? It wasn't fair.

I became bitter to all who had normal
children. This feeling was based on the normalcy of others, which accentuated Daniel's
disability.

Another painful experience was telling
others. A problem was that others attempted to
console us by telling us how it could be worse.
For us at this point in our lives this was the
most terrible thing that could have occurred.
We desperately wanted and needed someone
who could identify with our feelings and respond to our needs.

As a mother my feelings toward Daniel went
through some changes. I found myself afraid to
love him. I guess this was a means of protecting
myself. Also the image of injections was
repulsive, but I was able to overcome it. During
this time a persistent thought was why did it
happen to us? One family out of 10,000. A
critical factor in our being able to survive these
difficult times was our ability to talk to and
support one another. We cried, shared, and
grew together. This was a challenge we knew we
had to face together or it would eventually
destroy us.

As time passed we began to separate Daniel
from his disability. He was a unique child who
was a part of our family. We feel the reason we
were able to do this was based primarily on the
fact that we did not know Daniel was a
hemophiliac until he was 6 months old.
Therefore we treated him as a normal child.
This time enabled us to establish our roles as
mother and father. We see these roles as compatible and supportive as well as necessary for
the growth and development of the child. The
reality of the disability became more apparent
when we had to go to Children's Hospital and

see other disabled children. This was a sobering
experience. We began to internalize that we
were faced with a life-long problem that would
not get better.

A multitude of implications began to surface: 1) problems with cutting teeth, 2) limitation in activities, 3) orthopedic concerns, and
4) pain. These were abstract considerations that
crystalized when Daniel had his first treatment.
The emotion of the infusion and the recollection
of having to hold him down are difficult for us
to recall. However, getting through the first
bleeding episode was an important developmental step because it proved to us that it could be
done.

Part of the difficulty we have with coping
with the disease is that we never know when a
crisis is going to occur. This is accentuated by
the fear in the middle of the night, the red tape
of the emergency room, repeating of the story,
different doctors. These are factors that intensify the experience and alter it from a reality of
living to a horror show.

During the past year and one-half our perceptions have been tempered by the input of relevant information, support of the Hemophilia
Association's self-help group, and exposure to
other hemophiliacs and their families who have
coped with the disease and who are well adjusted.

While we have shared a common experience, both of us perceive it differently. I as
mother tend to be optimistic; Rich as father is
still angry, although he hopes for new treatment.

At this time a major consolation for us is
that we are both convinced that Daniel will be a
well-adjusted child. We believe that through our
efforts we can help Daniel adjust to his personal
inconveniences by balancing them with a supportive family environment.

As parents of a hemophilic child it is amazing how you find yourselves making compari-

sons with other parents who have children who are "normal." The more children we meet, it seems the more normal they are. However, we recognize that there is more to the picture than superficial appearances and we are well aware of Daniel's other resources, which make him a joy. We were able to reach this point by having exposure to other families through the Hemophilia Society. This exposure enabled us to see how other families had adjusted. One mother in particular became personally involved with us. This was a most helpful experience for it was additional input from someone who knows what it is about. This is an important point because there are few people who can relate to the problems and fears of being parents of a hemophilic child.

In reflecting upon the quality of our relationship we must consider the period of time before Daniel's birth. The best way of describing it is that it was very positive. We were able to talk to one another, rely on and support each other. These abilities would play a significant role in the adjustment to Daniel as a child coping with hemophilia. The ability to support one another was needed in the crisis situations that surrounded Daniel's episodes. At this time there are many demands and strains created. The intensity of the stress is almost unbearable but we have developed the resources to take from and give to one another. As a result, the crisis does not become destructive.

In retrospect we initially had to learn to cope on our own since many of the interventions were not immediate. It would have been most helpful to have support the day we found out. As a result we have become active in the Hemophilia Society and are trying to heighten the awareness of the needs of others.

As a baby we could control Daniel and have things done to him. Now that he is older he is beginning to associate hospitals with pain. We are hopeful that future infusions will not be as painful.

As we think of the future we are concerned about how other neighborhood kids will treat Daniel. When he goes to school, will other kids be insensitive to him? This is becoming a very painful issue as Daniel becomes older and wants to play as other children do. We are struggling with our need to have him be as normal as other children, but there is a risk in the constant fear of injury.

A factor that has helped us cope with these issues has been our families, which have treated Daniel like any other child, but were aware of his unique needs. Another aspect of this process of adaptation is that we are able to be thankful for the fact that the condition is not terminal. Our only response to this is "How could we cope?" but as in all things you cope when you have to. There are other areas that have been affected by our situation and they are related to having other children. This is a very difficult issue to resolve. With Daniel we are delighted to have him as our son; he is a joy and a treasure. When we consider having other children, we are faced with issues such as: if it is a male, how do we respond knowing we could bring another potential hemophilic child into the world? During pregnancy, should we have tests done to determine the sex of the child and abort if it is male? What are the chances of a female being a carrier? These are very emotional issues, for we do not have any easy answer to them.

We are presently adjusting to an ongoing process that will test our resources, challenge us, and take its toll. Our hope is that we will be able to adjust to the new demands and provide Daniel with the support, understanding, and encouragement he needs.

CHAPTER **6**

PARTICULAR DISABILITIES AND FAMILY INFLUENCES

Paul W. Power and Arthur E. Dell Orto

This chapter explains the varied reactions of family members to a particular disease or disability. These reactions are carefully and extensively discussed in the three articles in this chapter. There are some specific causes why many patients do not make more progress toward feasible rehabilitation goals. Frequently the source for this lack of needed change exists within the family. This chapter includes many suggested causes for family maladaptation or successful adjustment in a disability situation. In becoming aware of these many possible reasons, the health professional can then choose particular goals for rehabilitation intervention. For example, if the presence of chronic stress within the family inhibits any efforts to assist the patients, then steps could be taken to alleviate this stress.

An understanding of the family influences that can affect the patient is in harmony with the material explained in the articles. Each article focuses on a specific disease. The illness can produce recurrent crises within the family simply because of the disease progression. When the prognosis implies a rapid deterioration, usually there is greater stress on the family. Without time for replenishment the family will face a variety of crises over a period of time. In a slow but progressive illness the disruptive effect to the family over a combined period of time can be less severe than in the quickly deteriorating diseases. Following the initial shock of diagnosis, and often the temporary confusion among family members, family life can become restabilized and living with the trauma an uninvited, but accepted, reality. Adaptation will be more difficult if there are deterrent forces within the family.

SELECTED FAMILY INFLUENCES ON THE DISABLED PERSON

Seven causes, each representing a possible family influence on the disabled client, are emphasized: chronic stress, secondary gain, lethal dyads, the family's level of functioning, information, expectations, and sexual concerns.

Chronic Stress

Jaffe (1978), in his article in Chapter 8, identifies chronic stress as a "pathway by which family relationships contribute to illness" (p. 333). The presence of continued stress in the family can seriously hamper the patient's adjustment, motivation, and willingness to respond to rehabilitation efforts. It also prevents a family from developing necessary coping mechanisms to deal with the living demands associated with a disability or chronic illness. In the stress situation, the family is primarily attempting to survive. The stress is generally characterized by anxiety, fear, frequent irritability among the family members, resentment, little hope of achievement for individual members or the family group, and a basic insecurity among the family members. All of these characteristics prevent change.

The origins of this stress are many. The patient's emotional reaction to the disability, the possible deviant behavior of the children, severe financial concerns, and the uncertainty generated by not knowing how much the illness will progress (e.g., multiple sclerosis, cystic fibrosis) can provoke stressful situations for family members. The following are examples of such situations: 1) A patient's anger over the debilitating effects of an illness can sustain constant tension in the family. 2) Children who are away from the home for unusually long periods of time cause anxiety in their parents. Such children may find it difficult to live daily with a parent who is seriously ill. 3) If the disability has brought to the family members new financial restrictions and the family is concerned about meeting their bills, resentment and anger are generated.

Secondary Gain

For many patients a disability becomes a way of life, a means to gain new attention. This often occurs if there has been little satisfaction with life or few achievements before trauma or the initial diagnosis. The disability or illness becomes a more acceptable way of identifying with others. Secondary gain occurs when family members shift roles in order to cope with the disability but exclude the patient from gaining new role responsibilities in the home. Many families feel that with a disabled family member they are actually "much better off" than before the disability onset. For example, family members may believe they are living only slightly above poverty level, but a disability occurs that brings them into contact with community resources, provides better family financial compensation than before the disability occured, and brings much attention from community workers. In these situations the family members feel their standard of living has been enhanced. If rehabilitation efforts mean that they will lose these newly gained resources, the family members will often block these attempts. From the health professional's perspective there is maladjustment to the disability, but from the family members' view they are coping very well.

Lethyl Dyads

In his article in Chapter 8, Jaffe explains lethal dyads as "couples who escalate each other's potentiality for illness by the structure of their relationship and the nature of their demands on each other" (p. 337). In other words, if the disabled person says "I am sick," the spouse may state "I am sicker." Another form of such interaction is when the person's severe illness forces the other family members to switch roles and assume new responsibilities. They resent the change and frequently show symptoms of illness. In these families adaptive measures to a disability are thwarted because the members are threatened too much by the needed shift in family duties.

Family's Level of Functioning

In Chapter 1 the different family life stages were discussed. Each stage brings certain tasks for family members and introduces the reality of change. For these tasks to be negotiated means that the family members have achieved a level of functioning necessary to effect the change. Families as a unit also have different levels of functioning. For example, the lowest level of family functioning can be characterized by disorganization in all areas of family life (Tapia, 1972). There is no orientation to the future, the family members are barely able to meet their physical needs, e.g., adequate nutrition, heat, and clothing, and are unable to utilize community resources and services. There is role confusion and no emotional support for the family members. In contrast, childhood families (Tapia, 1972) show some distortion of family roles but are more able to meet their needs for security and physical survival. They are also more willing to work together for the benefit of the whole family. Yet these families are unable to support the growth of their members or utilize effectively community resources. Adolescent families and adult families (Tapia, 1972) are capable of physical survival and of providing security for their members. They are able to utilize community resources and have the ability to confront some of their problems and to seek solutions. Adult families generally take more initiative in referring themselves to outside sources for help.

The family's level of functioning suggests how its members are able to adapt to a disabling trauma or utilize coping resources. The family that is continually disorganized and unable to provide for the emotional functioning of its members will find it too difficult to help the patient toward rehabilitation goals. A family that can use outside help effectively, is able to provide support to its members, and can actively look for solutions to problems will frequently be able to meet the adjustment demands associated with a disability or severely handicapping condition.

Information

Information refers to the understanding the family members have of the disability and the personal meaning of the illness to the patient. This knowl-

238   Power and Dell Orto

edge includes the physical aspects of a disease, the course of the illness, and to what extent each family member views the disease as actually disabling. A frank revelation of these facts pertaining to a disease will ordinarily cause shock, anger, and resentment. When the families and patients are told the important and appropriate facts of an illness at the time of diagnosis, however, they are given the opportunity to "work through" these feelings and eventually come to a stage of adaptation when they begin to resume the business of daily living. They are also given the chance to appraise realistically the situation in order to make future plans.

Uncertainty about the illness, however, generally causes apprehension and lingering fear of the unknown. It also inhibits the establishment of family plans that focus on adjustment, since often at the time of onset of a chronic illness there has been no consideration for total life planning. After becoming aware of the characteristics of a chronic disease, what complications would occur, and what are appropriate preventive procedures, the family may be able to deal with many periodic medical problems. In turn, this knowledge then can become the basis for their coping. For example, with many disabling conditions regular exercise greatly facilitates the patient's daily functioning. Family members can reorganize a part of their daily life to assist the patient in a treatment regimen. The assurance that the patient is attempting and doing something productive is a resource for the family and could alleviate their negative feelings about the disease. Through their understanding both the patient and family members can begin to adjust to the results of the disease and its impact on family life.

Certain families and patients will deny selected aspects of the disease. This denial usually softens the initial shock that occurs upon learning of the diagnosis and thus assists the patient in adjustment. However, persistent denial becomes destructive to patient and family welfare when it prevents necessary adaptive measures, as in persons who refuse to use a cane or a wheelchair when necessary.

Sick Role Expectations

Expectations related to the disability usually flow from the family understanding of the condition. For example, if the family incorrectly perceives that the illness causes a person to be different rather than just to act differently on occasion, they place the patient in too dependent a role before the condition warrants it. Their attitude prevents the patient from continuing many family duties, and often encourages the relinquishment of satisfying social activities.

Upon hearing information that emphasizes patient assets, family members begin to think more positively about the future, and thus contribute to family adjustment, since they want the patient to continue to function as optimally as possible for as long as possible. If the patient and family have received vague, uncertain facts about the illness, the patient often uses symptoms to punish significant people in the family. Uncertainty brings anger and fear, and the reactions to these feelings take the form of regression to an unwarranted dependent state, manipulation, and excessive demands from others within the family. The patient's unsatisfied expectations from the family result in anger and contribute to a deterioration of family relationships. Positive sick role expectations, namely, information that emphasizes productive and useful capacities, help the patient to focus on capabilities for the present and reduce that continued feeling of dread for the future.

Sexual Concerns

Although sexual concerns contribute to chronic stress within the family and are frequently the source of misinformation or low expectations, this area of the marital relationship should be viewed alone. Many traumas or diseases, e.g., spinal cord injury and multiple sclerosis, cause some impairment in sexual functioning. Unfortunately, most couples are hesitant to discuss sexual problems resulting from disability trauma. At the same time, health professionals have been reluctant to identify this area as a possible deterrent to rehabilitation goals. Hohmann (1972) believes that "In the past there has been a general feeling among professional staff that the less said to cord injured patients regarding sexual functioning, the better; and that repressive mechanisms should be allowed to take their course in stifling thoughts and preoccupations about sexuality" (p. 55). Yet sexuality is one of the marriage's major forces, one that guides and shapes patients' psychosocial rehabilitation (Cole, 1972; Bregman, 1978). In many families with a disabled husband the wives complain of excessive sexual demands from their husbands, or the men feel that their wives do not understand an apparent diminished sexual capacity. These complaints and perceptions generate a tension between the spouses that in turn causes them to become more easily irritated with other family members (Power & Sax, 1978). In such an environment it is difficult for family members to be a constructive influence on the patient.

ADAPTIVE AND MALADAPTIVE PATTERNS

Because of many negative influences from within and without the family, maladaptive patterns occur that affect the patient's adjustment. The family members can deny the reality of the deteriorative illness for so long that inclusive treatment considerations are ignored. They attempt to eliminate the disability/illness-related problem by ignoring the problem, and often the patient is ignored; or, because of certain predisposing factors, e.g., alcoholism or limited financial resources, family life is never restored after the onset of the trauma and the family becomes very disorganized. Because of family pathology the members may have to cope individually, leaving the patient alone while they attempt to survive. A chronic, deteriorative illness may eventually cause the spouses to divorce, although the authors believe that the disability may be just one cause of the marital break-up. Other maladaptive responses that can be exhibited by family members over an indefinite period of time are hypochondriasis, continual projection of angry feelings onto other members, extreme regression on the part of the children, a withdrawal from accustomed social interaction, or a rigidity that impairs role flexibility within a family. Yet what is important for health professionals to understand are the causes of these adaptive and maladaptive family reactions; to identify them is to become aware of what kind of intervention is needed. Rakel (1977) describes five criteria that Glasser and Glasser (1970) developed and that are applicable to a family's adjustment potential to a disability:

1. *Internal role consistency among family members*   Each family member has a conception of what is expected of him, and this should be consistent with what other members expect of him.
2. *Consistency of family roles and actual role performance*   The understanding of each individuals' role must remain the same and be performed as expected.
3. *Compatibility of family roles with community norms*   "The behavior of the group must be acceptable to the surrounding community in order to prevent undue external pressure" (Cohen, 1966, p. 265).
4. *Meeting the psychological needs of family members*   "The psychological, social, and emotional needs of all members must be satisfied in order to avoid frustration and internal conflict" (Cohen, 1966, p. 265).
5. *The ability of the family to respond to change*   Duvall (1974) believes that families best able to withstand stress and maintain balance show the following characteristics:
   a. They approach problems in a unified manner as a family.
   b. They have a nonmaterialistic orientation.
   c. The husband and wife frequently share tasks.
   d. They perceive the nature of the problem accurately.
   e. They have a democratic orientation, with diffusion of leadership regarding problem-solving tasks.

Families that can adapt positively and are able to make good adjustments share other features, such as effective and constant communication, flexibility of family roles, tolerance for individuality, marital adjustment characterized by satisfaction, happiness, and stability, social participation of wives outside the home, and ability to support each member's self-esteem (Rakel, 1977).

CONCLUSION

A serious illness or disability in a family can generate closer relationships among family members or it can fragment the family, causing such a state of disorganization that the family disintegrates. Early intervention by health professionals is absolutely necessary because they can be effective catalysts for successful coping and eventual adjustment. Recognizing that different illnesses or disabilities could have differential effects facilitates intervention.

The articles by Bray, Romano, and Lambert in this chapter identify the unique effects that different disabilities can have on family members. Mary Romano explains that the family response to traumatic head injury can be alleviated by denial, and this continues as the effects of living with the illness invade interpersonal family relationships. Denial is a persistent family reaction, and is a very different response from the responses of families experiencing a neurological illness observed by Gladys Lambert. Her discussion is directed more to the health professional. She believes that the helper can assist the family to cope with the members' ambivalent feelings about the patient. Grady Bray, however, describes a four-stage adaptation process to spinal cord injury. From his research he reports that increased rehabilitation success with the spinal cord-injured person will depend upon a better understanding of this adaptation process following the injury. With the other articles, Bray's work represents a distinctive contribution to the development of intervention approaches. He offers many suggestions in each stage on how the health professional can help both the patient and family. All three articles emphasize the family as an integral part of the rehabilitation process.

REFERENCES

Bregman, S. Sexual adjustment of spinal cord injured women. *Sexuality and Disability,* 1978, *1,* 85–92.

Duvall, E. M. *Family development.* Philadelphia: J. B. Lippincott Co., 1974.

Glasser, P., & Glasser, L. Adequate family functioning. In P. Glasser & L. Glasser (Eds.), *Families in crisis,* pp. 290–301. New York: Harper & Row Publishers, 1970.

Hohmann, W. Considerations in management of psychosexual re-adjustment in cord injured males. *Rehabilitation Psychology,* 1972, *19,* 50–58.

Power, P., & Sax, D. The communication of information to the neurological patient: Some implications for family coping. *Journal of Chronic Diseases,* 1978, *31,* 57–65.

Rakel, R. *Principles of family medicine.* Philadelphia: W. B. Saunders Co., 1977.

Tapia, J. The nursing process in family health. *Nursing Outlook,* 1972, *20,* 267–270.

REHABILITATION OF SPINAL CORD INJURED: A Family Approach

Grady P. Bray[1]

The impact of severe injury and disability extends beyond the injured individual to his family, friends and general society. As life-maintaining systems, emergency medical treatment, and medical technology are enhanced, the problems of the severely disabled are exponentially applied to society. One group included in the severely disabled, the spinal cord injured (SCI), increases at an estimated 10,000 cases per year (Hamilton, Muthard, & Turner, 1974). These newly injured SCI have a projected life span only 10 years less than the average person and an average societal cost of $181,320 for a lifetime of care (Smart & Sanders, 1976).

Clients with spinal cord injuries have been difficult and expensive to rehabilitate (Poor, 1975). Estimates vary on rehabilitation success with the SCI from 39 percent (Rusk, 1963) to 48 percent (Young, 1972). Traditional approaches have not been effective with the SCI, and the historical cost-benefit associated with rehabilitation has been assaulted by the sudden influx of these clients as a result of congressional mandates for services to the severely disabled (Public Law 93-112 & 93-516), increased public awareness of the severely disabled, increased longevity for SCI, and increased assertiveness and militancy by handicapped citizens.

To meet the needs of hard-pressed rehabilitation programs, new concepts and approaches to rehabilitation must be researched. One response to these needs is an emerging emphasis on the family as an adjunct to the rehabilitation process.

The implementation of family involvement in rehabilitation is relatively recent. In 1967, the Milwaukee Curative Workshop developed a project to demonstrate that focusing intensive family counseling on the family of stroke patients would result in the maintenance or enhancement of therapy gains following discharge from the rehabilitation program (Overs & Healy, 1971). However, follow-up studies revealed no significant differ-

Reprinted from *Journal of Applied Rehabilitation Counseling* 9(3), pp. 70–78, © 1978, with permission.

This research was sponsored in part by Grant #12-P-57897 from the Rehabilitation Services Administration, Department of Health, Education and Welfare, Washington, D.C.

[1]Assistant Professor of Preventive Medicine, University of Rochester School of Medicine, Rochester, NY. Dr. Bray was formerly director of research at the Georgia Warm Springs Hospital.

ences between experimental and control groups on the criterion measures of activities of daily living, social contacts, avocational activities and return to employment. Another "family focus" program was developed at the Stanford University School of Medicine. The Stanford program was based on the premise that the patient needing post hospital care could best be served by training the family in an environment closely approximating the home setting. The authors concluded "hospital care should look beyond the discharge date and prepare the patient and family with the skills and support necessary for optimum out-of-hospital living" (Davies & Hansen, 1974).

Nau (1973) reviewed family rehabilitation programs in which the family in toto, was treated as the rehabilitation client and concluded that family rehabilitation is a viable approach to resolving many different issues associated with severe cases of disability. However, a major disadvantage of family rehabilitation extended residential programs is a high initial cost, annually averaging from $1,200 to $2,500 per person.

Utilizing the best of these approaches, a family involvement program with emphasis on the spinal cord injured was developed in June 1976 at Georgia Warm Springs Hospital, Warm Springs, Georgia.

To be eligible for the research program, families had to have a member who: a) had received a traumatic spinal cord injury; b) was injured less than one year at the time of admission to Georgia Warm Springs Hospital (GWSH); c) was a Georgia resident; and d) agreed to participate in the research program. The admission criteria was later expanded to include traumatic SCI patients with a second or later admission to GWSH and/or greater than one year post injury.

A research team composed of psychologists, nurses, a physical therapist, occupational therapist, rehabilitation counselor, social worker, and two secretaries was formed to implement the family research program. The research team provides family and patient assessments, counseling, education and training beyond the standard operating procedures of the hospital. The research team is an adjunct to the regular hospital staff and is not designed to replace existing personnel. The focal point for the research team is the family and its influence on the patient's rehabilitation. Therefore, the team concentrates on the family and usually works with the patient when the family is present. Interactions between team members and patients without involving family members are designed to monitor changes in knowledge, attitudes or behaviors brought about by the routine hospital program for SCI.

All families agreeing to participate in the research program are scheduled for a family assessment within two weeks of the patient's initial admission to the Warm Springs Hospital. This assessment, or Session I, occurs during a two-day residency at the hospital. A wheelchair accessible cottage has been secured for family use during their research related visits. The cot-

Table 1.   SCI programmed teaching modules

Medical	Psycho/Social
Prevention of respiratory infections	Dependence vs. independence
Medications	Communications
Kidney and bladder stones	Reactive patterns in families
Autonomic dysreflexia	Developmental stages in SCI
Irrigation of catheters	Defense mechanisms
External catheters	Roles and role expectations
Skin care	Community resources
Diet and fluids	Basic human needs
Foot care	
Urinary drainage units	
Bowel management	

Physical/occupational therapy	Vocational rehabilitation
Body positioning	Consumer knowledge
Care of orthotics	Avocational activities
Range of motion exercises	Basic work habits
Transfers	Getting a job
Functional clothing	Holding a job
	Personal grooming
	Appropriate dress

tage has four bedrooms, a kitchen, two bathrooms, and a large living room area. Utilizing the cottage allows the family to establish routines and patterns typical of the home environment. This affords the research team the opportunity to evaluate family interactions and establish base line data.

There are three facets to the initial family assessment: a) knowledge and information; b) practices or behaviors; and c) family attitudes. To determine the family's information and knowledge of spinal cord injury, the research team uses structured interviews and check lists. Critical information needed by families with SCI was identified by the staff based on literature reviews, experience and pilot study research. Programmed teaching modules were developed for each of these areas (Table 1). The interviews and check lists are used to determine the family's functional level of information concerning these critical areas.

During the behavioral segment of the family assessment, the families are queried about the family routine and practices particularly as they relate to the patient. If the patient has been home prior to his admission to GWSH, the team develops a profile of interactions and behaviors exhibited by the patient and family during his stay with them. For those families with no post injury at-home experience with the patient, family routine and behaviors are identified and the family is asked to project how these behaviors will change once the patient returns home. Families are given problem situations or discussion topics, video taped, and behaviorally analyzed using a behavior coding system for the video tapes.

The third facet of family assessment identifies significant family attitudes from a psycho-social perspective. This includes family role assignments and assumptions, identification of the family myth system, the family power structure, the family's evolution in the adjustment to disability process, and attitudes of family members towards the patient, each other, work and disability. To identify the significant family attitudes, the research team used videotape analysis of family interactions, interviews, psycho and sociometric testing, and rating scales. Only minimal information is given to families during Session I. It is a phase for establishing rapport, collecting data, module pretesting and gaining insights into the family's dynamics and adjustment.

Upon completion of Session I, the research team meets to review their findings. A family profile is developed depicting the family's functional status in information, behavior and attitudes. After this profile is developed, the statistician reveals which families are experimental and which are control. Assignment to these groups occurs when the families agree to participate in the research program and is based on a table of random numbers to reduce the probabilities of a biased distribution.

Research modules needed by the experimental families are identified during further staffing by the team. A complete program for each experimental family is developed and the family is scheduled for Session II as soon as is medically feasible for the patient's participation in the program. Following identification as a control group, interactions by research team members with control families is limited to periodic re-assessment.

During Session II, experimental families receive three to five days of the counseling, education and training modules. The modules focus on four criterion areas: medical, social, psychological and vocational. Each module has a pre and post-test component for evaluation and immediate feedback.

Team members have functioned individually and collectively to present the Session II program without significant major differences in family responses. However, the most effective method to date has been a male-female diad, particularly with the psycho-social modules.

Whenever possible, the patient lives with the family in the cottage for the duration of Session II. Each family is encouraged to develop a living situation approximating their home environment. They generally establish home routines despite intermittent observation by team members which enables the researchers to observe problem areas, problem solving skills, role changes and patient reintegration into the family nucleus in a more naturalistic setting. Observations are made during assigned modules and informal team contacts throughout the family residency. The research team is on call at any time should a family request their services. Many significant breakthroughs for families have occurred during weekend, late evening, or night encounters with the research team. Therefore, team members have to maintain flexibility in work hours and schedules to accommodate research families.

Within two weeks of a patient's projected discharge, the family returns for Session III. The third session is a two-day review, re-evaluation and problem-solving program. Between the second and third sessions, the family is encouraged to identify problems related to the patient's return home. Intervention strategies for problem resolution are explored by the family and research team. The team models appropriate problem-solving techniques and families are assisted in developing more effective approaches to problem solving. Session III emphasizes "hands on" experience for those responsible for primary patient care while stressing independence for patients as they return to their families and society.

The research team will continue to evaluate families with spinal cord injured following the patient's discharge from the hospital. Within six weeks of the discharge date, two team members will make the first home visit. For these visits one position is always allocated to a nurse and the other will be filled on rotating schedule between the various disciplines represented on the research team. It is the duty of the rehabilitation nurse to give a complete skin examination on this first visit and collect pertinent medical information relating to the research modules presented to the families. During the first follow-up visits both subjective and objective data is collected on the patient's family members, and interactions within the family constellation.

At six months post discharge and thereafter, at yearly intervals from the discharge date, families are visited for re-assessment and evaluation. Long range effects from the family intervention program of counseling, education and training are identified, tabulated and coded for analysis.

EMERGING TRENDS

While it is too soon to draw definitive conclusions from the study, some trends have emerged from the available data on families with SCI. Four major stages have been observed in patients adapting to spinal cord injury (Table 2). Average duration and behavior characteristics for each stage were established through psychometric evaluations and behavioral observations. As with most research describing patterns observed in human subjects, the duration and behavior characteristics described for each stage are typical for the "average" SCI patient. Where specific numbers are used, the mean or average value has been determined based on the best data available. In applying this system to any SCI patient one should always allow for the uniqueness of the individual and consider the pre-injury personality.

Table 2. Stages following spinal cord injury

Patient adaptation			Family adjustment	
Stage	Phase	Average time for occurrence	Stage	Phase

I. Anxiety	A. Fear
	B. Denial
	C. Bargaining
	D. Depression
	  1. Impotence
	  2. Anger
		0–9 months post injury	I. Anxiety	A. Fear
				B. Denial
				C. Depression-anger turned inward
				D. Mourning

II. Accommodation	A. Mourning B. Resignation C. Compromise	10–24 months post injury	II. Accommodation	A. Compromise B. Reconstruction
III. Assimilation	A. Reconstruction B. Integration C. Acceptance	25 months to life	III. Assimilation	A. Reintegration B. Acceptance
IV. Reflux	A return to a former stage caused by a physical, psychological, social or economic trauma	Anytime		

The SCI patients were intrinsically motivated to proceed from one stage to another. The time required for this process depended primarily upon individual flexibility, the supportive services available to the patient, and the innate ability to modify oneself. Therefore, the term, adaptation, was selected to describe the process of change rather than adjustment which denotes the use of skill or judgment to bring things into proper relation. The proposed SCI adaptation process is similar to general coping patterns presented by DiMichael (1969), Kubler-Ross (1975) and Meuller (1967). It has been presented to professional, paraprofessional and lay groups involved with SCI at the Roosevelt-Warm Springs Rehabilitation Center and to rehabilitation counselors attending the Georgia Rehabilitation Association State Conference and APGA National Conference (1978). The process has been particularly beneficial during in-service education for rehabilitation and allied health professionals, counseling with families participating in the spinal cord injured research project, and orientation programs for researchers investigating the impact of spinal cord injury. The use of this model has facilitated staff communications, patient/family education, and programming within the rehabilitation center by providing a consistent frame of reference for the patient's progress.

STAGE I

The adaptation process is a lengthy one, often requiring two or more years for completion of the first two stages. Stage I, which lasts approximately nine months, has been labeled as the Anxiety stage. During this stage, marked variations in anxiety test scores occur (Figure 1). State, transitory but current, anxiety levels are initially higher for quadriplegics than for paraplegics.

This may reflect the greater threat to life associated with a higher level spinal cord lesion. SCI with cervical injuries display a noticeable decrease in anxiety from the third to the sixth month. Many appear to resign themselves to a fate often referred to as existing, but not really living, and rapidly become depressed.

Paraplegics with thoracic (T) and lumbar (L) injuries continually increase in state anxiety until approximately the sixth month. This continued increase in anxiety may be related to the level of expectation presented to the paraplegics by the allied rehabilitation team. The general concensus, based on the team's actions, is that paraplegics should be expected to do almost as much as a non-injured counterpart. Therefore, the program for these patients is often more physically intense during the initial phases of rehabilitation. Since greater expectations are placed on the patients, higher levels of anxiety occur. This differentiation, based on level in injury, is usually a hidden agenda for the rehabilitation team and few members appear

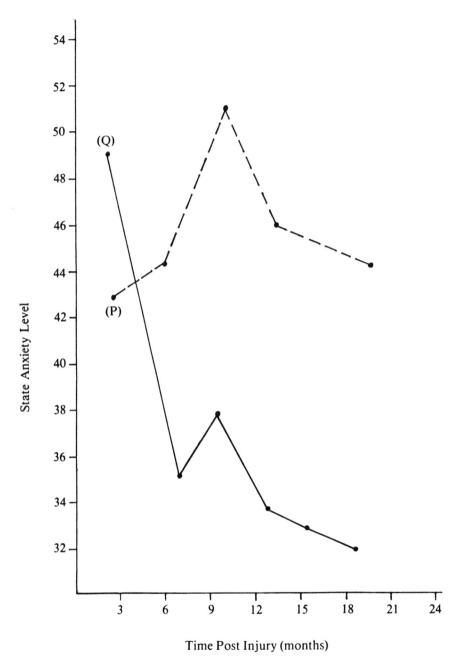

Figure 1.   Group Mean State Anxiety Scores for 120 SCI using the STATE-TRAIT Anxiety Inventory. Solid line, Quadraplegia; broken line, Paraplegia.

consciously aware of its role as they develop comprehensive plans for the patient's rehabilitation.

While differences between quadriplegics and paraplegics do occur in the onset and duration of stages in the adaptation process most major behaviors associated with a particular stage manifest themselves at approximately the same time for both groups.

Fear

Four phases occur during the *anxiety* stage. Fear is the first phase and initial reaction to severe injury. For most SCI this is the first confrontation with their own mortality. They are fearful of dying and want reassurance that they will live. The patient's fear manifests itself through an obsession with details; the patient is demanding and requires the constant presence of staff and family members for reassurance. These intense feelings of fear usually subside by the end of the first month, but a residual often remains as unresolved conflict, leading to free-floating anxieties and retarding the adaptation process.

Denial

Denial is the second phase experienced by the SCI patient. During this phase, the patient is aloof, often pseudo-optimistic, and independent. They use selective perception with great skill and seek those who reinforce their own beliefs. The denying patient is hostile, stubborn, and unreasonable. They perceive little benefit to be gained by complicated and annoying therapy or counseling since they are not as seriously involved as has been reported to them.

Denial is often reinforced by family members who experience most of the same stages as the injured person (Bray, 1977). Thus, the Denial stage is doubly difficult for an allied health and rehabilitation team. The patient should experience information consistency from all team members and a constant but low key reality orientation. The denial phase can be characterized by an ability to acknowledge the severity of the spinal cord injury.

Bargaining

Following denial, the SCI progresses to the third phase, *bargaining*. While in this phase, the patient will acknowledge that the injury is significant or even devastating, but often feels a remarkable recovery is taking place or complete restoration is inevitable. Many patients report religious or mystical experiences which indicate the time or place for recovery. Patients in Bargaining often exhibit long-suffering and conciliatory behaviors which reflect conditions of their restitution agreement (bargain).

Family and staff members find bargaining to be a pleasant respite since the patient is usually so cooperative and agreeable. They often succumb to a false sense of well being and may ignore signs of the acute stress evolving within the patient. During this pseudo-optimistic phase, many patients will be referred for vocational rehabilitation services since they appear to be doing so well. The VR counselor should be wary of any joint plans and programs developed in conjunction with the patient during this phase.

The staff working with a patient in Bargaining should orient the patient to functioning in a here-and-now mode. Statements such as, "Yes, you believe you are going to get complete return, but do what you can today and, if you get more return, we will work with that when it occurs," often encourage a patient to function within existing parameters of ability. Again, the positive change in Bargaining is, at last, an acknowledgement of severe injury.

Depression

The most acknowledged phase in the adaptation process is *depression*. During a two year period at Warm Springs, fifty-four percent of psychological referrals for SCI related to depression. Depression is operationally defined as impotent anger, but most SCI characteristically express their depression as either impotence or anger. The impotent type depression is quickly identified by both family and staff as classical depression. However, the angry depressed person is often labeled as non-cooperative or low in motivation by the staff and is simply confusing to a hurt and bewildered family.

Impotent

The impotent type depressed SCI is characterized by withdrawal, low motivation, manipulation, and passive-aggressive behaviors. They are overwhelmed by the magnitude of their injury and feel hopeless to cope with it. Many patients become self-destructive, and a greater frequency of decubitus ulcers is felt to occur during the Impotent Depression phase.

Anger

Another manifestation of depression is *anger*. These patients are overtly aggressive and hostile. They lash out at those closest to them, particularly family members. Angry depressed patients often move from one physical location to another as they quickly exhaust their welcome. Families soon search for placement alternatives, such as nursing homes, hospitals, evaluation or training centers. These patients feel hapless and see no positive future. They are critical of everyone around them, and the alienation they bring upon themselves reinforces their negative self-concept. Many patients accepted for vocational rehabilitation services during the subsequent phase of Depression due to a lack of motivation, non-cooperation or non-feasibility due to psychological factors.

STAGE II

The second stage in the adaptation to SCI process is *accommodation*. It is a time for reconciliation of differences, a realization of change within one's life style. The Accommodation stage lasts approximately fourteen months and is divided into three phases.

Mourning

Near the first anniversary of their injury, most patients experience the phase of mourning. The majority will have returned home and the reality of life with its myriad problems will slowly have emerged into the consciousness. Activities of daily life force the patient to acknowledge changes that have occurred because of the injury. At this confrontation with reality, the patient begins to mourn. Mourning patients prefer solitude and minimal activity. They should be encouraged to express their feelings of loss and sorrow. Mourning should be viewed as a positive process, and frequent opportunities should be provided to explore and express grief. Mourning is target-specific, that is, identifiable situations, hopes, aspirations, relationships, or goals are mourned individually as well as collectively. This phase should not be confused with impotent depression which is characterized by a nebulous, undifferentiated, helpless malaise.

Resignation

As the patient is able to mourn and release aspects of pre-injury life, stress is reduced and the phase of *resignation* occurs. During this phase patients are submissive, passive and repress most feelings. They yield to authority, are rather docile, and exhibit a purposelessness in behavior. They simply exist. Patients in this phase have released the old life style but have not established a new orientation to fill the void left by abandoned plans, goals, hopes and aspirations. These patients often express a general confusion and lack of meaning in their lives.

Compromise

Little internal impetus for change is produced during the resignation phase; however, near the end of the second year external pressures provide sufficient stress to produce an alternation in life styles. Many families have reached the limit of endurance and force the patient to explore more independent behaviors. Third party payee's and social agencies have exhausted most resources by this time and the patient must live with minimal supplementation or seek other support systems. As a result of these external stresses, the person moves into the Compromise phase. During the *compromise* phase the patient experiences strong competitive feelings. They perform "in spite of" their disability.

The patient in *compromise* makes concessions to the non-injured world but expects demands dictated by his disability to be met by general society. It is the most militant phase in the adaptation process. Since the patient in Compromise is assertive and involved with society once again, many members of the allied health and rehabilitation team view rehabilitation as complete. However, in terminating the process at this point, many patients are not assisted through the most personally rewarding stage.

STAGE III

Beginning the third year post-injury for an SCI is significant in many ways. Almost all physical return of sensation and motor control which will occur has taken place by the end of the second year. The fear of death has diminished to near pre-injury levels, and the psychological moment exists for the most intensive personal growth in the adaptation process. Stage III, *assimilation,* begins near the twenty-fifth month and continues for a lifetime. Assimilation is a stage for cultural incorporation of the SCI into an expanding society and the emerging of a new, personal gestalt for each SCI. It is a time of growth, challenge, and change which emerges in three phases.

Reconstruction

Reconstruction is the first phase of assimilation. It is a time for self-analysis, searching for meaning in life, and identifying components and behaviors which need changing. It is a dynamic, explorational process, and the most propitious phase for vocational evaluation. This phase can last from a few intense months to several years, depending upon the assistance available to the SCI.

Integration

Integration follows reconstruction and builds upon the direction developed during the intense personal evaluation. During integration, goals are identified, objectives and strategies implemented, and a marshalling of all personal reserves occurs in order to establish a life style deemed most appropriate by each individual. During this phase, the SCI feels constructive and positive. They initiate social and personal contacts where before they waited for others to initiate most relationships. They no longer view themselves as spinal cord injured people but rather as people with spinal cord injuries.

Acceptance

The final phase is *acceptance.* It can be compared to Maslow's self actualization. People with spinal cord injuries with the same feelings of value and worth experienced by all people, struggle to achieve the illusive prize of the totally "together" person. For the individual with SCI, as for all mankind, it is a struggle that separates.

STAGE IV

Perhaps the most devastating factor for the SCI in the adaptation process is the fourth stage, *reflux*. Reflux, a regression to an earlier stage, is not experienced by all patients but can occur at any time. It usually occurs as a result of serious physical (bladder infections, decubitus, impotence, etc.), emotional (divorce, separation, death, etc.), or financial insult.

When an SCI reverts to an earlier stage, he once again experiences each of the sequential stages before completing the adaptation process. The time for each intervening stage or phase is compressed, but each step is usually repeated in sequence before the person returns to the developmental level attained prior to the regression. Intensive counseling facilitates a rapid recovery and yields a much improved prognosis over patient isolation and self-initiated attempts at insight.

The SCI adaptation stages are not envisioned as mutually exclusive. Interfaces occur between the stages and the entire process is inalterably affected by the pre-morbid personality. However, a global assessment of the patient's status in the adaptation process should enhance program development and successful service delivery.

To determine the applicability of the SCI adaptation stages to program development, a review was conducted of all SCI enrolled in evaluation and training programs at the Warm Springs Rehabilitation Center during 1976 (Table 3). Sixty-two SCI entered evaluation/training (E/T) programs.

Based on the SCI adaptation stages, it was hypothesized that SCI patients injured less than one year would not be as successful in completing E/T programs as patients injured longer than one year, 17 or 68 percent did not complete E/T. The most frequent reason given for termination was low motivation or psychologically related problems. Less than half, 46 percent, of the patients more than one year post injury failed to complete an E/T programming. Medical complications and physical limitations were most frequently cited for early termination by these clients. A chi square analysis of the data indicates significant differences exist at the 0.09 level (Table 3). It is felt that with an increased sample size statistical significance should approach the 0.05 level; however, the 0.09 level has practical significance of its own.

One reason for our limited rehabilitation success with the SCI may be our attempt to enter the client into evaluation or training before he has had sufficient time to adapt to spinal cord injury. Based on interviews with rehabilitation counselors, many clients may be closed non-feasible only to return two or three years post injury with a sincere desire for vocational evaluation, training, placement or related services. Perhaps counselors should consider expending more time in counseling with SCI during the first year

Table 3.   SCI clients scheduled for vocational evaluation and/or training (E/T)

Time from injury to entry E/T	Clients completing E/T programs	Clients not completing E/T programs	Both
<1 year	8	17	25
>1 year	20	17	37
Totals	28	34	62

$X^2 = 2.94$* (* significant at the 0.09 level)

post injury and save the bulk of financial aid, wherever possible, for the later stages when the client is developmentally ready to challenge vocationally oriented tasks.

The preliminary findings from this research project indicate increased rehabilitation success with the SCI will depend upon a better understanding of the adaptation process following SCI and more effective use of resources available to rehabilitation counselors and their clients. At the conclusion of the project, a complete modular system of family intervention should have evolved with adequate documentation of its effectiveness and applicability for other rehabilitation settings. Hopefully, a more effective program for assisting people with spinal cord injuries in their struggle for comprehensive rehabilitation will emerge with benefits to the injured, their families and our society.

REFERENCES

Bray, G. P. Reactive patterns in families of the severely disabled. *Rehabilitation Counseling Bulletin,* 1977, *20*(3), 236–239.

Davies, A., & Hansen, R. A family focus program. *Family Process,* 1974, *13,* 487–488.

DiMichael, S. *The current scene in vocational rehabilitation of the disabled: An overview.* New York: New York University Press, 1971.

Hamilton, L. S., Muthard, J. E., & Turner, L. A. *Spinal cord injury in Florida: A pilot study.* Gainesville: University of Florida Rehabilitation Institute, 1974.

Kubler-Ross, E. *The final stage of growth.* Englewood-Cliffs, N.J.: Prentice-Hall, 1975.

Meuller, A. Psychological factors in rehabilitation of paraplegic patients. *Archives of Physical Medicine,* 1967, *43,* 151–159.

Nau, L. *Family rehabilitation: Viable human service delivery approach.* Paper presented at the American Psychological Association, Montreal, August, 1973.

Overs, R. P., & Healy, J. R. *Educating stroke patient families* (Vols. I, II, III). Final Report. SRS Grant RD 2537-P. Milwaukee, Wisc.: Curative Workshop of Milwaukee, July, 1971.

Poor, C. R. Vocational rehabilitation of persons with spinal cord injuries. *Rehabilitation Counseling Bulletin,* 1975, *18*(4), 264–271.

Rusk, H. A. *Specialized placement of quadraplegics and other severely disabled.* New York: Institute of Rehabilitation Medicine, New York University Medical Center, 1963.

Smart, C. N., & Sanders, C. R. *The cost of motor vehicle related spinal cord injuries.* Washington, D.C.: Insurance Institute for Highway Safety, 1976.

Young, J. S. *The cost of spinal cord injury.* Extracted from 1972 Grant Progress Report, SRS Grant 3367-M-70. Phoenix, Ar.: Southwest Regional System for Treatment of Spinal Injury, Good Samaritan Hospital.

FAMILY RESPONSE TO TRAUMATIC HEAD INJURY

Mary D. Romano[1]

From 1968 through 1972, we had occasion to closely observe the responses of thirteen families to traumatic head injuries incurred by individual members of their family units, as described in Table 1: these thirteen families include every traumatic head injury patient admitted to the Adult Rehabilitation Unit at the University of Michigan Medical Center within the period from May 1968 to June 1972. The length of contact varied, based on several factors: one patient was eventually institutionalized in a state mental hospital which precluded our followup; two patients sought ongoing care closer to their places of residence; and three patients were "lost" to followup when they or their families did not keep appointments. Our contacts with the remaining seven patients and their families extended from the point of inpatient admission through July 1972, i.e., periods ranging from seven months to slightly more than four years.

In all cases, the initial traumatic insult was followed by coma out of which the patients gradually moved, first to deep pain responsiveness and later to varying degrees of recovery albeit with physical and mental changes from their pretraumatic selves. The physical sequelae ranged from mild hemiparesis to profound hemiplegia; in one instance, there was a residual expressive aphasia. The mental sequelae ranged from a superficially inconspicuous affective euphoria with impairment in social judgement to marked impairments of old and recent memory, poor attention span, lack of impulse control, verbal perseveration, inappropriate affect, difficulties with voice modulation, and the absence of appropriate social judgement. In all cases, onset was sudden, with no prior warning. And, in all cases, patients' families had their first contact with the hospital social worker only after the patients were clearly past the point of possible demise, i.e., body processes had stabilized, and patients were showing some responsiveness to external stimuli.

What we saw, then, were families who had without preparation been informed that a loved one had been critically injured and might die. The families had found their injured members laid out in the very threatening intensive care situation, and the threat of the milieu itself was magnified by

Reprinted from *Scandinavian Rehabilitation Medicine 6*, pp. 1–4, ©1974, with permission.

[1]From the Social Service Department, Presbyterian Hospital, New York City, NY.

Table 1. Description of population

Sex	Age	Marital status	Etiology of injury Date of onset	Occupation at time of onset	Socioeconomic status of family
F	20	Single	Automobile (driver) 5/71	Factory worker	Blue collar, lower class
M	19	Single	Automobile (passenger) 12/70	University student	White collar, middle class
F	14	Single	Automobile (pedestrian) 4/68	Student	Blue collar, middle class
F	19	Single	Automobile (driver) 12/71	University student	Blue collar, middle class
M	18	Single	Automobile (pedestrian) 6/71	University student	White collar, middle class
F	18	Single	Automobile (driver) 3/70	Student	White collar, middle class
M	18	Single	Automobile (passenger) 8/70	University student	White collar, middle class
M	51	Married	Automobile (driver) 12/68	Gas station attend.	Blue collar, lower class
M	39	Married	Automobile (driver) 12/68	Telephone repair	Blue collar, middle class
F	24	Married	Automobile (driver) 12/69	Factory worker/ housewife	Blue collar, lower class
F	20	Single	Automobile (passenger) 1/72	Factory worker	Blue collar, middle class
F	34	Married	Automobile (driver) 3/68	Beautician/housewife	Blue collar, middle class
M	56	Married	Fall 8/69	Construction foreman	Blue collar, lower class

the gross unresponsiveness of the injured patients. Faced with this massive shock of seeing a family member quite healthy one minute and essentially "living dead" the next, all of these families responded with the understandable and expected denial: "Oh no, this cannot be true" as they were confronted with the possible loss of a significant other.

Ordinarily we would expect people facing such loss to deny it at first, but over time, we might also expect the denial to give way to anger ("It is not fair that this happened"), to bargaining for undoing ("If only this had not happened, then..."), and to grief for what has been lost. Such responses to loss have been clearly documented in the literature, by Kubler-Ross (1969), Garrett and Levine (1962), Crocker and Cullinane (1972), Goff (1970), and Schoenberg, Carr, Peretz, and Kutscher (1970) among others, in relation to other life-threatening illnesses, functional losses, loss of parents through death and/or divorce, etc. In the literature regarding responses of parents to premature birth or to the birth of children with anomalies, there are somewhat analogous responses to the critical events, as described by Kaplan and Mason (1966), Rapoport (1966), and other observers.

In our contacts with these families of head injured patients, however, we found relatively negligible movement past denial into anger, bargaining, or mourning losses, even when trained counseling help was available and even when families were engaged in family or group counseling processes. This very persistent family denial was manifest in several trends:

A. *Common fantasies* Regardless of the educational and socioeconomic levels of the families observed, several common fantasies predominated in family thinking about the patient. The most common of these involved sleep and was most typically verbalized by a father who said, "He is really sleeping now, but one day he will wake up and say, 'Hi Dad' ". It should be noted that the persistence of this sleep notion endured long past the point at which the patients had emerged from coma; in other words, the patients were in fact quite awake and at least responsive to some degree, but they were different personalities from their pretraumatic states. Similarly, families tended to fantasize the presence of measureable improvement when none had actually occurred, e.g., perceiving spasticity as voluntary movement. And there were a number of fantasies around the concept of will, such as, "She will get well because, after all, she has three children, so she must get well."

B. *Verbal refusals* Again typical of nearly all the families observed were continued verbal refusals, or denials, that these patients were any different than they had been prior to their injuries. While it seemed nearly inconceivable to hospital staff that families could deny the presence of the very obvious physical, mental, and behavioral changes of their injured family members, it was strikingly common to hear these families say, "He always did have a temper" or "His table manners never were too good" in the face of post-traumatic temper tantrums or food-smearing. We also observed families who allowed themselves to recognize one area of limitation, usually involving physical function, while maintaining denial of other limitations, typically those of mental functioning. Thus, for example, families might focus on patients' recovery of the ability to ambulate independently, each day asking us, "Is she walking yet?", without cognizance that, while walking might be physically possible for the patient, the patient's judgement was so impaired that (s)he could not perceive dangerous situations and might walk right into one. In a few instances, a family's skewed perceptions led them to allow the patient not only to endanger himself but the public-at-large, as when one father encouraged his son to drive the family car on public roads despite the son's very poor impulse control, depth perception, and judgement.

C.   *Inappropriate responses*   Even as months passed post-injury, family needs to deny often remained so great that they were unable to respond aptly to patient's needs, capacities, or behaviors. Limit-setting on expression of impulses, be they sexual or angry, was many times impossible for these families, apparently because a necessity for limits implied acceptance of disability where previously there had been none. When staff, for instance, suggested supplying means of contraception for judgmentally impaired, nubile female patients, it was not uncommon for families to irately declare, "She would never do something like that!", only to face out-of-wedlock pregnancies in patients within months after discharge. Similarly, in the face of patients' temper tantrums or other aggression, the most that many of these families could allow themselves in response was anxious laughter; they did not seem able to allow themselves to verbally or physically (when necessary) restrain the patient. Family inability to evaluate a patient's capacities realistically resulted in a broad range of overexpectations of the patient, in which families insisted that patients' life plans be resumed even when patients could no longer successfully function even in approximations of their old ways. Young adults were sent back to college despite shortened attention spans, impaired memories, limitations in ability to abstract, etc., and mothers were placed in positions of being responsible for households and young children when their tools to manage their responsibilities had been damaged.

For several of the families observed, there appeared to be marked anger used in the service of maintaining their denial and resulting in maladaptive responses not so much to patients but to hospital staff. Relatively few of these families could actually verbalize this anger toward the staff, usually through direct demands that they not be informed about the patients' conditions unless prognostication could be synonomous with total recovery, e.g., "We do not want to talk to you unless you tell us that he will be his old self, just as he was before this accident." More often, family anger of this sort took the forms of expressed belief that the staff was withholding positive information from them maliciously, by signing the injured family member out of the hospital against medical advice, by "shopping" from doctor to doctor in hopes of being told what they wanted to hear, or by sabotaging the injured family member's hospital program in conscious defiance of hospital staff.

It was our impression that the persistence of this denial in these families had grave repercussions both for the functioning of the families over time and for the patients themselves. For such families to live in denial of reality, even such a painful one, over a protracted period, it seemed that certain compromises in daily living became necessary; often family life became centered around the injured family member, defending his normalcy to society and consensually validating his normalcy among family members. This was frequently accompanied by a decrease in contacts with non-family members and, at times, by manifestations of emotional disturbance in those family members who might have moved to the point of relinquishing some of their denial. A poignant example of this involved a family where the patient's mother began to move out of the denial; the patient's father was unable to tolerate what he perceived as his wife's defection, and the ensuing marital conflict was great enough that the patient's mother again retreated into cheerful denial in order to preserve the marital relationship, joining the father in walling off the family from the outside world.

For the patient himself, family denial can serve well to maintain his own propensity to see himself as unchanged from his pretraumatic self. More problematic, however, are the situations in which patients are more able to see their own limitations than are their families. Receiving the family message of "you have to be fine" while themselves recognizing that they are not fine, these patients often feel that family love is irreparably lost from them as they are, and they experience a depression related not just to their physical and mental losses but to the loss of family acceptance as well. Often, however, the family prohibits its injured member from revealing any recognition of disability and attendant feelings, and this inability of the family to allow the patient to see himself realistically seems most commonly to result in at least some degree of denial within the patient of himself except as he was prior to injury.

Certainly the prevalence of denial in these families has a profound effect upon both in-hospital and societal rehabilitation of the traumatic head injury patient. If the families cannot accept even a most supportive confrontation with reality during the injured members' hospitalizations, then there seems to be even less likelihood of their becoming able to tolerate the confrontations between their denial and the community which sees the patient's physical and mental limitations as making him "different" indeed. Perhaps, threatened as communities may be at seeing physical handicaps, it is even more threatening to face the person who dresses peculiarly, cannot take full responsibility for his actions, and may act out impulsively, whose voice is not well-modulated, and whose manner moves quickly from euphoric to combative. Communities, in the face of this behavior, tend to demand the exclusion of the head injured individual from participation in usual community life, and this exclusion is seen as incomprehensible by the patient's family whose great need is to affirm and reaffirm the patient's normalcy. In our observation, most of the families tended to resolve this conflict by repeatedly insisting to the community that, if there were a problem, it lay in the community rather than in the patient, i.e., that it was the community that was abnormal, not the patient. Only three families resolved their conflicts by placing the individual outside the family unit, and in these cases, conflict within the family over the issue of denial remained after placement.

One can only conjecture, of course, as to why this phenomenon of long-term denial existed. Perhaps because each of the patients "awakened" once from coma, it was easy for families to continue to believe that they would wake up again; this would be fairly congruent with the "sleeping beauty" myth with which we are familiar from early magical thought. Perhaps, too, having had loved ones so close to death, with some of the anticipatory mourning inherent in that situation, families felt that they had to repudiate the mourning process, "to be glad just that he is alive", once the imminence of death had passed, even when the family member as he was pretraumatically was dead forever. And perhaps for these families, the fact of personality death, of the loss of those intangible factors that made each patient most human and individual to his family, is an even greater loss than body death, a loss so great that it is more than families ordinarily can bear.

REFERENCES

Crocker, A. C., & Cullinane, M. M. Families under stress: The diagnosis of Hurler's syndrome. *Postgraduate Medicine,* 1972, *51,* 223–229.
Garrett, J. F., & Levine, E. S. *Psychological practices with the physically disabled.* New York: Columbia University Press, 1962.
Goff, B. *Where is daddy?* Boston, Beacon Press, 1970.
Kaplan, D. M., & Mason, E. A. Maternal reactions to premature birth viewed as an acute emotional disorder. In H. J. Parad (Ed.), *Crisis intervention: Selected readings,* pp. 118–128. New York: Family Service Association of America, 1966.

Kubler-Ross, E. *On death and dying.* New York: Macmillan Publishing Co., 1969.

Rapoport, L. Working with families in crisis: An exploration in preventive intervention. In H. J. Parad (Ed.), *Crisis intervention: selected readings,* pp. 129–139. New York: Family Service Association of America, 1966.

Schoenberg, B., Carr, A. C., Peretz, D., & Kutscher, A. H. *Loss and grief.* New York: Columbia University Press, 1970.

PATIENTS WITH PROGRESSIVE NEUROLOGICAL DISEASES

Gladys Lambert[1]

> Sometimes it is not until residual impairments develop that the full implications of an incurable, debilitating disease become an emotional reality

Unlike the patient with an acute but transient illness, the patient with a progressive neurological disease is faced with an incurable, debilitating illness that may eventually lead to total physical dependency and a shortened life span. The long, slow, course of the disease causes overpowering anxiety in both the patient and his family, especially in those instances where other family members have had the same disease or where the patient knows other persons with the same diagnosis whose condition is more advanced than his. The dread of, and then the horror of, being unable to walk, feed oneself, get out of bed, and take care of one's toilet needs has been graphically described by articulate patients (Travis, 1966). As the patient becomes increasingly helpless and disabled, he and his family are called upon to make new and difficult emotional adjustments that frequently require social work intervention.

Progressive neurological diseases, which affect the brain and spinal cord, are primarily of unknown etiology. They vary in onset from early childhood and middle age to the later years of life. Multiple sclerosis, Parkinson's disease, and Huntington's chorea, a hereditary disease, are common in this group. Although symptoms vary with each disease, some fairly typical ones include involuntary irregular movements of the face, head, and hands; transient paralysis and weakness of extremities; instability of gait; and numbness and loss of sensation in various parts of the body.

BASIC CONSIDERATIONS

The patient with a progressive neurological disease is confronted not only with the normal stresses of living but with the additional problems and limitations inherent in his illness. The adjustment he makes depends to a large extent on his previous level of social functioning, the nature of the illness and its meaning to him, the existence of significant others who rally around him and are available to help, and his access to concrete resources. These

Reprinted from *Social Casework,* March, pp. 154–159, ©1974, Family Service Association of America, with permission.

[1]Social worker, University of Rochester Medical Center, Rochester, NY.

factors, when applied to the patient, can provide the social worker with psychosocial diagnostic clues to the patient's coping potential and can serve as the basis for formulation of a treatment goal and plan.

The patient with a satisfactory life adjustment prior to illness is more likely to cope adequately than a person whose previous adjustment has been poor or at best marginal. In evaluating the preillness level of social functioning, consideration should be given to the nature of the patient's previous family and social relationships and the extent to which these have been sustained and positive. His performance in such roles as spouse, parent, and worker provides clues about previous adjustment.

The physical limitations of a progressive neurological disease invariably interfere with the patient's performance of his previous role responsibilities. In our culture the husband carries primary responsibility for providing the family income. When he is the patient, the family is threatened with a loss or reduction of income and frequently a lower standard of living. For many men, the role of provider is a source of both status and deep personal satisfaction. Having to relinquish this role can result in a loss of self-esteem, a feeling of inadequacy, and an accompanying depression. Such reactions are culturally reinforced by the value our society places on productivity, self-reliance, and physical strength, particularly for men.

The patient who is a wife and mother may find it increasingly difficult to handle responsibilities attached to these roles. If she is the mother of an infant or young child, she may be unable to lift him or otherwise minister to his physical needs. Housework may become increasingly difficult. However, the reaction of each patient to these limitations will depend on the meaning they hold for him. Jeanette R. Oppenheimer (1967) points out that some individuals and families gain new satisfactions in the patient role because it serves to meet long-existing but previously unfulfilled needs. For many patients, however, the reverse is true. In his role as a patient, the individual may expect to be considered helpless and deserving of sympathy and tender care; he may anticipate that others in the family will take on protective functions and attitudes. These actions and attitudes, however, do not always come spontaneously from family members, who are charged with his care while simultaneously being affected by his abdication of his customary role. They may resent the onerous duties placed on them and the patient's release from his own duties.

The patient's ability to cope can be greatly influenced by the support and encouragement of friends and family. If the patient is married and has relatives who can share some of the responsibilities of the overburdened spouse, the adverse repercussions of the illness on the marital relationship are often less excessive. However, the too-ready response by the family to the patient in his new role may create further problems for him as he experiences the loss of a role that had deep meaning; he may feel no longer needed or valued (Oppenheimer, 1967). When there are no family or friends, or the relationship is extremely poor, the patient may rely heavily on the social worker for help in coping with the problems confronting him.

The availability of resources in the community can alleviate some of the more concrete problems facing the patient and his family and allow time for long-range planning. These resources may include various programs—frequently financed through medical insurance and local welfare departments—that provide for physical care of the patient at home and care of young children in the family. Although such programs exist in many communities throughout the country and render valuable help, they do not adequately meet the needs of the patient with a progressive disease because the help offered tends to be time-limited whereas the patient's needs often are not. Commercial programs which do not have this built-in limitation are usually prohibitive in cost for most middle-income families. In addition to the need for long-term home care services, community respite programs would be invaluable in offering temporary physical and emotional relief for families from care-taking responsibilities. Unfortunately, many communities have not yet addressed themselves to the long-term needs of this patient group.

Sometimes the problem faced by the patient and his family is not a lack of access to concrete resources but rather a reluctance to accept what is available. Applying for social security disability benefits and other forms of assistance may symbolically represent an admission of disability and dependency which neither the patient nor his family is yet ready to face.

TREATMENT IMPLICATIONS

The social worker in a medical setting is in a particularly good vantage point to intervene and help the patient and his family begin to cope with emotional and social aspects of a progressive neurological disease and prevent family dysfunction. Because the patient frequently visits a clinic or hospital for treatment of his illness, he is accessible to the worker. For some persons it may be less threatening to accept help with psychosocial problems in a setting which has medical treatment as its primary function.

If the patient and his family are to be helped to cope with a progressive neurological disease, it is important that the social worker not be overwhelmed by the disease process itself and that he keep the medical diagnosis in its proper perspective. The diagnosis should be viewed as a source of clues to the possible areas in which the patient and his family may need help.

In treating the patient, it is essential that the social worker provide opportunity for him to express and clarify feelings about his illness. Those in his immediate environment, his family and friends, often feel threatened by such expression and may overtly and covertly prevent him from doing so. The expression of feelings can liberate emotional energy needed to cope with the changes and limitations in his life and lessen his need to displace anger and frustration onto family and the medical team. Irving N. Berlin (1956) notes that he has known a number of seriously handicapped neurological patients for whom the continued opportunity to express their feelings about their handicap, without an attendant show of anxiety, helplessness, and hopelessness from the therapist, has helped them to focus their attention on the realities imposed by their handicaps and to proceed to do what they could to earn their own livings, to be productive, and thus to be more satisfied with themselves and happier despite severe and incapacitating handicaps.

Since the patient's feelings are never completely resolved and often need to be dealt with during various stages in the progression of the illness, it is extremely important for the worker to be aware of his own feelings about the illness and to bring these under conscious control. Unless he is able to do so, he will be less prepared to help the patient with his feelings.

The patient's use of denial in coping with his illness, particularly when it is first diagnosed and during its early stage of progression, is fairly common and has been much discussed in the literature (Abram, 1969). Denial can serve a useful purpose and should not be questioned unless it interferes with the patient's treatment and makes it impossible for him to handle reality problems precipitated by his medical condition. The use of denial is a signal that the patient is not yet emotionally able to face his illness and all of its implications for him and his family. Each patient has his own timetable for acceptance.

CASE ILLUSTRATIONS

The following case summary illustrates early intervention of the social worker, initiated to help a patient with multiple sclerosis express and clarify feelings about his disability and begin to cope with his situation.

Multiple sclerosis generally afflicts the patient during the most productive years of his life, between the ages of twenty and forty. The fatty substance called myelin, which acts as a protective covering for the nerve fibers of the spinal cord and brain, disintegrates, thereby blocking and distorting nerve impulses which control speech, vision, movement, and balance. Although early symptoms may disappear, over the years they reappear in more severe forms, resulting in paralysis and often urinary and bowel incontinence.

Mr. B, aged thirty-four, married and father of five children aged seven years to twenty-one months, was referred to the hospital social worker by his physician because of Mr. B's concern about his family's income during his hospitalization. He was hospitalized following the onset of blurred vision and paralysis of limbs. The tentative diagnosis of multiple sclerosis was confirmed. Nine years earlier, he had experienced transient visual difficulty and at that time there was conflicting medical opinion as to whether he had multiple sclerosis. Mrs. B, a full-time housewife and former registered nurse, was expecting their sixth child. Two years earlier, when Mr. B accepted a research position with a pharmaceutical company, they had moved into a new community, leaving behind relatives and friends.

Mr. B was an intelligent, capable young man who took pride in his role as husband and provider for his family. Mrs. B derived gratification from her role of wife and mother. In the marital relationship, she appeared maternal and more dominant, with no desire to work outside the home.

The worker saw Mr. and Mrs. B during and after hospitalization to help them adjust to his illness and its repercussions on their life. There was periodic consultation with Mr. B's physician and the nursing staff regarding his medical condition, prognosis, extent of impairment, and capabilities. This information was essential to the worker in helping the B family plan realistically for the future. Mr. and Mrs. B were given the opportunity to express their feelings about Mr. B's illness. Mr. B reacted to his diagnosis with depression and verbalized fear of becoming dependent on "public charity." He expressed disapproval of disabled people he had known who lacked initiative and expected others to take care of their needs. Such feelings reflected his own conflict and anxiety about dependency.

After leaving the hospital, Mr. B returned to work for approximately eight weeks. However, a subsequent exacerbation of his condition, resulting in further weakness of limbs and unsteady gait, made it impossible for him to continue working. Although eligible for veteran's and social security benefits, he initially denounced each as charity and was only able to accept these sources of income when a representative of the Veteran's Administration pointed out that he should consider the needs of his family. The social worker, recognizing Mr. B's need to deny his dependency needs, supported his rationalization that he had decided to accept help only because of his concern about the needs of his family. The family was able to manage on a reduced income chiefly as a result of their ability to economize.

Mrs. B, faced with her husband's illness as well as her pregnancy, avoided discussion of her own dependency needs. Because of her nursing background and experience, she understood a great deal about Mr. B's illness. Although she generally used strong intellectual defenses, she expressed a sense of loss and anger toward Mr. B for permanently depriving her of some aspects of companionship which he had not fully gratified previously. She recalled her own fondness for dancing and her attempts to prod him into dancing with her. Now, because of his condition, there was little possibility that he would ever be able to dance.

Looking ahead to the future, Mrs. B expressed the philosophy of enjoying to the fullest each day spent with her family. She used casework help to handle reality problems resulting from Mr. B's illness. The worker responded at the level Mrs. B sought and gave her advice and guidance about procedures and requirements for social security benefits and temporary public assistance. Mrs. B expressed a sense of shame in having to accept the latter and needed an opportunity to discuss her feelings and receive support from the worker before proceeding with the application.

In anticipation of Mrs. B's confinement, the worker helped her to consider various alternatives for the care of the children, and she was able to ask a relative to help. Following Mr. B's discharge from the hospital, both partners experienced some difficulty adjusting to his presence at home all day. The noise of the children distressed him and he expressed his feeling that his wife was not strict enough with the children. She complained that he was underfoot frequently and began to explore possible outside activities which would take Mr. B out of the home for a portion of the day, since he was ambulatory with the aid of a cane. Mrs. B, who had a retarded brother, suggested Mr. B volunteer his services at a local center offering day care activities for retarded children. Mr. B became enthusiastic about the volunteer experience, and the worker encouraged him to discuss his role at the center, supported his involvement, and gave recognition for his contribution to the children at the center who needed his interest and help. When Mr. B again saw himself as a productive person and when his self-esteem increased, the couple's relationship also improved.

As this case illustrates, a progressive neurological disease has emotional implications, not only for the patient but for his family as well. Sometimes it is not until the patient develops residual impairments that the full implications of the illness become an emotional reality. Since all relationships contain some ambivalence, the negative, resentful feelings of the patient's spouse and other family members are bound to increase as the patient becomes increasingly helpless and dependent on their care. Because they recognize that the patient is not responsible for his condition, they often feel guilty about these feelings; they then may become rejecting or depressed and overprotective of the patient. By helping family members express their ambivalent feelings without responding in a judgmental way, the social worker can help them cope with their responsibilities in a way which is constructive for family and patient.

The patient's increasing helplessness may upset the previously established balance in the marital relationship. A frequent area of difficulty is the change in the patient's ability to meet the needs of his spouse. Highly vulnerable are those marriages in which the ill spouse had played a protective nurturing role toward a highly dependent spouse. The increasingly disabled spouse may also be unable to meet the sexual needs of his partner or to fulfill his own. The nature of the couple's companionship frequently undergoes a change. Some previously shared social and recreational activities may need to be modified or curtailed and other substitutes found.

The following case illustrates the role of the social worker in sustaining a couple during the acute and terminal stages of the wife's progressive illness and prolonged hospitalization.

Mrs. R, a thirty-one-year-old married woman, mother of six children ranging in age from twelve years to seventeen months, was hospitalized because of a severe exacerbation of multiple sclerosis. She was unable to walk or sit upright in a wheelchair. She could not feed, bathe, or dress herself and was incontinent. Mrs. R's condition had been originally diagnosed shortly after the birth of her youngest child. Since then she had been hospitalized for brief periods but had been able to resume her normal activities as wife and mother.

She was referred for help to the hospital social worker by a staff nurse because of the concern Mrs. R expressed regarding care and supervision of her children. Mr. R, a construction worker, had been at home recovering from a back injury but was now ready to return to work.

This was the second marriage for both Mr. and Mrs. R, whose first marriages had ended in divorce. The present marriage had been plagued by long-standing differences over disciplining the children, especially the three older ones who were born during Mrs. R's first marriage. She was extremely protective of them and saw Mr. R as too strict and rigid. The two children of Mr. R's first marriage lived with his ex-wife in another state. Despite this area of tension in their relationship, they had positive feelings for each other. They shared common goals, had middle-class aspirations, and were buying their own home.

The social worker explored with them various alternatives for the care and supervision of the children and helped obtain a homemaker from the county department of social services. Later, the three children of Mrs. R's first marriage went to stay with their paternal grandmother who lived nearby. When the homemaker was placed in the family, Mr. R returned to work. The worker maintained periodic contact with the county department of social services throughout the seven months of Mrs. R's hospitalization. There was a sharing of information regarding her condition and the family's adjustment to the homemaker.

Mr. R, a rather passive, dependent man, had relied on his wife to make decisions regarding the family, and he continued to do so, with her acquiescence. To the worker, he showed considerable sorrow over her illness and he expressed his dependency on his wife by complaining about the lack of comfort and care when the house was run by the homemaker. The worker recognized his longing to have Mrs. R recover and return home to him.

Mrs. R, an intelligent, determined woman, displaced her anxiety about her illness onto continuing anxiety about the children. Under the increasing stress of her condition, complicated by a pulmonary embolism, she became quite paranoid for several weeks. She suspected her husband of poisoning her, transmitting a venereal disease to her, and seducing her ten-year-old daughter. There was no evidence to substantiate these suspicions, which subsided once her condition improved.

There was a change in social workers when, after three months of hospitalization in the neurology division, Mrs. R was transferred to the rehabilitation unit. Although Mrs. R's illness resumed a downhill course with a poor prognosis, she was able to spend some weekends at home with her family. Before the weekend visits began, the worker visited the home to evaluate its adequacy and determine the kind of equipment Mrs. R would need.

Both partners continued to use denial and to express hope in coping with Mrs. R's poor prognosis. They formulated plans for their future together in anticipation of her recovery and return home. Mrs. R continued to focus on the needs of her children. She was concerned about the academic performance of the eight-year-old daughter of her first marriage who was in a classroom for emotionally disturbed children. The worker conferred with the school personnel and shared pertinent information about Mrs. R's condition, interpreting the needs of the family.

The worker consulted frequently with members of the rehabilitation team regarding the changes in Mrs. R's physical condition. Because there was no improvement in her ability to function, the worker began to help Mr. R to consider the chronic care needs of his wife. Because of his dependency on Mrs. R and because he saw placement as essentially an unloving act, he was insistent on taking her home when discharged. However, as her condition further deteriorated, the focus shifted to helping him face the imminent loss of his wife.

After Mrs. R's death, Mr. R came to see the worker and talked about his wife's death and the plans he had made for the care of the children, following consultation with the county department of social services. The children of Mrs. R's first marriage were to remain with their paternal grandmother. Two children of his marriage to Mrs. R were to live with his mother in another state and the remaining son, a first-grade pupil, would continue to live with him. He had arranged to have his cousin supervise the child while he worked.

SUMMARY

Because of the difficulties which patients with progressive neurological diseases and their families must face, they often need the help of a caseworker periodically during the course of the disease. The worker can help the family to cope with the members' ambivalent feelings about the patient while helping the patient to clarify his feelings and maintain a sense of self-worth and dignity. This task is exceedingly challenging in a society that places a high premium on self-reliance and productivity.

REFERENCES

Abram, H. S. Psychological responses to illness and hospitalization. *Psychosomatics,* 1969, *10,* 218–223.
Berlin, I. N. A review of some elements of neurology. II. *Journal of Social Casework,* 1956, *37,* 493–500.
Oppenheimer, J. R. Use of crisis intervention in casework with cancer patient and his family. *Social Work,* 1967, *12,* 48.
Travis, G. *Chronic disease and disability,* pp. 111–112. Berkeley, Cal.: University of California Press, 1966.

CHAPTER 7

TERMINAL ILLNESS AND THE FAMILY

Paul W. Power and Arthur E. Dell Orto

Terminal illness represents a devastating reality for both the afflicted person and the family. Individuals who are experiencing a life-ending disease usually show many strong emotions, such as shock, anger, helplessness, and a need for hope. Kubler-Ross (1969) and Giacquinta (1977) have documented the many emotional stages that people can go through during a terminal illness. The reactions of the family members can parallel those of the patient, because confronting terminality is generally just as difficult. Living with a family member who is suffering from a fatal illness frequently creates a crisis situation for family life. This chapter explores these traumas and some of the determinants of the family reaction, and indicates many of the ways that family members cope with a person who has a terminal disease.

DETERMINANTS OF FAMILY REACTION

There are many reasons why family members react as they do to the stress of a terminal illness, including the nature of the marital relationship, the family's characteristic way of dealing with stress, the nature and strength of the family's values and beliefs, and their ability to utilize effectively varied community supportive services. One of the strongest determinants is the reaction of the patient to the fatal illness, because often how the patient handles the disease decides how the family members will cope. For example, a person who continually remains angry and resentful can generate added tension among the family members. A demanding patient can arouse anger within the family.

The reaction of the family can also be gauged by the needs of the terminally ill person. Gammage, McMahon, and Shanahan (1976) believe that patients have the need to talk with someone about their feelings and fears,

273

to be listened to and acknowledged, to maintain self-worth and dignity, and to maintain some environmental control. Cassem (1974) refers to competence, concern, comfort, and communication when discussing the needs of the fatally ill person. Many families, because of poor communication patterns among family members or inadequate resources to deal with stress, may not respond to these patients' needs. A lack of response precipitates further emotional difficulty for the patient and consequently brings added tension for family life. For example, an adolescent child slowly dying of leukemia needs to feel that people care and are most anxious to communicate with him. If for some reason such attention is not given, the young person may become very angry and could show it by varied forms of acting out.

One of the strongest determinants of the family reaction revolves around the issue of disease-related information. If, as so often happens, family members maintain a conspiracy of silence between themselves and the ill person, much family tension usually results. Although most of the people involved with the patient will have confused feelings concerning the dying process and the person's eventual death, a neglect to alleviate this confusion will create added anxiety. Many patients and their families do not want to know the truth, but continual avoidance of learning the necessary facts related to the illness, and then not appropriately sharing such information with each other, generally prevents the family members from gaining necessary family support. If the health professional cooperates with the family in the conspiracy of silence, information that really belongs to the patient is withheld from him. Failure to provide the information to the patient's family also can lead to a decrease in the quality of their relationship in the time remaining, "since tensions and fears felt by the patient are not understood by those close to him" (Rakel, 1977, p. 375).

Consequently, if a family has the capacity to face a crisis as a unit, each member providing the other with support, comfort, and strength; if the parent-child relationship is characterized by respect and affection; and if a family can manage its difficulties appropriately, then the family will have stronger resources to cope with the trauma of terminal illness. On the other hand, if there are strained, alienated, fragile, or borderline marital adjustments, and if a terminally ill person has harbored feelings of rejection and hostility, then the family will usually have much more difficulty in handling fatal disease.

REACTION OF THE FAMILY

Depending upon the nature of the loss and many determining factors discussed previously in this chapter, the family members will show many reactions to the fatal disease of the patient. Their response usually begins with shock, a "why did this happen to us" feeling. Often the shock is replaced with a form of denial, a belief that the family member is not going to die. Denial of the diagnosis appears to be strongest in the first few weeks after the person has been informed about the illness (Cassem, 1974). Then denial may take many forms, such as the family members predicting that the patient is going to last much longer than statistics predict. Although they don't deny the nature of the illness, they deny the rate at which it is progressing. A common and more subtle way of denying occurs in those family members who remain ignorant of the patient's condition. Delay in making necessary family changes because of the medical condition of the ill person is a frequent behavioral form that denial takes. The most harmful manifestation of family denial is the well-known "conspiracy of silence." Cassem (1974) prefers to label it "deception," because those families who practice it tend to make heavy use of denial. Denial may become a necessary coping mechanism for many family members until they are able to marshall their own resources for adjustment to the trauma. However, when the denial becomes a deception or jeopardizes necessary family adjustments, then this obstacle should be broken down. At these times the family members will need some help in changing their attitude.

There is usually a trend for denial to decline as a person gets sicker and approaches death (Cassem, 1974). With anger, anxiety, and a feeling of helplessness, the family confronts the reality that the person is going to die. Grieving becomes more intense, sadness descends upon the family, and the family members need the opportunity to ventilate their feelings. Such ventilation allows the family to alleviate anger, guilt, fears, and resentment. Many families need to be reassured that these feelings are natural and that they are doing all that is possible for the person. Gammage et al. (1976) explain that it is even normal to desire the death of a loved one to occur soon to relieve the person's pain and suffering. If family members are able to express their emotions before death, acceptance is more easily facilitated.

When a family member is dying, the strength and resilience of family relationships are taxed severely. The stress is heightened when the dying process is prolonged. Arndt and Gruber (1977) report that the uncertainty about when death will occur leaves the family with the feeling of being in limbo, "enduring the strains of current hardships while attempting to prepare for painful changes, knowing neither when these changes will occur nor exactly what sequence of events to anticipate" (p. 42).

In living with the dying family member the family faces tasks that always are painful and sometimes make contradictory demands. While caring for the dying person, the family should continue to interact with the patient. This interaction is often emotionally difficult because of their own struggle to deal with the impending loss. Also, the total family is attempting to prepare for the final separation that death will bring and for a future without the family member.

As the family member slowly deteriorates, often fatigue and resentment increase within the family. New responsibilities must be assumed and economic pressures may also burden the family as expenses increase. Often, anger at the dying person and then the accompanying guilt only add to the family members' mounting frustration over demands that threaten to become intolerable. The family environment becomes even more tense if the patient and family cannot interact in an open, honest way. Strain is placed on family members when they must withhold knowledge of a poor prognosis from the patient. Orcutt (1977) believes that closure of communication is most frequently observed among families where there is the intense stress of dying. Closure tends to be linked with avoidance as the individual family member's mode of coping. Unfortunately, the dying member who supposedly does not know he is dying cannot participate in family planning and role reassignments, which causes him to feel alone. On the other hand, when the family members can interact in an open, honest manner, and have become accustomed to being sources of support to each other, the disease trauma is handled more appropriately. Many families become closer in this period of severe stress.

The reaction of the children to the dying family member depends upon their age, maturity, ability to comprehend and integrate the meaning of the illness, and the stability of family life. Many children, realizing that the family member is seriously ill, begin to feel abandoned, angry, and alone, and handle these feelings through varied forms of acting-out behavior. Behavioral problems may occur at school and home, or the child may spend an unwarranted amount of time away from the family with friends (Power, 1977).

When the dying family member is a child, usually the shock, denial, anxiety, grief, and fatigue are more acute. Death is generally unwelcomed under any circumstances, but the terminal illness of a young family member brings a distinctive depression and a unique form of grief. The depression has its foundation in an anger at seeing a young life being taken away. The particular relationship of the sibling for the ill child will be most important. The parents can harbor much resentment, and often project this anger onto health professionals. If the caring responsibilities for the ill child are extensive and very demanding, necessitating frequent absences of one of the parents from the home, then role responsibilities may have to be changed. This can create a burden for other family members, as well as being continually fatiguing to the principal caring person.

The grief in families with a dying child is typified by the pain of losing a life that has been enjoyed for so few years and the realization that possible future happiness with the remaining young person will never be. The family gradually feels helpless, because the members feel an overwhelming desire to do everything possible for the child but know that their efforts will never be enough. Hostile feelings are frequently mobilized in the parents, and such emotions may be related to feelings of guilt, futility, and helplessness.

Although certain reactions from the family can be highlighted, the response from the family members will still be unique. Each family has its own way of coping with a stressful situation. Some will confront the crisis whereas others will show, for as long as possible, avoidance behavior. Some will be able to discuss the medical event with each other in a frank, open way, whereas others will be too threatened either to learn necessary disease-related facts or to discuss them with the patient.

Knowing how the family reacts is important for the health professional, because such an understanding provides a focus for helping intervention.

HELP FOR THE FAMILY

A more detailed treatment of a model that can be utilized with families who face a terminal illness is discussed in Chapter 12. There are specific helping considerations for the family with a terminally ill patient. These factors center on two points: attending to the needs of the patient and providing the family during this crisis with a sense of competence, especially after the person has died.

Earlier in this chapter the needs of the patient were summarized under the words competence, concern, comfort, and communication (Cassem, 1974). The patient usually looks to the family for the fulfillment of these needs. Once the inevitability of death is recognized and accepted, the patient enters a stage of resignation and quiet expectation. It is the final adjustment in preparation for death, and a time when the greatest fear of the dying patient is that of suffering alone and deserted. Saunders (1976) sums up the needs of a dying patient with the words of one patient: "Watch with me." The readiness to listen and the personal caring contact are comforts that cannot be matched by modern medicine procedures. Hope is also necessary for the patient to limit the magnitude of despair. It is a hope conveyed by the family and health professionals that something unforeseen may occur. Even when death is near, the patient can hope for a measure of happiness during the time that remains.

Patients with a terminal disease need to feel they are still in control of their life as much as is possible, and family members can help them to maintain the freedom to make choices and assume responsibility over as many aspects of their existence as possible. The family can also help the ill family member to take care of financial business, or encourage him to complete a cherished project.

The family needs to maintain its sense of equilibrium. Wijnberg and Schwartz (1977) suggest two sets of tasks for family members during the experience of a dying family member. If they are achieved a sense of competence can perhaps be gained. One involves the family members helping the dying patient by their physical presence, by interpreting the patient's emotional reaction to the illness, and by giving the person a sense of self-respect from the conviction that they value him for what he has done or for his personal qualities. The other comprises helping the family members to cope with the disruption of their own personal life. To attain this goal much support can be provided to the family, such as feedback to the family members on how well they are doing under their burden and grief, mobilizing social networks, and helping the family members to maintain their other family responsibilities while still allowing them to meet the dying patient's needs.

The family may still need help after the death of the family member. In a protracted illness the family has already paid dearly emotionally, physically, mentally, and financially for many months. Having been convinced that the progression of the disease and the extent of the patient's disability invariably leads to death, they waited for the end. Now there is fatigue, and the family shows a need for emotional support and for someone who understands their loss. Recovery for the family members requires the strengthening of relationships with others who are also close and have a significant meaning in one's life. Often an increase in communication and involvement with these individuals compensates for what was lost. Recovery for the family also depends on the manner of death, the suddenness with which it occurs, the length of the illness before the death, the age of the deceased, the amount of suffering experienced by the patient, and the stability of the family.

CONCLUSION

The family has a necessary role to play in the care of the dying patient. Terminal illness is a family trauma whose burden can be lightened when the family members can gather their resources to provide comfort to the ill person and help this individual to achieve as much satisfaction as possible in the remaining days. Living with a terminal illness is a stressful time; perhaps the most appropriate intervention at this time is to help the family stay intact and to assist the members to ease their own grief.

The following articles in this chapter highlight a few of the relevant questions about the family and terminal illness. In describing a study in which the authors explored how the family changes in response to long-term illness, Pauline Cohen, Israel Dizenhuz, and Carolyn Winget report on how the terminal disease affected children. They emphasize the value of communication among family members and provide many suggestions for the health professional when the family communication is poor. Dr. Krant, Beiser, Adler, and Johnston's article explains an intervention therapy for helping the family cope with the events of the terminal period. It is a unique helping approach which takes the family as the central focus of need in the hospital system, both during terminal illness and after a death has occurred. All of the material presented in this chapter underlines the belief that the family can play a significant, supportive role in the care of the terminally ill.

REFERENCES

Arndt, H., & Gruber, M. Helping families cope with acute grief and anticipatory grief. In E. Prichard, J. Collard, B. Orcutt, A. Kutscher, I. Seeland, & N. Lefkowitz (Eds.), *Social work with the dying patient and the family,* pp. 38–48. New York: Columbia University Press, 1977.

Cassem, N. H. Care of the dying person. In *Concerning death: A practical guide for the living.* Boston: Beacon Press, 1974.

Gammage, S., McMahon, P., & Shanahan, P. Learning to cope with death. *The American Journal of Occupational Therapy,* 1976, *30,* 294–299.

Giacquinta, B. Helping families face the crisis of cancer. *American Journal of Nursing,* 1977, October, 1585–1588.

Kubler-Ross, E. *On death and dying.* New York: Macmillan Publishing Co., 1969.

Orcutt, B. Stress in family interaction when a member is dying. In E. Prichard, J. Collard, B. Orcutt, A. Kutscher, I. Seeland, & N. Lefkowitz (Eds.), *Social work with the dying patient and the family,* pp. 23–37. New York: Columbia University Press, 1977.

Power, P. Chronic illness and the family. *International Journal of Family Counseling,* 1977, *5,* 70–78.

Rakel, R. *Principles of family medicine.* Philadelphia: W. B. Saunders Co., 1977.

Saunders, C. Living with dying. *Man and Medicine,* 1976, *1,* 227.

Wijnberg, M., & Schwartz, M. Competence or crisis. In E. Prichard, J. Collard, B. Orcutt, A. Kutscher, I. Seeland, & N. Lefkowitz (Eds.), *Social work with the dying patient and the family,* pp. 97–112. New York: Columbia University Press, 1977.

FAMILY ADAPTATION TO TERMINAL ILLNESS AND DEATH OF A PARENT

Pauline Cohen,[1] *Israel M. Dizenhuz,*[2] *and Carolyn Winget*[3]

The experience of the staff of Cancer Family Care, a community-based agency providing counseling on nonmedical problems to families of advanced cancer patients, led to an interest in learning, in a more systematic way, the adaptive and maladaptive processes utilized by families.

This article describes a study jointly undertaken by the department of psychiatry at the University of Cincinnati Medical Center and Cancer Family Care. The purpose of the study, which was funded by the University of Cincinnati, was to increase knowledge regarding the effects of the chronic stress of catastrophic illness on middle-class families, in which a parent died of cancer. Staff members were particularly interested in learning more about the adjustment of children because they had observed a reluctance on the part of families to discuss with the children the seriousness of the parent's illness and impending death.

Because the loss of a parent can produce emotional problems for a child (Furman, 1974), it seemed important to learn more about how the prolonged illness and death of a parent affected children. It was hoped that with this knowledge more effective methods of intervention could be developed.

The prolonged illness of a parent means that certain role responsibilities can no longer be managed as they have been in the past. How changes are made will be influenced by the family pattern of functioning—how roles are defined, how tasks are assigned, the stage of family life, and the patterns of communication. More information is needed to determine the nature of the changes that occur, and what helps families to manage transition in ways that promote healthy postdeath restabilization.

Through the study, staff hoped to learn more about family changes in response to longterm illness and death at several nodal points: at the time of diagnosis; at the point where it was learned the patient was terminally ill; at death; and following death. Further, staff wished to learn what support sys-

Reprinted from *Social Casework,* April, pp. 223–228, ©1977, Family Service Association of America, with permission.

[1]Executive Director, Cancer Family Care, Inc., Cincinnati, OH.

[2]Associate Professor of Child Psychiatry, Department of Psychiatry, University of Cincinnati Medical Center, Cincinnati, OH.

[3]Senior research associate, Department of Psychiatry, University of Cincinnati Medical Center, Cincinnati, OH.

tems were utilized in managing these changes at each of the nodal points. Support systems were conceptualized as any individual or professional activity or institution which was of help to the family in coping. Support systems were classified as internal and external. A family utilizing internal support systems relied primarily on family structure. External support was viewed broadly to include extended family, neighbors, friends, professional caretakers, as well as community agencies and institutions.

The authors believed that future patients and families would benefit from this study, that it would provide information that would increase the effectiveness of support systems, and that it would provide knowledge that would be of help to professional people in their work with this population. This latter aspect was important because both surviving spouses and children who have lost their parents have been identified as vulnerable to physical and emotional breakdown (Murray-Parks, 1972; Furman, 1974).

THE STUDY POPULATION

The group surveyed were middle-class families who had received service from Cancer Family Care. These families are helped to work out coordinated home care plans for the patient. Originally, fifty families were to be included in the study, but in reviewing cases, three families had moved, two families had no surviving spouse, and in three families, the patient was still living.

The executive director of Cancer Family Care, sent a letter to the surviving spouse in forty-two families, describing the purpose of the study, inviting them to participate, and stressing that their participation would be helpful to other families faced with the terminal illness and death of a parent. The surviving spouse was prepared for a call from a research interviewer who was a social worker with a rich background in clinical practice. Of the forty-two families, twenty-nine agreed to be interviewed. Of the remainder, one was unable to be reached, two had moved from the area, one had died, and ten refused to participate. Of these ten, three were women and seven were men. All of the men who refused to participate had also resisted counseling. Two of the women had been ambivalent about their contact with the agency, and one had used service appropriately, but did not want to participate in the study because she thought it would upset the balance the family had achieved.

METHOD

Subsequent to the receipt of the letter, the research interviewer telephoned each surviving spouse. This telephone interview was planned as a bridge to preparing the family for the research interview. To this end, questions about the process of the study were answered, and its purpose was clarified. The telephone interview was also used for the mutual benefit of the parent and the interviewer, in that considerable fact sheet data and information about the family situation were obtained. Where possible, the family interview time was scheduled during this call. Most interviews were held during the late afternoon or evening to accommodate the family. Interviews with twenty-nine families were held. Seventeen were with surviving husbands, and twelve with surviving wives. Six parents were interviewed without children, the children being too young, at work, or away. Two parents explained that a child was unable to participate because of emotional factors.

Instruments for Data Collection

Four instruments were devised for data collection. *Form One* had largely to do with demographic and medical information. Completion of part of the first questionnaire had been effected during the telephone interview. Its major purpose was to secure data on the family composition, social economic position, and stability, as evidenced by continuity in significant patterns and changes in residence, employment, and financial adjustment. Family experiences with medical sources of support were sought, particularly experience in communicating with physicians.

Form Two supplied the interviewer with a semi-structured format for the family interview, and dealt with issues of family functioning at the nodal points of the crisis. In using the semi-structured family interview, the interviewer sought to clarify the ways in which the family functioned, the changes that occurred, and the support systems utilized at the various nodal points. In order to evaluate the risk factor, the family was asked to discuss illness, accidents, problems in school adjustments, or in social adaptation with respect to the nodal points.

Form Three, which the family members were asked to fill out individually, provided an opportunity for each family member over the age of eight to contribute freely his or her experience and viewpoint with reference to the illness and death of the parent. There were twenty-five items, including multiple choice questions which could be checked, and sentence completion items. This questionnaire was devised with the idea of encouraging individual family members to express their own reactions if they were hesitant to voice them during the family interview. For, during the interview, the strategy called for focusing on the death of the parent or the spouse, and then moving backward and forward in time to assess the type of change and adjustment that occurred for the family and the individual, and the support systems used at varying times.

Form Four was a brief clinical description of the family written by the interviewer. These were reviewed and rated independently on six scales by two raters, a psychiatrist and a social worker.

Data Analysis

All data were coded and punched on a series of IBM cards. Computer programming was utilized for the results reported. Data were combined to form indices for the following variables: socioeconomic status, residential stability, job stability, use of the employer as a support, and index of financial stress. Data were also combined to construct special measurements for the assessment of variables central to the hypotheses to be tested, namely, free flow of information, the use of support systems, postdeath restabilization, index of family change, and classification of centripetal or centrifugal families.

RESULTS

The first hypothesis to be tested was that a free flow of information within a family facilitates the use of support systems. Neither the pooled data nor the clinical data showed that the communication patterns of the family have much to do with how a family utilizes external support systems such as schools, agencies, friends, clergy, and so forth. Utilizing the clinical data and the average of the two raters, however, there was a significant correlation between the free flow of information and utilization of internal support systems.

The second hypothesis to be tested was that postdeath restabilization was facilitated by previous experience with death. Although the data tended to support the hypothesis that restabilization is facilitated by previous coping with death, it failed to achieve significance by the Chi square test. Postdeath restabilization showed a significant correlation with the effective use of external support systems such as agencies, institutions, and individuals outside the nuclear family. Postdeath restabilization was related both on the clinical ratings and the pooled data to free flow of information. The more family members were able to communicate with one another, to share information, and to share in decision making, the greater the likelihood of an effective adjustment during the postdeath period.

There were a number of findings with respect to the woman patient that were of interest in view of the relationship between the free flow of communication and postdeath restabilization. Work by family sociologists points out that the female adult is the expressive leader, and plays the integrative role in the family (Parsons, Bales, Olds, et al., 1955). It is of interest that in the authors' study, those families where the patient who died was the mother were significantly rated lower in communication patterns than those in which the father died. This finding suggests that in view of the wife-mother's role as family communicator, professionals working with these families need to help with the transfer of this function to other family members. This task may be made more difficult to another finding of the study, namely, that there was a significant difference, based on gender, whether the patient was informed that she or he was terminal. In twelve of the seventeen female patients, 71 percent, either no one discussed the terminal nature of the illness, or family members were unsure that such a discussion had taken place. In contrast, when the patient was male, he was often explicitly told of his status. Twelve men, 67 percent, knew that they were terminal. This finding takes on more significance when one considers that the quality of family relations after death is correlated with the free flow of information. Of the eleven families who reported improved family relationships after death, nine had been classified as having a free flow of information. Families rated as open in communications were more flexible about changing roles, and experienced less difficulty in postdeath restabilization. It assumes even greater importance because significantly more of these families reported more difficulties in managing household tasks during the postdeath period when it was the female, rather than the male who died. There was also a strong trend toward increased illness of family members during the terminal period if the dying person was the mother, rather than the father. These findings strongly suggest that professionals working with families where the patient is the mother, must reexamine their approach and develop strategies that help open up alternate channels of communication prior to the death of the patient. It also suggests that professionals need to concentrate more on the preventive mental health aspects of work with the family of the dying patient. An emphasis in this direction would mean a shift from focusing primarily on the patient's illness, to being more concerned with how the patient's illness is affecting family functioning, to what extent they are being helped to adapt to the current situation, and how this adaptation prepares them for future functioning. This shift in focus does not mean ignoring the patient, but suggests that professional caretakers could be more innovative in working with the patient and other family members in mapping alternate paths of communication and family functioning.

The third hypothesis tested was concerned with characterizing a family as centripetal, or inwardly centered, as contrasted with the centrifugal family, which tended to reach out in its effort to adapt. It was hypothesized that families with centripetal tendencies would be less likely to utilize external support systems than those characterized as centrifugal.

Of the twenty-nine families participating, nineteen were classified as centripetal, ten as centrifugal. Contripetal families did not differ from centrifugal families in the sex of the patient who died, length of illness, socioeconomic status, religion, residential or job stability, or length of service from Cancer Family Care. The findings strongly support a position completely opposite to the one hypothesized. The findings showed that the more inwardly directed the family, the more likely it was to make effective use of external support systems. Centripetal families also tended to rate significantly better than the centrifugal families on the effectiveness of postdeath restabilization. No family classified as centripetal listed the physician as helpful at the time of death. By contrast, one-half of the families classified as centrifugal responded with "physician" to the open-ended question, "What people were helpful at the time of death?"

Additional Findings

As previously noted, the authors had observed a reluctance on the part of the family to discuss the seriousness of the parent's illness and impending death with children. The findings of this study support this observation. There is also a difference in when, and by whom, both adults and children are informed about the impending death.

Ninety-eight percent of the surviving spouses learned that the patient had cancer at the time of diagnosis. In contrast, about 50 percent of the children under eight learned about the diagnosis during the terminal period, and a few learned after death. The spouse was usually told by the physician. In no instance in the eight to fifteen age group, and in only two cases in the sixteen to twenty-eight age group, was the family member told by a physician that the parent would die. Children between eight and fifteen were less likely to think death was possible at an early stage than parents and older children. Children in both age ranges are quite similar in the proportion who guessed about death, and in those who heard it from one of the parents. For the patient-parent, the task of informing his children of his impending death is painful. He grieves over not being able to see the child reach maturity, and he also has to cope with his own feelings of guilt about not being able to complete his task as a parent in rearing the child. Expressed reasons for not informing the child are fear of breaking down in front of him or her, or of being unable to deal with a strong show of feelings on the part of the child.

The authors' experience points out that even families who describe their communication as open find it difficult to discuss the nature of illness and impending death of a parent. Parents are often unable to recognize the clues given by children indicative of their anxiety—their wish to know what is going on, and what is going to happen to them.

In response to the question as to who helped them most, for those in the younger age group, most often mentioned was the surviving spouse, while the older children turned to a friend. For the surviving spouse, an agency, usually Cancer Family Care, was most frequently mentioned, although other relatives were also seen as an important resource.

The responses to the question as to who was most bothered by the illness, indicated that none of the older adolescents or young adults saw himself as most troubled by the illness. Yet, they were overwhelmingly concerned with their own adjustment to the death of the parent. They viewed the terminal period as a time when support seemed inadequate. Twenty-three older adolescents and young adults believed more help was needed. This finding also correlates with self-reports of "the hardest time for me." Over 50 percent of the family members reported that the terminal period, the actual death, and the funeral, were the most difficult times. In response to the question: What was the hardest time for the family? the terminal period was seen as most difficult for family functioning, although the young children termed it equally with the time of death.

In discussion of the need for more help at the various nodal points, 33 percent felt they could have used more help at the time of diagnosis, and this proportion increases for the terminal period. For the older children, the terminal period was the time when the care seemed most inadequate. It is likely that this period is felt by the older adolescents and young adult children to be a time of additional responsibility at the very point at which energy is being drained into grief and mourning. The younger children reported the terminal illness and the time of death as critical periods when they needed more help.

These findings strongly support the thesis that families experiencing terminal illness and death of one of their members are under a great deal of stress. As Colin Murray-Parkes points out, they are more prone to physical and mental breakdown (Murray-Parks, 1972). It also points, as does the work of Furman, to the vulnerability of children to the death of a parent (Furman, 1974). It suggests that support systems that are in touch with these families, such as physicians, clergy, teachers, and community agencies, must become sensitized to their needs and develop skill in helping them through this critical period. The healthy spouse is often a key person in these situations, much in need of help because his knowledge of the potential threat to the family's integrity usually begins earlier than it does for the children. Also, he or she is the person looked to most often to provide support to the patient and other family members. If the surviving parent is a man, he may, as the study indicates, have been dependent on his wife to act as the communicator in the family, and may be ill-prepared for the role in which he now finds himself. Because of stereotypes in our society with regard to sex roles, it may be hard for men to request help when it is badly needed. Perhaps one way in which helping professionals can learn to reach out is to become less disease- or patient-oriented, and more adept at focusing on the kinds of adaptation and change that occur in families in order to accommodate to long-term illness and death.

In this regard, it should be of interest to look at the material this study produced in response to the question about when the respondent's life and the family life changed most. Thirty-six, or almost 50 percent of the seventy-eight respondents to the individual questionnaires, gave the same response to both items. For example, if one reported the period of diagnosis was the period when life changed most, one also felt this was the period when family life had been most affected.

Sixty-six percent of the children said there was little change in their lives at the time of diagnosis. Over 50 percent of the parents reported minimal changes at time of diagnosis. For all groups, those reporting "no change" declines steadily from diagnosis to the time of death. There was a rapid rebound for the younger children during the postdeath period. Older children showed more areas of change than younger siblings, and the parental group showed the most areas of changed functioning in the postdeath period.

For teen-agers and young adult children, social life was the area most changed—27 percent at the time of diagnosis, 48 percent during the terminal period, and 68 percent at the time of death and the funeral. Unlike the parents, where changes in social life remained an area most affected even during the postdeath period, older adolescents and young adult children showed a marked trend toward resumption of previous functioning in social activities.

The parent group reported a steady increase in health problems through nodal points, with some lessening of changes in this area during the postdeath period. In response to the question whether the family was back together again, almost 70 percent felt that restabilization of the family had taken less than six months. However, 33 percent of the families did not respond. Only two of the fifty-two who did respond felt that restructuring had not been accomplished.

SUMMARY

Although this study is limited, it has produced data which increase understanding of families faced with the terminal illness and death of a parent. It has pointed up the value of open communication among family members in coping with the crisis at all nodal points, but particularly with respect to postdeath restabilization. It has made the authors aware that women patients, who are often the family communicators, are less informed about being terminal. Thus, it is important for caretakers in a variety of support systems to develop strategies to deal with this situation, and help families develop alternative paths of communication.

Because centripetal families made better use of external support systems, and were more successful in achieving postdeath restabilization, reaching the centrifugal families who may be equally in need of help must be examined.

Most often, families reported the terminal illness and the death as the most difficult time, and the time during which most changes took place. It is important that external support systems be apprised of this situation in order to increase their helpfulness to these families who have been identified as high risk. Further, it is essential that attention be given to the interface between professional caretakers and other support systems, both formal and informal.

REFERENCES

Furman, E. *A child's parent dies.* New Haven, Conn.: Yale University Press, 1974.
Murray-Parkes, C. *Bereavement.* New York: International Universities Press, 1972.
Parsons, T., Bales, R. F., Olds, J., et al. *Family socialization and interaction process.* Glencoe, Ill.: The Free Press, 1955.

THE ROLE OF A HOSPITAL-BASED PSYCHOSOCIAL UNIT IN TERMINAL CANCER ILLNESS AND BEREAVEMENT

Melvin J. Krant, Morley Beiser, Gerald Adler, and Lee Johnston[1]

The management of patients with fatal illness, especially in the late stages of their lives, has become the subject of much concern in the past decade. Multiple articles have appeared in health related, as well as in general publications, concerned with different facets of the dying experience. Descriptive words such as loneliness, isolation, and despair are now in common parlance, as are such psychological terms as denial, bargaining, and acceptance. Institutional medicine's concerns have grown as more people die in hospitals and nursing homes. For people with long term chronic and fatal illness, the hospital is not just the place where they die, but is the major support system during the last months to years of life.

The after effects of a death on survivors have also been receiving considerable attention. Death may come suddenly and unexpectedly, or after a prolonged and chronic illness, resulting in different bereavement patterns in survivors. Such patterns are influenced by age, direct kinship relationship, personality characteristics of survivors, and other psychologic and socioeconomic factors. In a broad sense, a death and consequent bereavement exposes survivors to potential deterioration of mental, social and physical health (Parkes, 1965a; Maddison & Maddison, 1968; Lopata, 1970). Increased mortality due to heart disease, suicide, and other disorders have been noted, as have serious depressive states and psychosis, and such derangements as alcoholism, extensive drug use, and inappropriate behaviors (Parkes, Murray, & Fitzgerald, 1969; Birtchnell, 1970; Parkes & Brown, 1972). Work and school problems, as well as increase in anti-social actions, have been recorded (Bonnard, 1962; Paul, 1974).

Visible grieving is scarcely acceptable today as a social requisite, and an exhibition of grieving beyond the initial days after a death is given little tolerance by middle class American society. Most bereaved, after an intense week or so of open community and family support, are usually left on their own, with proscriptions against 'carrying on too long'. The intra-psychic and interpersonal problems in bereavement behavior are poorly understood by most health professionals, although some excellent reviews of grief and bereavement exist in medical literature (Parkes, 1965b; Averill, 1968). In

Reprinted from *Journal of Chronic Diseases 29*, pp. 115–127, ©1976, Pergamon Press, Ltd., with permission.

[1]All from Tufts Psychosocial Cancer Unit, New England Medical Center, Boston, MA 02130.

general, medical support systems for the bereaved do not exist in our communities.

The clinical course for many cancer patients, and for their families, is marked by chronicity, gradual deterioration of function, dying and bereavement. The patient with non-curable cancer is usually offered multiple treatments in the form of surgery, radiotherapy, chemotherapy, and immunotherapy, each of which present the patient with an opportunity for improvement and may extend his survival, but which also bring problems of invalidism, long term hospital stay, toxicity and protracted dying. The manner in which an individual patient, and his family, deal with the realistic as well as symbolic implications of the illness is seldomly explored in the hospital, unless grossly abnormal behavior calls for psychiatric consultation. An analysis of the coping mechanisms in patients and their families is rarely part of the medical workup. Mitigation of the psychological consequences of prolonged illness and dying, for both the patient and for his family, are not standard strategies in our modern hospital support systems. And after a death has occurred, the hospital support system, which frequently has operated satisfactorily for many of the physical, as well as some of the psychosocial needs of the patient and the family, is almost universally withdrawn, leaving the survivors more or less on their own.

The Tufts Psychosocial Cancer Study Unit was formulated some eighteen months ago, supported by a grant from the National Cancer Institute, to study patterns of interaction between family, patient, and the larger society including the health care system, in the terminal phases of cancer, and to relate these patterns to bereavement outcomes in the years following the death. The Unit developed a study of intervention therapies, to test the hypothesis that a carefully designed effort directed at helping the family cope with the events of the terminal period, and with the post death months, would have a favorable effect on health patterns manifest during that time, and in the subsequent years.

This report describes some of the intervention principles which have emerged from our work to date. We will not attempt to statistically document the effectiveness of intervention, since the controlled study will require several additional years of observation before such evaluation is possible. However, we are convinced that families are extremely grateful for the interventions offered. The Unit as it now exists is primarily a research unit, and not a service unit. The research orientation has required that the patient and family understand that they are contributing to data collection before they enter the study. It is only after data has been accumulated and a randomization into control or intervention groups has been effected, that about half of our families are offered intervention as a service. However, we feel that a description of the intervention process might be of help to other hospital groups attempting to assist in the problems faced by terminal patients and families.

DESCRIPTION OF UNIT

The Psychosocial Unit consists of three full-time psychiatric social workers, two full-time research assistants, and a full-time clinical research psychologist. In addition, the project director, a medical oncologist, spends 30% of his work time in the Unit, and two psychiatrists devote one day, and a half day, respectively to the supervisory support of the social workers and to weekly group meetings. The Psychosocial Unit is housed in the Department of Psychiatry, although the social workers maintain a direct liaison with the Departments of Social Service in the three hospitals in which the work is conducted. A direct relationship has been established with the Oncology Units at three hospitals (Tufts New England Medical Center Hospital, Lemuel Shattuck Hospital, and the Youville Hospital). Patients are acceptable to the study if the following criteria are met: a) expected survival of six months or less, b) patient and first-degree blood relatives are in the Boston area, c) patient and family speak English and can effectively communicate with the medical staff.

When a terminally ill cancer patient, under the care of the staff of the three hospitals, is identified both he and his next of kin are contacted by one of the social workers, either by letter or by telephone if an outpatient, or by a direct visit to the bedside if an inpatient. A home visit to the patient or to the family members, or to both, is conducted. If the patient and the family members accept our invitation to participate in the study, a semi-structured interview is conducted with the patient and with family members. The questionnaire elucidates medical experiences to date, expectations of patient and family, feelings regarding self and others in relation to the illness, thoughts about dying and about future. Information is gathered as to how the patient, or family members, view the health vulnerability in survivors, and the patterns of communication in the family are detailed. Following the open-ended interviews, a battery of psychologic tests are administered by the research assistants. In all, approximately 3–4 hr of interviews and tests are required.

We often are unable to interview and test all primary members of a family. Where children and young adolescents are present, one or the other parent may specifically exclude contact with them. Elderly parents have been kept at a distance from the interviewers. We have often waited several weeks before a spouse, or sibling, would complete the research materials, for all our desired data cannot be collected in one sitting. There have been a number of families and patients who have rejected our offer to participate outright, or having started the project, have dropped out before completing the data.

After the initial interview is completed, the family is randomly assigned to an intervention or a non-intervention group. The intervention group families are then offered the services of the same social worker who conducted the initial evaluation. These interventions begin prior to death, and continue through the time of the death of the patient to a point in time six months following. The non-intervention group is not seen from the time of randomization until the first follow-up 6 months post-death. Evaluations of health, mood and social functioning are documented with family members in both groups at 6, 12, and 24 months post-death.

Upon assignment to the intervention group, data is reviewed by the entire study unit, and coping styles, personality structures, previous experiences with loss, present patterns of interaction between patient and family members, and social resources available to this family are assessed. We attempt to judge patterns of 'vulnerability' in family members, as well as potential assets. An intervention program is designed to ameliorate disturbances in the family psychosocial system, and to promote healthy adaptations. There is a periodic reassessment of the interventive processes. At no time do we suggest any alteration in established hospital services, although for the intervention group, we attempt a close alliance with the medical and paramedical staffs in working through problems.

To date, intervention has been extended to 28 families, totalling 88 family members. We have concluded interventive therapy (six months post death) with 7 families, totalling 22 people. We have conceptualized our interventive efforts to date into a schematic set of principles, and they are presented as follows:

THE PRE-DEATH PERIOD

Establishing a Relationship

Although obviously necessary, it has not been easy to establish a working relationship. In part, this has been true because of our research orientation. While it may be true that many individuals facing death, their own or that of an essential family member, are in a state of panic or disorganization, this does not mean that they are either eager to participate in a research project, nor 'trust' psychological help, nor anxious to share thoughts with strangers. Individual patients, or family members, may be too caught up in the day by day unfolding of events, or in the denial of the essential problems, or defending against exposing their pain, to allow probing into their affect by an outsider. They have, not infrequently, seen the social worker as an agent of the hospital coming to pry into their affairs, especially financial affairs. Many people equate social workers with 'welfare' and feel insulted by the contact. But when the social worker can function as a resource person to assist in a specific concrete task, such as mobilizing a service, or acquiring a needed hospital bed for home use, a relationship is greatly enhanced. Once established, the relationships have proven stable and ongoing, and have extended easily and naturally into the post-death period.

Opening Blocked Channels of Cognitive Communication

Although the existence of a fatal, if not terminal, illness in general, is known to both patient and adult family members, such knowledge is often not commonly shared between them. Participants in the drama are often left to struggle by themselves with a fragmented and frequently distorted view of the whole. Opening a blocked channel requires recognition of both general and specific difficulties by all involved. The intervention worker helps family members to search out needed medical and prognostic information by arranging a group conference with the medical staff. Because of time pressures, doctors usually avoid repeating explanations to multiple family members, and further seldomly check to ensure that the family member, or the patient, 'heard' and 'understood' the information offered. The intervention worker attends these conferences and helps the physician to understand the communication problems in the family, as well as helping family members to obtain an accurate picture of the illness status. While it is felt that denial patterns, for patients or families, are working adaptively, we help the medical staff to support them. Where we feel these patterns are disrupting family relations, or are maladaptive for appropriate medical care, we attempt to confront and adjust such responses.

We not infrequently deal with people who have a life style of not sharing with others in the same family. When illness appears, they may wish to play the same game. Sometimes, the implication is that keeping quiet about the truth 'protects' the others. At other times, avoiding the issue is a way of maintaining control, or not facing the shame and strain so often assumed in the physical and social failing associated with illness. We do not push family members into sharing the information with each other, but to help them conceptualize the gains and losses of the position they assume.

A particular spouse confided to the intervention worker that she suspected 'the worst' about her husband. However, she was sure that her husband was not aware of the seriousness of his condition. She lived in a constant state of anxiety and apprehension that her suspicions might 'slip-out'. In order to ensure against this happening, she studiously avoided talking with any of her husband's doctors or nurses. Even though she would have liked to know what to expect, she used ignorance as a shield behind which her knowledge could be hidden. She avoided discussions with her husband about deaths of friends, illness in friends or family, and any situation which might intimate how ill he was, even if only by association. The avoidances meant that she had to virtually avoid her husband, but it was not surprising that she expressed all sorts of fantasies as to what was really happening to him.

Facilitating the Mourning Process

Being sick, and living with sickness, requires considerable readjustment on the part of the patient and on his family. Both the patient and his family give up certain expectations in life. As death approaches, the process of relinquishing expectations continues, and although not easy, a mourning process is set in motion. For mourning to proceed, a person must face his feelings in relationship to alterations in the inter- and intrapersonal spheres. The sadness that is so essential in the mourning process may be minimized or denied by the patient, as well as by his family members, in order to stave off its pain. Guilt feelings from past experiences can block reality-testing. The giving up of cherished roles that have defined one's self-esteem can lead to marked feelings of unworthiness, with resultant depression. As new roles and new demands are placed upon various family members, anger and confusion can easily result. Long term and continual ministering to a sick individual can produce great resentment, which frequently cannot be admitted as 'allowable'. On the other hand, the realization of the 'abandonment' inherent in dying often times produces feelings of fear and anger, although such emotions are usually poorly acceptable, leading to further guilt feelings, and tendencies to deny reality. There is even a tendency to idealize the individual who is about to die. The inability to accept the various emotions related to dying blocks the capacity for early anticipated mourning, and also results in displacement of anger and resentment to other family members, to medical staff, or inwardly against oneself.

An assessment of the manner in which previous deaths in the family, such as parents or siblings, were handled by the patient and his family, often helps to determine coping styles, and gives insight as to both unresolved tensions, and expected ways that the present loss will be handled. In helping family members, as well as the patient, come to grips with present realities and the associated intense feelings, an appropriate mourning, which often times helps the supportive living care go on, is encouraged.

Where sadness seems minimized or absent, we have helped a patient and family focus on detailed memories of their past lives together. Such focus often helps tap the sadness they have been avoiding. We have helped patients and families adjust their insights on anger, and have legitimized anger at the entire loss process. We attempt to explore feelings of 'wishing to run away', feelings of 'wishing it were all over with', and similar concerns that are often times felt by family members, but interpreted to be evil and unacceptable. In only one of our cases to date, we have found a patient and spouse who have actively been supportive to each other through mutual denial of what was happening: each was able to acknowledge apart from the other that they were aware of the seriousness and irrevocability of the illness, but preferred to maintain 'denial' with each other.

Good-Bye Saying

Facilitating 'anticipated' mourning, and opening cognitive and affective communications, frequently expedites a process, which we have often observed, that can be called 'saying good-bye'. Saying good-bye is the summing up of the life together with the other person, and the sharing of last wishes for the future. Sometimes permission may be sought for remarriage, or an attitude explored as to where and how a survivor should carry on. Questions of working, of moving from the shared home, of forgiving quarrels with other family members, can be explored. Frequently, 'good-bye' saying is acknowledging that one has been a good spouse or a good son, or that one has been truly loved in the now-to-be changed relationship. In cases where this unfinished business has not been attended to, the bereaved survivors often report being haunted by doubts regarding questions they wish had been asked when there was still time to do so. The 'last words' of a dying person have always been given strong social, if not legal, force. Thus a positive good-bye expression of approval, of caring, and of forgiveness, has extraordinary validity and meaning for survivors.

Catalyzing Interactions with Psychosocial Support Systems

In critical times, family members often group together to offer mutual help and support. When this does not happen, it is often due to one of two reasons: a) families may be so ridden with dissension that regrouping is blocked, b) the resources of the family unit are already so strained, that supportive help for each other within the family nexus is impossible. A major interventive effort has been to help heal old family wounds, often by individual counseling, but also by catalyzing face to face meetings during which opposing expectations, old grievances, and mutual suspicions can be aired. Since the worker often takes the initiative in setting up these meetings, and stresses a common goal of helping the dying patient, people frequently feel that they can attend, even though considerable risk exists between them in the family, without appearing to look like they are losing face, or giving in.

These solidarity-promoting meetings are often the prelude to the more task-oriented activities that will be carried out. We are well aware that complicated intra-family problems, especially long-existing interpersonal and inter-generational difficulties, cannot be solved by short term meetings of this nature. We see such meetings as smoothing over enough surface dissention to allow for family regrouping for care-giving and care-taking. In such sessions, factual information about the status of the patient, particularly medical information, can be shared, and some realistic guidelines regarding prognosis and expectations can be reviewed.

In several chronically unsupportive families, the added emotional, physical and financial problems of illness becomes not a rallying point, but a disintegrative force. In such situations the intervention workers have struggled to put the families in touch with support systems in the general community. Family members are often unaware of certain benefits for which they are qualified, or do not have the capacity to cut through interfering red tape. A community such as Boston has many organizations and institutions capable of delivering services, such as transportation to and from the hospital, home care services, financial support services, and the like, of which patients and their families are often unaware. There have been occasions where existing breeches with spiritual and religious agencies have been rectified when the intervention team has brough a family member together with a sympathetic priest or minister.

Fostering Individuation

In the emotion-laden pre-death period, it is not unusual to see relationships so intensified, that one might speak of 'fusions' taking place. Individual needs and desires of patient and survivors are no longer clearly differentiated. In one case, a woman formed a close symbiotic relationship with her daughter who was dying of lung cancer. The worker noted that the mother was behaving as if she had no identity of her own. She neglected urgent health problems which required immediate attention even though realistically her daughter did not need her full time care. The intervention worker discussed this behavior pattern with mother and daughter openly and candidly. They worked as a group of three to resolve such issues as a) helping the mother come to terms with the fact that she, as an individual, would go on living after her daughter died, b) that even though the mother-daughter relationship was close and important, the mother had a necessary identity of her own, with a set of needs and attributes which demanded recognition in their own right. The mother was able to liberate time from her caring role without feeling disloyal, to attend to her pressing medical needs which were satisfactorily resolved.

Role Rehearsal

A death often spells a drastic shifting of roles, for at least some of the survivors. Widows may be forced to assume financial and legal responsibilities for the first time, and widowers may be called upon to fulfill effective and caring relationships with their children which they had formally relinquished to their wives. Such role changes may be catastrophic if people feel inadequate to the task, or may present a new opportunity for personal growth and satisfaction. When there is an opportunity for rehearsal for new roles, prior to the actual assumption of these roles, we believe the chances of a positive outcome are increased. Thus, a wife during her husband's illness may begin to take driving lessons, learn about the business, assume some financial responsibility, take steps to assure that the will has been properly drawn up, insurance is properly tended to, and so forth. Some of these behaviors obviously require that the individual be able to separate his/her needs from the caretaking needs of the sick family member, without an inhibiting sense of disloyalty. Such behaviors also require that a sense of reality-testing has been supported, and that denial and blocked communication have been worked through.

Steps in this direction often go slowly, and expected survivors may begin to take on such new role behaviors only after extensive discussion of the meaning and implication of these new roles with the intervention workers. Frequently, of course, a dominant-dependent relationship between husband and wife may have existed to gratify the needs of both individuals. Taking on new responsibility in such a situation may be extremely difficult, given the nature of the relationship of the past.

DEATH AND ONE WEEK POST-DEATH

The moment of death and the immediate period thereafter, is a time when the bereaved receive maximum attention and support from the family and community. Formal intervention work is usually neither possible nor desirable at this time. However, our intervention team members frequently attend the wake and/or funeral of the deceased. This practice was not formally agreed upon by the Psychosocial Unit, but evolved naturally as a consequence of the relationships established with the families in the pre-death period. The worker's presence during these events has always been welcomed, and frequently the worker has been greeted with expressions of deep gratitude, and frequently astonishment that professionals would take the time for such a personal gesture. From the worker's point of view, a personal and meaningful relationship has often been established with the deceased during the pre-death period. The workers themselves feel the need to mourn, and have found that attendance at these rituals helps them personally, as well as serving to reinforce their bond with the survivors.

THE POST-DEATH PERIOD

In most homes, a week or two after a death, the relatives begin to depart, condolence callers drop away, and survivors begin to be more on their own. The bereaved are left with a past that has ceased to be and a present in which the wounds of loss and grief are still fresh. Our interventions during the post death period continue for approximately six months.

Maintaining the Relationship

The continuity of contact with intervention workers has been meaningful to many survivors, allowing interaction to proceed in a fruitful fashion. The bereaved speak of the importance of . . . 'just knowing there is somebody to talk to'. Survivors confirm the meaningfulness of the antecedent relationship between the deceased and the social worker, but it is necessary to re-establish an intervention contract with survivors. Many bereaved expect that hospital-based services will terminate now that the 'real patient' is dead.

Facilitating the Mourning Process

The sustained relationship with the worker is utilized to help family members grieve. Even when significant pre-death anticipatory mourning has existed, a death as an absolute event elicits intense response. Once again, feelings of sadness may need facilitation in order to be expressed. Whereby prior to the death, a survivor was kept busy in visiting the dying patient, and attending to patient-oriented needs, the termination of that activity enforces the growing realization that a loss has actually occurred. Acknowledgement of fears of being alone, or of feeling inadequate to the task of reintegration, can be helpful. A survivor may be uncomfortable with the anger felt towards the hospital system, and towards other family members and may need help in discussing such feelings.

Guilt feelings may interfere with effective mourning. The patient may have died in the hospital rather than at home, as he would have preferred, arousing feelings of betrayal. A survivor may feel that he or she was not always as available, patient, and supportive as he might have been during the terminal phase. A survivor may well have been harboring thoughts of wishing the individual dead before death occurred, and now finds the recollection of such thoughts intolerable. Survivors have even expressed the guilt of responsibility for the cancer itself. Guilt of this nature can readily intensify the pain associated with grieving.

The worker who has helped the family in anticipated grieving before the death, and who knows some details of the previous relationship between the deceased and family, is in an excellent position to help the post-death mourning process ·by touching on remembered incidences. Acknowledgement and expression of the sadness and the pain of the loss can be facilitated. Considerable tact must be present, for the sadness may be too painful at times, and survivors may wish to turn away from continuous open confrontation. Recollections can put someone in touch with their sadness, but may also help to place anger in some perspective. Anger against the dead may be extremely difficult to acknowledge and great tact must be exhibited by the therapist. Anger may sometimes be acknowledged by helping an individual look more realistically at his guilt feelings and simultaneously to assess the reality of loving, caring feelings as well as real or imagined omissions, in relationship to the deceased. On more than one occasion, remembering has taken the form of repeated reviewing of the events of the illness and the circumstances of the death. Such 'repetitious recollection' although obsessive in style, is not necessarily pathologic. Such recollections may be a way of achieving a sense of perspective and a mastery of the event itself, and is encouraged when it appears.

Imparting Factual Information

Survivors sometimes report experiences which leave them to suspect their own sanity, such as momentary feelings that the deceased is alive, or recurrent dreams and illusionary experiences in which a chance noise is misinterpreted as the deceased's actual footsteps. Not infrequently, frank hallucinations appear. It is useful to inform survivors that such feelings and experiences do occur, and can be expected, and are not a sign of insanity. An opportunity for a survivor to express doubts regarding his sanity when such events are repetitive is provided. Survivors are frequently helped to realize that not only are such experiences common, but that they do pass with time. An opportunity is provided for full amplification of the experience, and the associated emotions, which are clearly unique and highly personal to the individual suffering.

Questions such as 'contagiousness' and the role of heredity can be explored. The belief that the cancer was acquired from some misbehavior or omission on the patient's or family's part needs, on occasion, to be explored. Factual and objective information, from both the intervention worker, and from the attending physician, are very important.

Symptoms in the survivors occasionally emerge which may be seen as part of an identification with the deceased, mimicking aspects of his terminal illness. Pains and feelings of discomfort in various parts of the body similar to anatomic areas involved by the disease are not uncommon. Troubles with swallowing, defecation, eating habits, and the like, are not unusual during these months after a death. We attempt to review these complaints and symptoms in relationship to the mourning process, and to help an individual survivor understand the evolution of such symptomatology. Where medical workup seems indicated, this is arranged for, but the primary locus in symptom manifestation, namely in the psychologic rather than in the primary somatic sphere, is kept in focus.

Catalyzing the Psychosocial Support System

Psychosocial support from friends, family, the clergy, and others in the community are particularly important during the post-death period. The intervention workers help survivors lean on others, and facilitate the entry of other individuals in the family and community nexus into the world of mourning. In addition, many greater Boston communities have established organizations such as Widow-to-Widow Programs and Parents Without Partners. Especially towards the end of the period of intervention, the worker, if she feels the group is appropriate, helps the survivor to pick him/her self up to attend meetings.

Reinforcing the Process of Individuation

Survivors often idealize the dead person, particularly in the immediate post-death period. A woman may attribute her whole reason for being to her husband, and all the social success and achievements of the family to his efforts. The deceased may be seen as one who could do no wrong in his lifetime. In such cases, the workers emphasize the survivor's own accomplishments and capabilities regarding such matters as raising children, managing a household, work performance and so forth. His or her own needs, assets and liabilities are highlighted in order to reinforce a unique sense of identity. This process, touched upon in the pre-death period, frequently needs re-exploration and continued reinforcement. One of the widowed survivors felt that she was incapable of making decisions regarding her teenage son. Some months after the death of his father, the youngster was pressuring his mother to release some of the husband's insurance money so that he could purchase a car. While she felt reluctant to do this, she also felt powerless to take a stand on the issue. One day, while her son was pressing his argument, a towel hanging near the stove in the kitchen suddenly caught fire. The widow interpreted this as a message from her husband that she should not accede to the boy's request, and with that she ended the matter. The worker in this case was able to help her look at the entire process as one in which her own desire in the matter had been transformed into a concrete action. While the 'sign' from her husband helped catalyze the final decision, she was helped to understand that she was in fact gaining confidence in her own competence as a 'taking over' of attitudes and skills which derived from her husband.

Understanding Loneliness

The period after a death is frequently a lonely time, especially for a spouse. As with other affects already discussed, it is supportive to simply be able to share with another what it is like to feel so lonely. It has also been of importance to highlight this particular emotion because of its unique ramifications. Survivors not uncommonly misinterpret the action of others. A casual remark by a male neighbor or a fellow employee may be perceived as a flirtation, and an expression of sympathy as a frank sexual advance. But just as important, in their loneliness people are vulnerable to the predators of our civilized societies. People are extremely susceptible to cajolery during this time, and can be talked into buying things, or into other commitments, that they later regret. One aspect of dealing with loneliness has been to help survivors test reality. Is what they heard actually an invitation or an iron-clad promise, or because of their need, do they introduce something into the situation which does not really belong there? By exploring the emotion and providing some measure of comfort, the workers have been able to help survivors deal with such questions, and to ease them back into productive relationships with others.

Exploring Major Decisions

It is not infrequent that a bereaved individual will seek to resolve painful confrontation with memories of the deceased by making a major decision which changes her/his life position, such as moving from one place to another, quitting a job and taking on another, or dropping out of school permanently. Such actions may result in distasteful or actually sorrowful consequences. Carefully exploring the reasonings that have led to the decision has helped an individual to postpone 'running' too quickly into a major change in role or life status. The converse has also been seen, namely that a decision that should be made is delayed inappropriately. However, acting slowly on major decisions, taking time to review more carefully and thinking the consequences through, often times result in a more gratifying outcome. Because certain decisions may be made to assuage guilt, or to run from painful thoughts, a bereaved person may not voluntarily discuss such thoughts. Therefore, inquiry as to possible plans regarding major changes is tactfully made rather than waiting to be told.

The Search for an Explanation

Most, if not all cultures, deal with death and its reasons, and this is sometimes formalized as religious dogma. The search for an explanation can also be a quest for responsibility, as opposed to suffering a feeling of helplessness in the face of fate. In our study group, the search for an answer almost always takes place. Explanation may take the form of blaming either the patient himself, his doctors for inadequate attention, caring or skills, or other family members. The intervention workers run the risk of becoming the object of blame. One of the widows in our series accused the social worker of hastening her husband's death because she had discussed the issue of dying with him. Such accusations require patient, but persistent explanation if long-standing, inappropriately directed anger, which can interfere with later health-related behavior, is to abate.

DISCUSSION

Changes in the nature of family structure and residential patterns, in the format of health care delivery (few community-based physicians, more full-time hospital physicians), and in the technical treatment of disease, have resulted in marked alteration in both the manner in which, and the place in which, an individual dies, and in the support structure offered to the bereaved. The enormous growth in medical technology has tended to accentuate disease oriented care as opposed to person oriented care. Hospitals are remarkably efficient places for the management of disease states, but often times do not consider family members as essential primary targets for concern and intervention when a fatal illness, and especially when a terminal period, envelops a group. The nature of the hospital system is such that family members play an entirely secondary role to that of the patient, but even so, suffer a sharp discontinuity in their relationship with the institution when the particular family member, as patient, dies. The absence of appropriate strategy that centers on family members as primary health care concerns results in rather hit-or-miss relationships being established between medical forces and families during an illness, and a total absence of organized health care for survivors after death. The exception, of course, is found where the family has had a long term relationship with an interested private practitioner. Such an individual physician often times participates in family concerns during the bereavement period. Unfortunately, fewer and fewer of such relationships seem to exist, and are notoriously absent in large urban areas.

Although the program described in this paper is essentially a research project, the data derived to date leave us with the firm impression that families as a group, and as individual members, benefit considerably when they are taken as a central focus of need in the hospital system both during terminal illness and after a death has occurred. The intervention strategies that we have elaborated in both the pre-death and post-death periods are not presented as the definitive concept. The notion of pre-death and post-death continuity seems valid. The hospital, the place where so many individuals now experience their terminal illnesses as well as their moments of death, is the natural place in this twentieth century for a family oriented care program to be constructed, and the dearth of out-reach care for the bereaved in most communities suggests that a hospital-based on-going service after a death is a logical extension in community concern.

Although there is a concept in crisis intervention literature that people who are experiencing an extraordinary event or series of events in their lives can often benefit from the availability of appropriately trained intervention workers, (whose primary purpose is to help a person cope with the paralyzing or overwhelming consequences of the event) our data indicates that many families experiencing a terminal illness are frequently unwilling to talk to a research worker, and may be just as unwilling to accept professional help. This may be due to a 'defensive' posture, or because of a suspicion of professionals who want to deal with feelings and personalities. (The majority of our families are lower middle class, urban dwellers.) It is also quite possible that many families do not need any help. Because of lack of understanding as to what psychosocial help can really do, psychologic or social support is not frequently requested by the patient, or by his family. Reaching out provides a potentially more favorable therapeutic-intervention opportunity.

The loss of an important and central family member can produce serious health dislocations, as frequently in the physical sphere as in the psychologic and social spheres. Developmental psychologic maladjustment looms as a threat for any child or adolescent who loses a parent, either by sudden death, or through prolonged illness. Similar problems concerned with the quality of life, if not specific mental and physical derangements, hold for adults as well. There is a great need to identify those factors present in family members of all ages which make them 'vulnerable' to poor bereavement outcomes at various time intervals after a death. However, there is not firm evidence today that presently employed psychosocial interventions for a family in a dying experience will prevent or ameliorate serious health consequences. Experiences with intervention techniques need to be gathered. The purpose of this communication is not to elaborate on the pathologies associated with bereavement. Rather the purpose is to structure a series of interventions which can be viewed, criticized, and hopefully challenged as to their applicability for care-giving.

Bereavement may be a normal consequence of life, but that is not to say that people undergoing the experience are necessarily healthy. Grief in bereavement is a marked dislocation from normal health and people in the midst of deep grief experience a multiplicity of psychologic and physical features which may spontaneously heal, but which can go on to permanent disorder. In this sense, services directed at such individuals are interventive and therapeutic and not only preventive. As third party health insurance carriers extend their coverage of psychologic aberrations, treatment of the bereaved on an outpatient basis should well qualify for such coverage.

Clearly many family members will be able to tolerate the loss of a loved one without great consequences. If a death is more appropriate, in the sense that it comes to an older citizen, those children have grown and have generated their own families, and who have ceased to be the central pivotal individual in the lives of those around him, the likelihood of consequent psychopathology is diminished. However, one can never know what is appropriate and what is inappropriate without studying the interactions occurring in the family in relationship to the terminally ill individual.

At this point in our work, we are unable to conclude that six months of therapy after a death, in which the worker and the family member meet one to two times a month, for an hour or so, is sufficient. We have worked with several survivors who require much longer treatment and of a more intense nature. In such situations, it is our approach to find appropriate ongoing support. The task of reconstruction as a widow or widower probably only begins around six months to a year after a death has occurred, and such reconstruction may require the help of community agencies, such as Widow-to-Widow Programs. Professional resources should remain available to such individuals who have a need for them.

The physician is essential to a family-centered effort of this type. It is essentially for his services that the patient and the family have come. His guidance and advice in the matter of interventive help during this period of losing and bereaving can be crucial. In their training, many physicians feel that they have inadequate skills, and inadequate time, to deal with the many psychologic and social issues in patients and their families. A trained staff dealing mainly in these areas, especially with family members, can be of significant assistance when the physician emphatically grasps what they are trying to do. It is our hope that physicians will come to appreciate the deep 'pain' associated with fatal and terminal illness for family members, as well as the patient, and will harness resources to help such individuals.

REFERENCES

Averill, J. R. Grief: Its nature and significance. *Psychological Bulletin,* 1968, *70,* 720–748.
Birtchnell, J. The relationship between attempted suicide, depression and parental death. *British Journal of Psychiatry,* 1970, *116,* 307–313.
Bonnard, P. Truancy and pilfering associated with bereavement. In S. Lorand & H. Schneer (Eds.), *Adolescent, psychoanalytic approach to problems and therapy.* New York: Paul H. Hoeber, 1962.
Lopata, H. Z. The social involvement of American widows. *American Behavioral Scientist,* 1970, *14*(1), 41–57.
Maddison, D., & Maddison, V. The health of widows in the year following bereavement. *Journal of Psychosomatic Research,* 1968, *12,* 297–306.
Parkes, C. M. Bereavement and mental illness. I. II. *British Journal of Medical Psychology,* 1965a, *38,* 1026.
Parkes, C. M. A classification of bereavement reactions. *British Journal of Medical Psychiatry,* 1965b, *38,* 1–26.
Parkes, C. M., & Brown, R. J. Health after bereavement: A controlled study of young Boston widows and widowers. *Psychosomatic Medicine,* 1972, *34,* 449–461.
Parkes, C. M., Murray, V. B., & Fitzgerald, R. G. Broken heart: A statistical study of increased mortality amongst widowers. *British Medical Journal,* 1969, *1,* 740–743.
Paul, N. Psychiatry: Its role in the resolution of grief. In A. Kutscher (Ed.), *Death and bereavement.* Springfield, Ill.: Charles C Thomas Publisher, 1974.

PERSONAL STATEMENT ......
Geraldine

A MOTHER'S DIARY

February 3, 1974   Discovered a lump in
her breast. Went to Strong Clinic in University
of Rochester for 6 weeks of radiation after a
lumpectomy, which was treatment prescribed.
Her husband insisted on driving her himself, a
200-mile trip daily. I volunteered while I was
there for a short while, but he rejected my offer. When I left, they took their son, who was
young enough to nap during the trip. They were
very optimistic, took it in their stride, and were
certain—after much investigation—that they
were following the correct course.

September 6, 1975   Discovered a lump in
the left side of her neck in the lymph node—
diagnosed as malignant. They were in the midst
of moving from Waterloo to University of Michigan and reacted in panic: Should they leave
Rochester Strong Clinic who knew her case? Go
immediately on chemo and radiation? Was the
lumpectomy versus mastectomy the right
choice? They had signed a lease for their house
in Ann Arbor and had rented their house in
Waterloo. Money and contracts on both sides.
After much consultation and opinions, her records were sent to Michigan and they were told
to sit tight. Several different opinions were offered. In September she had an ovariectomy to
slow down hormones.

October, 1975   Came to New York City
and went to Sloan to two doctors recommended.
One said chemo and radiation. One said sit tight
and watch. They followed his advice, to sit tight.
They were extremely worried, and she and
Frank read everything on cancer they could
find. They both realized chemo and radiation
were devastating and felt it was the last thing.

November, 1975   In Ann Arbor started
chemo. Was feeling better health wise, tired but
not bad, and was very optimistic about the
chemo and was glad they were doing something.
She hated to think of the cancer she had in her
body. The lump in her neck did not change, but
I think another small one appeared. She tolerated the chemo well and, after 1 week in the
hospital, was on an outpatient basis. After the
second week, they took a blood test and found
the white blood corpuscles very low and discontinued the chemo until they could be raised.

December, 1975   Developed pneumonia—
hospitalized. I visited, and when I left, my other
daughter, Bonnie, left California, her friends,
and her courses toward her master's in remedial reading and stayed with Geraldine. On December 15 Bonnie and Geraldine came to New
York. Geraldine was not well, had to be assisted
in walking—weak and dizzy. Before her visit,
about the middle of November, Pat and I,
through various means and a thousand telephone calls, were able to find a doctor and a
place where we could get Laetrile. They could
not find a doctor or nurse who would show
them how to inject the substance in Michigan.
Finally, a nurse showed Frank, and he had to
do it. When Geraldine came to New York, I had
to do it. It was very difficult to plunge a needle
into her buttock, but she insisted and felt sure
it would help. Meanwhile, Frank had at least
two or three different cures—cloves especially
grown, every vitamin imaginable, only natural
foods processed at home, gold—anything from
all over the world he could use. Spent nights in
the medical library reading. Could, in fact, tell
doctors about new treatments and ideas on
cancer.

After arriving in New York, got progressively worse. Frank was in Ann Arbor. We
blamed her intense dizziness and nausea on the
Laetrile. She was so weak we had to feed her.
Every night she seemed a little better, and then

we would bathe her (Bonnie and I—Bonnie
stayed all that time) and try to feed her and felt
she was getting used to the Laetrile. We were in
touch with Frank, but he did not realize how
very sick she was, and I hesitated to put her in
the hospital until he arrived. He arrived
December 24 and realized she was very bad.
Christmas Day was no day to go to a hospital, so
we went December 26—diagnosed as a brain
tumor. Treatment—radiation to reduce the
tumor and cortisone. Result—loss of hair, moon
face, but felt less dizzy and was able to go to the
bathroom by the time she left.

January, 1976   Back to Ann Arbor and
rehabilitation for loss of muscle and use of
hands. Needed wheelchair to get around.

February 15, 1976   Got pneumonia, followed by urinary infection, strep throat—white
corpuscles very low. Very sick, at least 6 weeks
in hospital in Ann Arbor.

Everyone very worried. I visited several
times, as did Bonnie and Frank's parents. Someone was always at the hospital. One had to stay
with Paul, so we were needed. Frank tolerated
the intrusion. He desperately wanted to do it
alone. Geraldine was very despondent and expressed the wish to die at home. She spoke of
dying, which I listened to but tried to point out
that she had youth, good genes, and desire to
live on her side and not to give up. She really
wanted to fight the hateful cancer and tried
hypnosis, psychiatry, charismatic movement,
plus a lot of faith in a relic of Mother Seton she
had gotten from a nun in New York and prayer.
She really had a very strong will to live, but I
think knew she would not. She was sad at leaving Paul and knew Frank would be famous
someday and wanted very much to help him
achieve greatness. She also worried about who
would take care of us when we were old. I let
her talk, but tried to reassure her.

May 7, 1976   I visited Ann Arbor for
Mother's Day. Bonnie was still with her. On Fri-

day she was extremely weak but lucid. On Saturday, seemed very relaxed, drifting, sort of knowing something and not telling. We blamed it on the codeine in her cough medicine. Went to bed Saturday, and Sunday 7 am were unable to get any response. She was sleeping peacefully. Called fire department and police department and brought her to the hospital. Geraldine was in a coma for 5 days and died May 14.

IMPACT ON US AS PARENTS

Pat could not talk about it. He had to go out to the cottage for a few days and be alone. It was not until about 7 months later (New Year's Eve) that we really cried together. Bonnie would not talk about it either. I felt much better talking and would discuss it with anyone who would listen. I was very sensitive to people's reactions and could tell if they were interested. I cried alone a lot but on the whole did very well. I did what I always did. Went out, worked, and just kept going. I felt a little angry, bitter, and jealous of other mothers who had their daughters. Geraldine and I were extremely close. Could discuss anything, and I depended on her a lot for advice. I knew she was very happy and secure, and we both enjoyed our visits to each other. That I miss the most. I also used to feel guilty. While she was so sick, I was an old woman and was dashing at work, running for trains, and enjoying life, and once expressed a wish that we could change places. She got angry and said this was her life and the way it was meant and everyone is entitled to his own life. I still miss her dreadfully, still cry at very odd moments and am reminded of her a couple of times a day. At first I had her pictures all around the house. Very soon I think I will put the one on my dresser away. It hurts too much to look at it. I know I will never be the same. I was always a very happy person, accepted everything without

question, and felt life was great. Now I think
life can be cruel; not for myself only, but
there's war, disease, corruption, government,
etc., and I wonder what's it all about. Everyone
has problems and troubles. A part of me died—
it could be my lust for life. Pat seems to be coping very well. I know he misses her and loved
her very deeply and would have done anything
to make her well. She loved him equally, as
Frank said very often. I asked him if he wanted
to help me write this, and he said he couldn't.

HOW I COPED WITH THE ILLNESS

I coped with the illness by being very optimistic. I never gave up—even till the very last minute. I prayed desperately and was very certain a
miracle would happen. I kept thinking positive
and what I would do to help her get better. I
was able to take care of her, doing the most delicate tasks while she was sick, and felt I was
helping her to get better. Prayer kept me going.

HOW GERALDINE COPED

She coped the same way, I think. She knew
Frank and Paul needed her and often said
Frank was keeping her alive. She had a very
strong will and always got what she wanted—
the lead in a play, queen of her prom, dean's
list in college, and not least, Frank, whom she
felt was the most desirable catch of all. So she
was certain—most of the time—she could in her
own way lick the cancer. She meditated, wished
it out of her body, did everything the doctors
told her to do, and prayed fervently. She often
said she was going to lick it. But, of course, at
times she was very depressed, lonely, and sad,
and said she was not afraid. I know she seriously thought of suicide and asked me to forgive her if she did. But she felt it might in some
way hurt Paul. She knew how much we were all

hurting and she wanted to hasten the agony.
She was not really in pain, but the mental anguish was terrible.

Speaking of mental anguish, that is the part
that hurts me the most. I knew it was with her
and Frank night and day. All the hopes and despair. I would wake up at night, suddenly, and
know her mind was frantic—so was mine. Mental suffering is worse than physical.

WHAT WOULD I HAVE DONE DIFFERENTLY?

I hate to answer that question, but I would have
been more insistent of her having a mastectomy
versus a lumpectomy. They were so sure by all
they had heard and read (it is done extensively
in Europe) that the lumpectomy was as good.
Really, I keep telling myself they were right. I
think it had spread by then, because the in-
fected lymph node was on the other side.

The pain does not mellow. I feel as sad and
lonely now as I did then. It is always there at
the pit of my stomach. People say time heals. I
don't think so, neither does Frank. It is always
there and pops up many times a day when I'm
least expecting it. A song, a dress, or a flower
can bring a memory of Geraldine. I just try to
get over it and know life keeps going on and I
cannot inflict my feelings on others. Everyone
has their own hell. Perhaps this is part of mine.
If it is, I have fared pretty well. I'm very fortunate to have Bonnie and Kevin and Pat, who
love me very much and I them. I thank God
for that.

RECOMMENDED READINGS FOR SECTION II

Borden, W. Psychological aspects of stroke: Patient and family. *Archives of Internal Medicine,* 1967, *57,* 689–692.

Currier, L. The psychological impact of cancer on the cancer patient and his family. *Rocky Mountain Medical Journal,* 1966, February, 43–48.

Dell Orto, A. The role and resources of the family during the drug rehabilitation process. *Journal of Psychedelic Drugs,* 1974, *6,* 435–445.

Dyk, R., & Sutherland, A. Adaptation of the spouse and other family members to the colostomy patient. *Cancer,* 1956, January-February, 123–138.

Foster, R., & Lomas, D. Anger, disability, and demands in the family. *American Journal of Orthopsychiatry,* 1978, *48,* 228–235.

Halman, M., & Sutinger, J. Family-centered care for cancer patients. *Nursing,* 1978, *8,* 42–43.

Kanof, A., Kutner, B., & Gordon, N. The impact of infantile amaurotic familial idiocy (Tay-Sachs disease) on the family. *Pediatrics,* 1962, January, 37–45.

Marshall, J., Rice, D., O'Mera, M., & Shelp, W. Characteristics of couples with poor outcome in dialysis home training. *Journal of Chronic Diseases,* 1975, *28,* 375–381.

Netsky, M. Dying in a system of "good care": Case report and analysis. *Pharos,* 1976, April, 57–61.

Prichard, E., Collard, J., Orcutt, B., Kutscher, A., Seeland, I., & Lefkowitz, N. *Social work with the dying patient and the family.* New York: Columbia University Press, 1977.

Rynearson, E. The acute brain syndrome: A family affair. *Psychiatric Annals,* 1977, *7,* 590–593.

Sibinga, M., Friedman, C. J., & Huang, N. The family of the cystic fibrosis patient. *Journal of Thanatology,* 1971, *1,* 223–228.

Tyzenhouse, P. Myocardial infarction: Its effects on the family. *American Journal of Nursing,* 1973, June, 1012–1013.

Watson, P. A family centered ostomy rehabilitation program. *Critical Care Update,* 1977, September, 5–17.

Williams, A. Perceptions of nursing care: Effects of written and verbal instructional methods on families of head injury patients. *Heart and Lung,* 1978, *7,* 306–312.

Wishner, W., & O'Brien, M. Diabetes and the family. *Medical Clinics of North America,* 1978, *62,* 849–856.

HELPING SKILLS AND THE FAMILY

Much of the material in this section presents and illustrates a helping model for intervention with families of the physically disabled. The implementation of this model presumes knowledge of material discussed in the previous chapters. More specifically, it assumes that the health professional understands the many family influences that possibly can determine the direction and course of rehabilitation for the disabled family member.

As the chapters in Sections I and II explain, such influences are many and diverse. Family strengths can greatly enhance the disabled person's rehabilitation efforts. Such family capabilities as the ability of family members to communicate openly with each other, utilize appropriately community resources, show congruences in role relationships, fill in for each other and assume different functions as needed, provide each other with a sense of family belonging and provide the patient with moral support and ego encouragement in various endeavors could be positive forces during the rehabilitation process. At the same time, family weaknesses, e.g., chronic stress, misinformation about the condition, a family life-style that reveals an inadequacy to meet family members' needs, low expectations for the patient in the home, the inappropriate, continued reinforcement of the patient's unwarranted dependency needs, poor communication patterns, and isolating the patient from the affairs of family life represent deterrent factors that can affect the person's response to rehabilitation intervention. Combined with the family strengths and weaknesses are the emotional reactions of family members that result from the disability experience. How each family member responds to the particular trauma can frequently have a strong influence on the patient's treatment progress.

The personal statements of Sabine and Ted found in this section emphasize the importance of these influences, and show how these factors can shape the style of family intervention. Sabine and her husband lost three children who were multiple malformed at birth. With the realization that in these circumstances modern medicine was unable to help them, they felt overwhelmed. They found in their own relationship and within the extended family needed reassurance and support. They also discovered that parents can be helpers to health professionals, and they offer suggestions on how this can be accomplished.

The story of Ted is an account of how each family member contributed to Ted's gradual recovery. It contains many questions that family members have during this particular trauma and stresses that the entire family has a need to "recover." In looking back on how they coped during the many difficult months, they reflect on their difficulties and on the hope they gave each other. Family strengths were the stimuli for the continued energy needed by the family members during Ted's rehabilitation.

The knowledge of what happens to families experiencing a chronic illness or disability, and how they can affect their member's rehabilitation, is necessary information for the health professional, but the application of this knowledge requires specific skills. Both knowledge and skills are required for an effective, family treatment approach. The chapters in Section III identify the many skills that are needed by health professionals when they are working with families and their disabled family member. These helping skills can apply to many different disability-related situations. The family in crisis, the family in bereavement, the family attempting to adjust to a long-term chronic illness, and the family experiencing a "reflux" after an adaptive period present their own adjustment challenges and each demands some modification of a basic family helping approach. This basic intervention style is outlined in Figure 1. The concepts of "exploration," "understanding," and "action," as well as the main components of the exploration phase, e.g., attending and listening, are provided by Anthony and Carkhuff (1976), who have formulated an effective interpersonal counseling model. The authors of this volume use these main concepts to develop a family helping approach.

An added assumption for the implementation of this material in Section III is that health professionals have the opportunity within their job responsibility to work with the family, even if only briefly. Attention to the family may be an extended function beyond their identified disciplinary skills and tasks. To include the family in rehabilitation efforts frequently means more duties for the helper. This involvement may also imply that the health professional has to convince appropriate supervisors of the need for this intervention. In itself such convincing requires certain skills: assertiveness, ability to identify the importance of the family, and showing how one's primary job duties will not be seriously compromised. When this is accomplished, and the helper understands the role of the family in rehabilitation, then skill application can take place.

REFERENCE

Anthony, W., & Carkhuff, R. *The art of health care.* Amherst, Mass.: Human Resource Development Press, 1976.

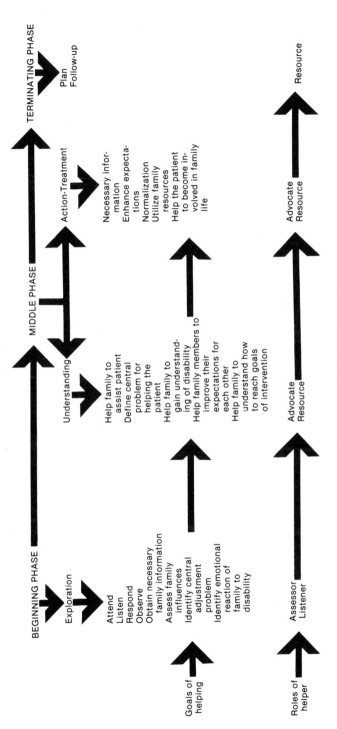

Figure 1. A family helping model.

315

PERSONAL STATEMENT ......
Sabine

As the mother of four children, I have been in an unusual position of giving them life and having three of them die. Both my husband and I have had to face many personal tragedies in our life, such as other personal losses and living through the ravages of war. However, coping with three disabled children has been the most demanding challenge of our lives.

My husband and I met in 1953 and were married in August, 1960. Our first child, a very healthy 9-pound baby girl, was born in 1963. A second child, a boy, was born in July, 1965, and was a relatively small child at 6 pounds and a few ounces compared to our girl. He had extra digits on his hands and feet and no sucking reflex. That is all they were aware of at that time. This baby died after 6 weeks. The diagnosis was the baby died of liver malfunction. At that time we decided to have another child as soon as possible. Our third baby was born in August, 1966, and had the same symptoms as the second child. He also had extra digits, cleft palate, microcephalus, paloric stenosis, and no sucking reflex. Those were the apparent problems. He, also, was only 6 pounds. The baby stayed 3 weeks in the Faulkner Hospital and went over to Floating Hospital. There he was diagnosed as being a child with Smith-Opitz syndrome. This syndrome was recently recognized and it was not known yet that there had been one case in our family already. People believed it could happen only to males and the chances were 25% per pregnancy to a couple like us. Apparently my husband and I have the same gene pattern, which only is known to happen in 1 out of 100,000. The chances of having another child like this, again, is only 25%. The baby was released to our custody after a month at Floating,

and we did not need help. We fed the baby by
gavage through the nose directly into the
stomach, which was not easy but certainly to be
learned how to do. From there on the baby
needed 24-hours-a-day attention. For example,
every 2 hours there was a feeding of 1½ ounces
of formula, and I took up the job for almost a
year before I realized that I was close to a nervous breakdown. Not because of emotion toward or against the child, but primarily lack of
rest coupled with the demands of the rest of the
family. At that time my mother-in-law asked us
if she could take over the duties and have the
child transferred to her apartment in Berlin,
West Germany. There he was well taken care of,
made very little progress, remained spastic to a
very high degree, grew tall but did not gain
weight, and became difficult to handle for this
elderly lady. But the love she gave to her grand-
child made her bear the inconvenience and
hardship she went through. Due to her care,
our son lived 6 happy years. He died in May of
1972. He was the oldest recorded child with
such a syndrome. After his death, we decided to
take another chance, and we had a baby in January, 1973. Again, the baby had the same syndrome. This time the child was a female. She
looked normal at birth except for the extra digits, not quite as pronounced a cleft palate, and
maybe microcephaly. She looked very much like
our first girl, who was normal, and at that time
we made the decision, which was not easy but
most probable best for all, including the first
child who was 10 at the time, to place the baby
into an institution. She went from Womens Hospital in Boston to a state school for a short stay,
since they tried to use her for research, and we
did not approve. From there we brought her to
an excellent small nursing home for young children with multiple birth defects. At that time
we made a point that she should have the best
of care but no heroic efforts should be made to
prolong her life, which obviously was done in

the first year of life to our third child. We did
not tolerate any more research on our children.
She lived 11 months, dying in December, 1974.
The diagnosis was pneumonia by food particles
in the lung, which unfortunately can easily
happen with children fed by gavage.

In looking back on our ordeal, I realize that
we helped the doctors, nobody helped us. We
helped them in learning more about the syndrome by our wanting to help medicine to discover why it occurred. The only thing I think
wasn't done quite right by the doctors was how
they told us what was wrong with the third
child. After having had one child already who
died, I think the doctors should have been more
sensitive in breaking the news to us and not
like in our case. Within 5 minutes after birth
the doctor unbundled the baby and said this
and that is wrong and the child will never be
normal and most probably would have been better if it hadn't been born, but that is how it is.
In other words, so live with it! That was the only time I lost my cool and it took about a week
to recuperate and accept that this could happen
to us, since both of us are very healthy people
and we never thought we might have any problems in having healthy children. The doctors
and hospitals were generally very uncooperative
in providing us with the records of our children. Also, I think it was insensitive and unpro-
fessional for personal opinions, such as "cute
baby" and "peculiar looking," to be entered on
records. Only strict medical information should
be put down.

Another difficult area for us was that we
got criticized not only from friends and neighbors but relatives after we had one abnormal
child to make the decision to have more children. We more or less ignored their feelings. We
thought we have to make up our minds and do
what we think is best for our marriage. Both
my husband and I love children tremendously
and were not willing to give up after having one

or two abnormal children. One reason we tried for a third child hoping it would be healthy was that the other two had died and we felt we could start all over. Nothing would have been more rewarding as having a healthy baby. We proceeded to live a normal life and didn't blame each other for having just one healthy girl. It seemed to be that everything was combined in our firstborn. She is healthy, very bright, pleasant. She combines what we could look for in four children into one. So we are grateful we have her.

What was most difficult was the realization that with all the recent advances in medicine, nothing could be done to alter our personal situation. We were most fortunate to have one healthy child, which has been a stabilizing factor in our lives. However, having lost three children places an increased burden on us, since we are very concerned about the health and safety of our surviving child. What would we do if something happened to her? How could we cope? The way we have resolved this is to recognize that, in spite of tremendous stress and strain in the past, we have been able to survive and cope. Therefore, we attempt to live our lives as fully as possible rather than constantly worrying about what may go wrong.

When we think about what we have been through, we recognize that it would have been impossible to survive if we did not have the support and understanding of one another as well as several friends and family members who were able and willing to help in times of need.

The constant physical care of our third child and the emotional drain that accompanied it was too much for any one person to bear. As parents of the child, we initially felt that it was our total responsibility. However, we soon recognized that it was more responsible to accept help rather than be unrealistic. Having lived with this experience and getting to know many other parents of disabled children, we feel that there are many things that could be done to initially ease the burden and reality of the situation. Most important to us would be the sensitivity and awareness of the medical profession to the emotional impact of having and caring for a disabled child. While there have been many excellent physicians and nurses who have worked with us, too often the busy schedule and high level of activity in medical facilities does not provide the opportunity or sensitivity required in responding and supporting parents in crisis.

Another area that was very difficult for us was attempting to find out those persons and resources who could help us during our time of crisis. It was most difficult having to phone and visit many agencies who seemed to be caught up in policy, procedure, and red tape, rather than personally responding to our needs. Reflecting upon our life, it is clear that the reason we were able to survive was because we had the ability to do so and we made the decision that we would not be destroyed by our problems.

However, we recognize that even though three of our children have died, we still live with the impact of that experience. This is where parents who have lost children need a great deal of support in resolving the many issues that will remain for many years, such as should they adopt or how can they learn to modify the feelings about what has happened so they can live as full a life as possible.

Both my husband and I recognize that our losses have taken their toll. We support one another, cry together and alone, and attempt to look ahead. Most important, we try to appreciate what we have rather than be bitter about what we lost.

CHAPTER 8

APPROACHES TO FAMILY INTERVENTION

Paul W. Power and Arthur E. Dell Orto

To help a family adjust to the impact of a chronic illness or severe disability requires diagnostic skills and an appropriate course of action after an assessment has been made. Often the patient does not achieve feasible rehabilitation goals because the health professional overlooks the importance of the disabled person's total environment as an influence upon treatment, or does not identify accurately the problem in this environment and is unaware of what to do after a positive or negative family influence has been understood. The authors believe that assisting the family to facilitate the patient's own adjustment, as well as helping the family itself to cope with the disability situation, calls for a distinctive helping approach.

The following pages contain a discussion of the goals and theoretical assumptions of this approach. Some implications of family therapy are provided. Because of their distinctive orientations, many family therapists make a substantial contribution to intervention during physical disability. In addition, a family assessment model is presented. With an adequate knowledge base obtained through the use of such an assessment, the helper will be able to assist the family more effectively.

INTERVENTION GOALS

Four goals are suggested for the health professional when assisting the family to help their disabled family member lead a more satisfying life. Each goal implies that during the helper's intervention efforts the family members can be assisted to adapt to the disability, and they also are being provided with specific knowledge and skills to help the disabled person. The goals are:

Providing the family with a sense of competence. The presence of a severe disability may increase anxiety and guilt for family members as well as reinforce feelings of worthlessness and helplessness. Because of the disability the family feels stigmatized, which in turn creates an atmosphere of inferiority. An intervention approach should aid family members to alleviate these feelings and to assist them to regain or develop control of their lives, individually and collectively. The development of such control represents the creation of new, positive family influences on the patient. Competencies to help achieve control include: 1) Communication—the ability of family members to express to each other their emotions, ideas, beliefs, and values, and to do so openly and freely (Otto, 1975). It also includes the capability of listening with empathy. 2) Flexibility—the willingness of family members to make necessary shifts in role responsibilities and to adapt to changes caused by the disabling condition. 3) Providing an atmosphere of belonging to each family member, namely, having the ability to give warmth, affection, and understanding frequently to each other. It includes giving responsibility to the patient for appropriate home duties and a voice in family matters, and extending support to each other in times of difficulty. If patients feel that the family is behind them they will be encouraged to be more productive. 4) The ability of the family to solve problems and make decisions. 5) The existence of mutual respect and recognition of the individual's self-worth, as well as the use of family meetings when plans, tasks, and problems are discussed jointly. 6) Participation in local, social, cultural, and school organizations and activities. This implies the family's ability to maintain and build friendships and relationships in their neighborhood, school environment, or vocational setting. 7) The capacity to seek and accept help when needed. Help might be sought from agencies, organizations, individuals, or professional sources. 8) Maintaining close and productive relationships with members of the extended family (grandparents, in-laws, relatives), where geographic proximity allows.

Assisting the family to normalize relations with each other and, as much as possible, with the patient.   All too often the family makes such severe adjustments in its daily life that it is living in a continuous state of serious disruption. Frequently this disruption causes the patient to be treated so differently that patient dependency and regression are stimulated. Normalization is an effort to provide appropriate patterns of living for the patient and all the family members. It includes normal expectations from family members for continued activities and maintenance of customary role responsibilities. Normalization does not eliminate the possibility, however, that many families will have to become re-oriented to the reality of the disability in their midst. For family members the problem is usually not the actual disease or disabling condition, but how to cope with it in every critical period of their lives.

One way to achieve family normalization is through appropriate coping efforts in the context of the family's own living environment.
Developing a renewed awareness by family members of their own resources and strengths. A disability situation often clouds an individual's perception of personal and family assets that can be used for adjustment purposes. For example, the basic emotional health of the family, the strength of the marital relationship, and the value and esteem that each member places upon the rights, aspirations, and needs of other members are often overlooked in a disability situation, but they can become important resources in time of family difficulty.
Creating a corrective, supportive, emotional experience for the family in which their mutual needs and feelings are recognized and acknowledged. This may include the need to deal with feelings of loss because of the disability condition of the family member, the need for emotional support from within the family, and the need to find social outlets apart from the family. Frequently the losses experienced by the patient, e.g., those caused by physical restrictions or loss of a regular job due to illness or disability, are overlooked by other family members. The disabled person may be hesitant to talk about personal losses because he perceives that other family members will not understand. Instead, these feelings are suppressed or the patient reacts to this family unresponsiveness by exaggerated dependency or continual irritation with others.

Of course, there may be additional family goals, depending on a specific disability or length of a chronic illness, but the achievement of these four goals by the family will represent a constructive reinforcement in the patient's life.

THEORETICAL ASSUMPTIONS

For a rehabilitation approach to be effective, there are certain underpinnings to an intervention with families of the disabled. They are assumptions that can both determine the way a particular family is helped and facilitate the attainment of the intervention goals stated in the beginning of this chapter. These assumptions are also convictions that arose from the author's past experience in working with families of the physically disabled.

1. Rehabilitation effort directed toward the patient and family is a joint venture shared by the helping professional and the family members. If the patient, family members, and professional worker share their energy and resources, it will intensify patient and family interest in their own contribution to the success of adjustment. In other words, the family is an integral part of the helping process, and most patients can-

not be treated in isolation. If they become a partner in rehabilitation efforts, the family members generally develop more willingness to work with each other. This is particularly true when family members choose between competing goals and values as they attempt to cope with the reality of a serious disability. The degree of consensus that develops among family members regarding the ranking of family goals can be a crucial factor in the family's ability to deal successfully with adjustment demands. What often fosters this consensus is the mutuality that has already been established between the worker and the family.

2. There will be predictable points of family stress in those affected by a disability or chronic illness. Each of these periods must be examined individually, because each can bring unique problems. For example, the birth of a congenitally disabled child or the diagnosis of a serious disease immediately after a trauma can cause blame, suspicion, fear, doubt, and guilt. The hospital stay, the convalescent period, or the time before a child with a disability arrives home can create anxiety and fear among family members. As disabled children mature and go through the preschool and elementary school years, reach adolescence, and then become adults, they will encounter specific difficulties. Problems can be created when disabled adults return home because new caring responsibilities may force family members to assume different functions in the home.

3. The basic instinct of people under stress is to hold to previously proved patterns of action, whether they are effective or not. A family reactive pattern will usually not vary too much from the way that family members have responded in the past. Health care professionals should make an effort during family assessment to understand these past adjustment styles; this will be helpful in establishing an intervention program.

4. Rehabilitation is generally a process of teaching persons to live with their disability in their own environment (Treischmann, 1978). Treischmann (1978) believes that the key to coping with one's disability is to receive enough satisfactions and rewards to make life worthwhile. When reinforcements for the patient are withdrawn from the family environment, the patient may feel isolated and become reluctant to respond to treatment efforts, or may become more manipulative in attempts to gain attention.

5. Family members will usually go through a grief-loss process after the birth of a congenitally disabled child or after the diagnosis or occurrence of a trauma or disabling condition. The way the family responds to the loss can be influenced by past losses and separations, the patient's age and sex, cultural and social attitudes toward loss, and current supports or stresses to the bereaved family. This grief is usually a normal reaction and, although it is draining, it can be a renewed opportunity for family adjustment.

IMPLICATIONS OF FAMILY THERAPY

Both the expansion of family theoretical knowledge and the continued development of treatment approaches have provided a valuable resource for professional workers when they are assisting a family with a severe disability. The variety of family therapeutic modalities allows the helper to select an approach that is appropriate to a personal, philosophical orientation and the particular family situation. Of the many relevant family concepts, the authors of this book identify three that are in close harmony with their own objectives of family treatment:

1. A family changes when its conception of itself and its ways of thinking changes (Ackerman, 1958). It changes by members learning to relate to each other in new ways, and then making changes that seem appropriate. To stimulate this change the therapist must determine the family's feeling level and create a new set of ways of acting and relating within the family. The responsibility for this change is with the family, not the therapist. Ackerman's beliefs have a direct implication for families of the physically disabled. Many families have trouble adjusting to a physical illness situation because of either incorrect or inadequate disease-related information. Also, the impact of the disability could have caused guilt, shame, and added anxiety. The family members begin to relate to each other in different ways, a difference that builds continued tension and serious disruption of family roles. The family often has to learn again how to relate in more positive ways. To achieve this, family members must learn new skills.

2. The family is held together by mutually reinforcing patterns and its goal is the nurture, support, and direction of its members (Satir, 1967). Satir (1967) believes that the family is the system in which various physical and emotional needs are met at different levels. This is especially true in families experiencing a physical disability or chronic illness. Situations that create new needs for family members include the patient facing slow deterioration or a changed body image, the family's involvement in physical treatment demands, and the limitations imposed on family members because of a person with a physical disability. Satir emphasizes the necessity of attending to these needs, and focuses on the identification of the mutually reinforcing patterns within a family. Unfortunately, such patterns are often lost when responsibilities change during the family adjustment process. If they are not lost, they may become obscured by new anxieties of coping with the new realities of living with a disabled family member.

3. "As a result of therapy,... changes are made in the set of expectations that govern its members' behavior" (Minuchin, 1974, p. 111). For families of the physically disabled, the key word is *expectations*. As family members attempt to adjust to the presence of a disability in their

midst, expectations often change for the patient and for each other. Many of these are necessary, such as those related to daily treatment demands or the patient's physical limitations. For example, a patient may not be expected to share in many family duties, or the mother of a disabled child may be expected to devote much of her time to caring demands. Family members may reorganize duties to compensate for caring demands, but the patient usually becomes angry when family members assume duties that the patient's physical condition permits him to carry out. Anger and lowered expectations contribute to family disruption and, more seriously, gradually cause family disintegration.

These selected tenets from three family therapists are part of the framework of a family helping approach. They indicate a direction to the health professional's intervention efforts. As stated many times in this book, the primary objective for the helper is to assist the patient to adjust to a disability or chronic illness. The family is viewed as a necessary agent for that goal. Another component of this intervention is a flexible, comprehensive, family diagnostic model.

A DIAGNOSTIC MODEL FOR FAMILY ASSESSMENT

In order to be effective in helping a family, health professionals should understand the dynamics that are unique to each family life. A diagnostic model includes this information, and focuses on more detailed characteristics of a family. It can identify those areas of family life that may be negatively influencing the patient's adjustment, and, in turn, indicate those factors in the family constellation that could promote the adaptation of family members. Family assessment can enable health professionals to expand the internal and external resource potential of the family unit (MacVicar & Archbold, 1976), and can assist them to determine what information the patient and family need to cope effectively with the illness condition.

The following outline is a suggested family assessment model that has been used by the authors for many years. The model itself is extensive, and parts of it can serve as an outline when taking a family history. To be utilized effectively the health professional must adapt it to the particular disability situation. More than one family meeting will be necessary to collect much of this information.

I. Family Demographic Data
    A. Age and sex of family members
    B. Occupation of spouses and family
    C. Educational background of parents and siblings
    D. Ethnicity

E. Religion
F. How many family members contribute to the family income?
G. How long has the family lived in its present location?
H. Are relatives living nearby and available in time of crisis?
I. Who pays the bills in the family?
J. Does the family have medical insurance coverage?
K. What are the family plans for the future concerning:
    1. education
    2. vacation
    3. retirement
L. Current major expenses of the family
M. Any previous family psychopathology?
N. What is the primary role of the patient in his family group? Is the patient left out from family planning, for example?
O. Is there a serious family problem, e.g., alcoholism? How is it vitally connected with the patient's medical or rehabilitation problem?

II. Communication Patterns in the Family
A. Is there open hostility among family members?
B. Do the family members appear to provide emotional support for each other? How is this support given?
C. What activities do family members share together?
D. Who dominates the family discussions? Who most frequently contradicts the dominant influence?
E. Do all family members express their opinions readily or is someone the spokesman for the family?
F. Do individual schedules permit much time together at home as a family?
G. Communication of feelings toward the disabled person
H. Description of sibling relationship
I. Present family areas of satisfaction

III. Division of Labor in the Family
A. Role of parents and children in family before illness/disability: what is to be done, who is to do it, and who takes leadership in deciding on allocation of tasks
B. What kinds of things are people expected to do around the house?
C. Which family members work together?
D. As a result of the disability, have family roles remained flexible or rigid? What role shifts have occurred?

IV. Extent of Family Members' Outside Socialization and Access to Social and Cultural Experiences

V. Health or Illness
- A. Do family members have regular clinic or doctor appointments?
- B. Any previous serious illness/disabilities in the family? If so, what are the family members' feelings about their experiences with doctors and hospitals?
- C. General attitudes toward pain, disability, treatment plans, or a specific illness: for example, do family members believe that the particular illness is amenable to treatment, or that treatment will lead to better health?

VI. Characteristics of the Disability/Illness
- A. Type of disability/illness
- B. Age of patient at onset of disease
- C. How is the person limited emotionally, physically, and intellectually?
- D. The suddenness of onset of illness/disability
- E. What do the family members and the patient understand about the nature and implications of the illness/disability?
- F. Attitudes of significant others toward the illness/disability event
- G. Family members' perception of the future limiting aspects of the patient as a result of the chronic disability
- H. Has there been a realignment of family goals?
- I. Has there been a change in the social needs of family members?
- J. Family members' references to past areas of satisfaction, including previous successful experiences with crises
- K. Is there a great deal of guilt, shame, and feelings of inadequacy among each family member?

VII. Impact of Disability on the Family
- A. On the regular performance of duties within the home?
- B. On the activities of family members outside of the home?
- C. Do the family members identify any continued adjustment problems resulting from the illness/crisis?
- D. Are community agencies used?
- E. Expectations of family members for each other:
  1. Toward household duties
  2. Maintaining social contacts
- F. How have the family members accepted the financial restrictions, if any, imposed by the illness?

Summary: Information
1. Appraisal of the residual health of the family relationships
   a. What areas of the marital and parental interaction and shared functioning are least damaged?
2. Appraisal of the damage of the relationships, resulting from the adjustment to the illness/disability

a. Does it threaten to engulf all major aspects of the marital and parental interaction, or are its effects relatively circumscribed?
b. Are there clear signs of a push toward isolation, disintegration, or regression in the family relationships?

CONCLUSION

There are many challenges in implementing a helping approach with families and patients of families who are living under the impact of traumatic illness or disability. Effective intervention by a health professional means providing a rehabilitation plan that is responsive both to the family's influences on the patient and the needs of the family. This approach is based on the helper's awareness of specific intervention goals, what is going on within the family, and the perspectives gained from family therapy that give a focus to family implementation. Frequently the first step in any family approach is for the health professional to have the job opportunity to provide such assistance. Often this demands a reorientation of the staff to the importance of the patient's psychosocial needs for rehabilitation goals.

The following articles in this chapter highlight this perspective. Dennis Jaffe identifies several family influences that can deter the patient's rehabilitation and also mentions the patient's emotional reaction to a chronic illness as a family obstacle to adjustment. He discusses the necessity of using the patient's immediate environment for treatment efforts, and explains a family therapy program that can be adopted by health professionals in a variety of work situations. Bruce Peck, in examining the relationship between illness and the rehabilitation process, draws upon selected case studies to emphasize the importance of the family's involvement. From his clinical practice he has found that when rehabilitation goals of one family member are not achieved, it usually means that other family members have some disruptive effect on the patient. Both articles show the value of exploring the many family influences affecting the disabled family member. These authors believe that rehabilitation must be a family affair.

REFERENCES

Ackerman, N. *The psychodynamics of family life.* New York: Basic Books, 1958.
MacVicar, M., & Archbold, P. A framework for family assessment. *Nursing Forum*, 1976, *15*, 180–194.
Minuchin, S. *Families and family therapy.* Cambridge, Mass.: Harvard University Press, 1974.
Otto, H. A. *Family strengths and their utilization in marriage and family counseling.* Beverly Hills, Cal.: Holistic Press, 1975.

Satir, V. *Conjoint family therapy*. Palo Alto, Cal.: Science & Behavior Books, Inc., 1967.

Treischmann, R. *The psychological, social, and vocational adjustment to spinal cord injury: A strategy for future research*. Final Report. Los Angeles: Easter Seal Society of Los Angeles County, 1978.

THE ROLE OF FAMILY THERAPY IN TREATING PHYSICAL ILLNESS

Dennis T. Jaffe[1]

As a family therapist, I look at human problems—whether psychological or physical—within the context of a person's most intimate relationships. In a decade of work I have seen how the family has a central role in the creation, maintenance, and alleviation of every aspect of human difficulty.

To mention the importance of the family in creating psychological disorders such as schizophrenia, depression, phobias, and sexual dysfunction, or in creating physical illness, is not to neglect or negate the presence of psychological or biological factors lying within the individual sufferer. Rather, taking the family perspective acknowledges that the individual is also shaped and molded by environmental factors.

The family is the most central and potent external force not only in shaping the individual personality and its difficulties but also in the expression of physical illness. Therefore, family therapy supplements other approaches to physical illness and psychological difficulty by considering that the family environment, which might add to the problem, may also be a key factor in overcoming it.

Family therapy is a style of psychotherapy, taught in most psychiatry departments, in which the primary patient or treatment unit is not the individual but the whole family. The aim of the therapy process is to change the way the entire family works together. Changes in patterns of family interaction have a clear and observable effect on many individual symptoms of distress.

For the first years of my work in family therapy, I stayed within the psychiatric section of the hospital, working with families containing individuals who had serious psychological difficulty. Then in 1974 I began to wonder whether chronic physical illnesses, many of which were termed psychosomatic, might to some degree also be the result of family processes. If so, people with physical illness might respond to family therapy.

I knew, for example, that psychosomatic illnesses were remarkably resistant to medical treatment at the symptom level. Some people come to

Reprinted from *Hospital & Community Psychiatry 29*(3), pp. 169–174, © 1978, American Psychiatric Association, with permission.

This paper is based on a presentation at the Conference on Psychosocial Innovations in Medical Practice, held February 25, 1977, in Los Angeles.

[1]Director, Learning for Health Program, Center for Counseling and Psychotherapy, Santa Monica, CA; and Adjunct Assistant Professor of Psychiatry, School of Medicine, University of California at Los Angeles.

clinics repeatedly with vague and diffuse complaints, while others can be relieved of their acute symptoms but continue their stressful life styles, which set them up for future difficulty. The situation is similar in psychiatric clinics, where family therapy has proven helpful. Certain behavioral and emotional difficulties, which had been difficult to treat with either drugs or individual psychotherapy, were overcome when the whole family became part of treatment and the ways that family members interacted were explored.

In my experience there is a clear connection between physical illness and psychological or family distress. Initially, I began to talk to medical patients and to their family members sitting in the hospital waiting room about what was happening in the family before the illness, how they did things as a family, and how illness affected them. I found them eager to talk, and most felt that their relationships, family history, and conflicts were indeed important factors in the current illness. Yet few of those concerns were communicated to the physician, who was not attuned to such dimensions and did not consider altering family relationships as a goal or aspect of treatment.

My own role evolved from the conversations with patients' families. I saw myself as a partner with the physician, as one working with the family factors. Just as the physician's role was to alleviate symptoms by intervening at the individual's biological and physiological level, my role was to help the family change the parts of their lives that contributed to stress, hindered rehabilitation, or led to conflicts that were likely to become expressed as physical illness.

While every physician knows that emotional, environmental, and other stress factors are significant in creating illness, medical training does not currently offer the physician any tools for altering family conditions, other than caring concern and common sense. Any member of the medical team—a psychologist, nurse, social worker, aide, or technician—can be trained in a few months to offer rudimentary family therapy. For it to be effective, however, the physician must learn enough about family treatment to support and reinforce the work of other team members. It is my hope that the use of family therapy in treatment of physical illness will not simply be confined to the psychotherapist's office, but rather will become an integral part of comprehensive medical care, taking place within the medical clinic.

DYNAMICS OF FAMILY ILLNESS

There are two interconnected pathways by which an aspect of family functioning can become part of a causal network, the outcome of which is some type of physical illness. The first pathway is through the stabilization and repetition of a dysfunctional behavior pattern. A common example is the family where a child is given sweets as a reward or as part of family gatherings. By learning to eat certain foods to excess because of their connection with love, warmth, and good feelings from other family members, a child begins a treadmill of dysfunctional family behavior that is probably transferred, in turn, to the next generation.

Many common family behavior patterns that bring short-term pleasure have long-term consequences that are destructive to health. I have observed many times that when an ill individual tries to change bad habits, the well-meaning but undermining responses of other family members—who continue to offer sweets, for example—effectively destroy his attempts to change. That process suggests the importance of altering family patterns to gain compliance with health regimens in situations where only one family member has become ill.

The second pathway by which family relationships contribute to illness is through the intervening variable of chronic stress. There are detailed accounts of how psychological, family, and social events can activate the body's stress response, which in turn is related to many forms of somatic illness (Pelletier, 1977; Jaffe, in press). Chronic stress, due to our personality patterns, relationships, and life styles, has been related to all of the most common and destructive illnesses today. Such aspects of family relationships as conflict, continuing anxiety, uncertainty, change, dislocation, or crisis create a stress response in the physiological system of each family member. That response, if not reversed, can help create or aggravate an illness, or make it difficult for treatment to overcome illness.

Between family processes and physical illness lie many intervening variables, such as constitutional predispositions, weak organs and body systems, personality make-up, individual ways of handling stress, and beliefs and expectations, which make it unlikely that any clear pathway can be found between a specific family pattern and a specific disease. Instead of looking for simplistic cause-and-effect pathways, the family therapist must look at the uniqueness of each family and how the specific history and patterns of relationship and attachment may lead to different physical consequences in each family member.

There has been little research on the relationship between family interaction and physical illness. In a recent review article, Weakland (1977) notes that "family somatics" has been almost entirely neglected since a pioneering review article by Jackson more than a decade ago. The results of most of the research have an unfortunate tendency to characterize family patterns as givens rather than as variables that can be changed. Yet family therapists have shown that even a relatively brief intervention (ten sessions) can alter longstanding family patterns.

My own work with more than 50 families in the Learning for Health program suggests that short-term family therapy can be a useful addition to the treatment process for many illnesses. In order to document its usefulness, review some of the literature, and suggest how individual families help create and complicate illness for their members, I will present accounts adopted from my work.

STRESSFUL LIFE EVENTS

A 30-year-old divorced woman with a young child has had three operations in the past year—for gallstones, for an ovarian cyst, and exploratory surgery—and was not recovering well from her last operation. She had recurrent pains, and was afraid of dying. Before this year she had no serious illness. She dated the onset of her troubles to her father's sudden death just two months before her first surgery. At the funeral she had a fight with her mother and younger sister and had not seen them since. She adored her father, whom she was much closer to than her mother, and she felt that her role in the family came about through her connection with him.

Between the first and second operation she broke off a long-term relationship with a man who was warm and loving to her, like her father. She was extremely upset and disoriented by her recent life changes, none of which had been addressed in her medical treatment. In talking to me, she began to explore her feelings about each of the changes in her family, and began to develop a new way of relating to her family. She was able to mourn her father's death, discover new ways to relate to the others in her family, and begin to think about having other deep relationships.

In addition to the stress and change in her external life, she was under pressure because of the way in which she interpreted the stressful events. Her personal reactions to them included feelings that she was somehow responsible, that she ought to have died instead, and that she couldn't live without her father. As she explored these feelings and changed some of her intimate relationships, she began to heal.

FAMILY EVENTS AND ILLNESS

Astute physicians have always linked family events to illness. Parkes and others found that widowers were five times more likely than norms would suggest to die soon after their spouses, often of the same illness (Parkes, Benjamin, & Fitzgerald, 1969). LeShan has reviewed scores of studies on personality, emotions, and family variables in relation to cancer, and he finds many studies supporting the association between cancer and loss of a person or object that is emotionally significant (LeShan, 1959, 1966). Thomas and Duszynski (1974) report on a prospective study of medical students that began more than 20 years ago. Their long-term data suggest that certain childhood family patterns can be linked with certain types of emotional and physical illness occurring many years later.

The definitive research on the association between stressful life events and illness comes from the work of Holmes and Rahe and their associates. They developed a scaling procedure to rate the relative degree of adaptation required for the common life events of an individual. The Social Readjustment Rating Scale is a list of 42 common events; each event has a weight of severity ranging from 1 to 100. At the extreme end, 100, is death of a spouse; in the middle, at 50, is marriage; and at the low end are minor traffic fines, vacations, and holidays.

They found in a series of studies that people, like the woman reported above, who have a number of serious life changes within a year—whether positive or negative—are at risk for serious illness. Their research suggests that any sort of adaptive change entails physiological stress, which may in turn lead to illness. Significantly, the majority of the important life changes on their scale are related to changes in family relationships (Holmes & Masuda, 1974). In my work I have found that even the anticipation of life events or changes can be a precursor to illness.

SECONDARY GAIN

Nearly all of us, when we were children, occasionally exaggerated a pain to stay home from school and received an unusual outpouring of affection and care from a worried mother. That is an example of what is termed secondary gain—a positive consequence of an otherwise negative condition.

Every physician observes how disability, chronic pain, and illness can bring a family member benefits and can excuse him from some responsibilities. It is my observation that secondary gain is present in a majority of illnesses and thereby contributes, probably not at a conscious level, to some people's reluctance or inability to get well.

A striking example of how secondary gain may affect illness came from the family situation of a woman with cancer. Her husband was suddenly transferred to a new office in a different city, and she had to leave her home of 20 years. During the same period, her children had been leaving for college. After the move it took her a few lonely years to make a place for herself. Her husband worked long hours during that time to earn another promotion. Finally she felt at home.

Once again, however, her husband announced that he had to move. She developed breast cancer. As a result of her treatment, he was unable to move. She did not respond to chemotherapy. During family therapy, she was asked what would happen if she got better. "We would move, and I would have to find a whole new set of friends," she replied.

I do not know how much the couple's subsequent agreement to stay in their current home, and the husband's decision to spend more time vacationing and doing things with her, had to do with her current remission.

After therapy, however, which involved airing her feelings about not being taken into account in decisions, she did better in medical treatment. The work of Simonton and Simonton (1975) offers many further examples of the association of secondary gain with poor response to cancer treatment.

Another aspect of secondary gain comes when one family member's sickness seems to be a way to compel attention, affection, care, or simply time from the mate or parent. Illness is often a part of family life in ways similar to alcohol. The ill person, like the alcoholic, is presumed to be helpless and infantile because he or she is "ill," and consequently gets a great deal of attention.

One of the most difficult aspects of family therapy is unraveling the sources of secondary gain in a family with an ill member. Yet in many cases where an individual becomes ill for no clear physical reason, maintains chronic pain, does not respond to treatment, experiences symptomatic recurrences after treatment, or simply does not return to health despite the success of medical treatment, secondary gain provides the key.

There are not only secondary gains for the ill person but also potential gains for other family members. For example, a sick child may keep a couple from having to spend time together, or help a wife keep away from her husband. Or nursing may be the most comfortable way for one spouse to show affection, so that person would encourage his or her mate to be sick as often as possible.

The many permutations of secondary gain all relate to its primary quality: through illness a person is able to exert control over other family members or get what he wants, without having to own up to the fact that that is what he is doing. It is not conscious, because the common assumption is "I can't help being sick; it's not my fault." Haley (1963) explores the effects of such denial of responsibility on relationships, and he offers guidelines for the therapist to help families to short-circuit these self-destructive pathways of communication.

I explore potential sources of secondary gain by asking questions of family members. First I observe that sometimes a person gains certain advantages from being sick, and then ask them to explore what they might be in their or their relative's case. Or I may suggest that they write a list of reasons why the patient became sick, and why he is remaining sick. Most people resist this approach at first, but with prodding are able to come up with reasons.

The suggestions made by some family members often lead other members to share the hidden feelings and reactions they have to illness, and to think of ways that they can be more honest in asking for what they need from each other. I have never found a family or an individual who could not identify secondary gains from illness. It is not that I feel it is wrong to receive secondary gain, but simply that most people can learn to receive the gain without the cost in terms of illness.

LETHAL DYADS

I have seen several examples of what I have named lethal dyads—couples who escalate each other's potentiality for illness by the structure of their relationship and the nature of their demands on each other. The emotional and personality patterns of each person seem to bring disaster to the other. It is not simply a specific personality or emotional make-up that brings on illness, but the personality that lives in an environment in which another person acts in a certain way. Unless the pattern of the relationship is changed, each member of such a dyad literally drives the other to chronic illness.

An example is a middle-aged couple, both of whom were seriously ill. The husband, an engineer, described himself as a workaholic. He had a serious coronary and had to work less. His wife was diagnosed as having cancer soon after. In family interviews, it turned out that the husband had always been the responsible one in the family, a role that his wife willingly agreed to. She grew increasingly helpless and dependent on his taking initiative and responsibility. His illness almost forced her to switch roles and take initiative. At that point she developed cancer, which in turn worried him and made him feel he had to be more responsible, to pay the bills, and to take care of her. He couldn't let down, but experienced new demands, responsibility, and worry.

Thus a lethal cycle was in motion. His illness seemingly resulted in part from his taking on too much and driving himself too hard. When he was forced to become dependent and reverse roles with his wife, she reacted by having a breakdown herself—in effect trying to get him back into his accustomed role. It was not a conscious process, but it was hard for me not to feel that their illnesses were connected with this interaction pattern. I helped them to do some things for themselves and to help each other. Each began to recover.

Hoebel (1977) studied coronary patients who continued to ignore risk factors like diet, exercise, smoking, and lack of relaxation and were uncooperative in their medical treatment. His assumption was that their wives could affect their behavior and help them to give up their dangerous activities. So he asked only the wives to participate in the program. In several sessions, he helped them see that, although their intentions were good, they may not have been meeting their husbands' medical needs. He helped them develop and put into effect strategies that encouraged their husbands to change. Without the husbands' cooperation, he was able to influence them to change simply by helping the wives change their behavior.

His conclusion was that health-threatening behavior in a family is due to interaction, and that family treatment can be successful even with the highly resistant or noncompliant patient. Hoebel suggests that noncompliance is a family problem, and is amenable to family treatment. He showed that lethal interaction in couples can be reversed. If spouses can lead each other to illness, they can also learn to help each other regain health. Hoebel has demonstrated a corollary of family therapy: since a family system is interconnected, a change in any one part or person, not necessarily the patient, can result in positive change in the patient.

> I tell prospective clients that my work is based on a hypothesis that psychological and family factors are important in illness and healing. I ask them to join me in an inquiry into the role of such factors in their illness.

I have found that any treatment regimen can benefit from work with the whole family, by promoting compliance and dealing with problems that arise as a result of caring for the ill member. Strauss (1975) suggests that the reaction of the family is the crucial determinant of the extent of rehabilitation from chronic illness. Also, as noted in the couple above, the illness of one family member creates stress and changes the family situation for the others, and may in turn lead them to illness. When one family member is seriously ill, all other family members are at risk to develop illness. That is why family-oriented physicians must be alert to the results of one family member's illness on the others.

THE CHILD AS A SCAPEGOAT

The most comprehensive application of family therapy to physical illness has been in the work of Minuchin and his colleagues (1975) with children with anorexia nervosa, abdominal pain, asthma, and diabetes. They observed certain family interaction patterns in those illnesses, created a theoretical model of how psychosomatic illness is created within families, and tested the model.

Of several factors Minuchin suggests as necessary for the development of severe psychosomatic illness in children, one is that the sick child plays an important role in the family's pattern of conflict avoidance and that role is an important source of reinforcement for his symptoms. The ill child is, in effect, a scapegoat whose illness takes up the family's concentration and focus, thereby allowing them to avoid some other conflict.

The way that the ill child short-circuits a parental conflict is illustrated by a family with an asthmatic child. Whenever the mother was angry at the father, she would confide in her ten-year-old son, telling him that he was the "only one who understood her." The father was cold and seemingly uninvolved in the family. The parents had no sexual relations. The mother seemed to put all her energy into her son, taking care of him and in a sense asking him to never leave her emotionally the way his father did. As the child felt the conflict and the responsibility of his role, he obeyed his mother by becoming weak, aggravating a hereditary predisposition, and developing asthma.

Ill children, whether as a consequence or a cause of their illness (probably a little of both), tend to be protected by parents, and develop few relationships with friends and achieve little independence from their family.

Minuchin's treatment strategy usually involves helping the child to become more independent from the family, and convincing the family to be less concerned, intrusive, and involved in the child's physical state. At this stage of treatment, the conflict or distance between the parents becomes obvious, as the child moves toward his friends. The parents' conflict must be addressed in the final stage of therapy. The parental conflict is not often obvious until the central focus on the child's illness is changed.

Following Minuchin's strategy, I helped this family accomplish several tasks. First, I tried to cut the secondary gain for the son by encouraging the family to send him to school and to play with friends. I had the physician reassure the family that he was not seriously ill and could be active without medical risk. That eased their anxiety somewhat.

Second, I tried to get the father to do more with his son. It turned out that both were interested in athletics, but the father had avoided them because he felt the son was not strong enough or interested. That suggestion helped the boy make contact with his father. The boy's attacks became less severe.

Soon I began to see the parents separately, and they began to see that they had very little to say to each other and spent very little time together. They also began to face the fact that their lack of sexual contact was hurting their relationship. They entered couples therapy to work on these issues, and the son's asthma receded from being a focus of their attention.

THE FAMILY THERAPY PROGRAM

My program, Learning for Health, involves applying to the area of physical illness family therapy techniques that have already been successfully applied to psychological difficulty. So far it has involved short-term individual, family, and group therapy—five to 15 hour-long sessions—as part of a comprehensive medical treatment program for a chronic physical condition.

My referrals come in almost equal numbers from individuals, their families, and physicians. The clients are often people who have had negative or inconclusive encounters with medical treatment and who want to explore psychological and family contributions to their illness. Since most of the clients have not had previous experience with psychotherapy, I do not feel that they are any more predisposed to believe that family factors are important than ordinary medical patients. However, they seek my help at a time when other approaches have failed and are eager to cooperate, as are their physicians. I tell prospective clients that my work is experimental, based on a hypothesis that family and psychological factors are important in illness and healing. I ask them to join me in an inquiry into the role of such factors in their illness.

While the work progresses differently with each couple or family, I have found that there are certain common elements that make up the total approach. They do not occur in any particular order, but they illustrate the range of activities that together fall within family therapy.

Family history. I always take a family history that includes how the family has developed over the last two generations, focusing on major events. I ask about illnesses and how the family reacted to illness; changes, transitions, crises, and scandals; personalities; and recent stress. I usually interview the couple or family together, focusing on each person in turn. Often I ask each person to write his autobiography between the first two sessions, to reflect on past factors that might contribute to illness. I also use a questionnaire that helps the family focus on their past in relation to their present concerns. That process takes from two to four hours, and often helps the family to make important connections without prodding or interpreting on my part.

Exploration of meaning of the illness. Whatever its physiological nature, I assume that an illness has a certain function, role, and meaning in the family. In asking how the illness is treated by the family, what it does for the ill person, and how it affects the family, I explore various secondary gains and also look for deeper symbolic significance of the illness for family members. Often the illness repeats a pattern of a generation earlier, such as an expectation that the ill person would die of the same disease and at the same age as a relative.

I ask the patient and other family members two questions repeatedly: why are you ill right now, and why did you first become ill? I let them find as many reasons as they can. My intent is to open discussion within the family that counteracts the common medical assumption that a person has nothing to do with his own illness. I ask families to explore the illness with the assumption that perhaps something they are doing, or have done, relates to its onset and severity. I let the family determine the relevance of their answers for themselves.

Education. Since my approach demands the active participation of family members, I need to educate them in an unfamiliar perspective on illness. Therefore, I give them some articles written by me and by others on psychological and family factors in medicine and on the relation of stress factors to illness. Each person also receives a personal health workbook and journal to focus his self-inquiry into illness. I also conduct classes in stress release, through meditation, imagery, or autogenic training, which I encourage all members of the family to attend. In addition, I furnish information about health habits and the role of behavior in maintaining health.

This remedial health education is one of the most meaningful and important parts of any total health program, although education is not traditionally conceived as part of either medical or psychological therapy. A discussion of readings on health can often precipitate important family insights about changes, and also is an important way to lead the family members to see that they are important to maintaining their health.

Contract to change. I help each family look at aspects of their interaction that they want to change, and support them in experiments to accomplish that change. At each session outcomes are evaluated, and subsequent steps planned. The relationship of all aspects of family life to the current illness are explored. I also make contracts with individuals to carry out changes, and work with family members individually when necessary.

System change. Following other family therapists, I try to change not only specific factors that may lead to illness but also general aspects of the whole family as a system. I have found that certain qualities of family interaction correlate with emotional and physical health. Those qualities include flexibility in sensing and responding to new situations; openness to and active seeking of information from friends, relatives, agencies, and schools; ability to express feelings so that other family members can respond accurately; and autonomy from the family so that each member can pursue outside interests and involvements.

Support group. I find that change can be maintained only when the environment supports it. Thus it is difficult for one member of a family to lose weight when other family members joke about it or bring home sweets. Changes in a family life style that support health and help individuals overcome illness are often hard to maintain. Therefore, I find that support groups, modeled after such groups as Alcoholics Anonymous or Weight Watchers, can be important in maintaining changes once they have been made. As a final step in therapy I like to see one or more family members participate in a support group or follow-up treatment. Health is not a one-time achievement; it must be actively maintained.

My clinical experience indicates to me that family relationships, behavior patterns, and the way that people respond to stressful life events are important causal factors in illness and health. As yet there are only rough theories and a few scattered clinical observations that move beyond the basic assumption that family dynamics are important to health. More research is needed to show the physician, therapist, or member of the health team that it is important to include family therapy in the treatment program. Through family therapy it is possible to affect family relationships and stress factors in a positive direction, toward greater health.

REFERENCES

Haley, J. *Strategies of psychotherapy.* New York: Grune & Stratton, 1963.

Hoebel, F. C. Coronary artery disease and family interaction: A study of risk factor modification. In P. Watzlawick and J. H. Weakland (Eds.), *The interactional view,* pp. 363–375. New York: W. W. Norton & Co., 1977.

Holmes, T. H., & Masuda, M. Life change and illness susceptibility. In B. S. Dohrenwend & B. P. Dohrenwend (Eds.), *Stressful life events: Their nature and effects,* pp. 45–72. New York: John Wiley & Sons, 1974.

Jaffe, D. T. *Healing from within.* New York: Alfred A. Knopf, in press.

LeShan, L. Psychological states as factors in the development of malignant disease: A critical review. *Journal of the National Cancer Institute,* 1959, *22,* 1–18.

LeShan, L. An emotional life-history pattern associated with neoplastic disease. *Annals of the New York Academy of Sciences,* 1966, *125,* 780–793.

Minuchin, S., et al. A conceptual model of psychosomatic illness in children. *Archives of General Psychiatry,* 1975, *32,* 1031–1038.

Parkes, C. M., Benjamin, B., & Fitzgerald, R. G. Broken heart: A statistical study of increased mortality among widowers. *British Medical Journal,* 1969, *1,* 740–743.

Pelletier, K. R. *Mind as healer, mind as slayer.* New York: Delacorte, 1977.

Simonton, O. C., & Simonton, S. S. Belief systems and management of the emotional aspects of malignancy. *Journal of Transpersonal Psychology,* 1975, *7,* 29–47.

Strauss, A. A. *Chronic illness and the quality of life.* St. Louis: C. V. Mosby, 1975.

Thomas, C. B., & Duszynski, K. R. Closeness to parents and the family constellation in a prospective study of five disease states: Suicide, mental illness, malignant tumor, hypertension, and coronary heart disease. *Johns Hopkins Medical Journal,* 1974, *134,* 251–270.

Weakland, J. H. Family somatics: A neglected edge. *Family Process,* 1977, *16,* 263–272.

PHYSICAL MEDICINE AND FAMILY DYNAMICS:
The Dialectics of Rehabilitation

Bruce B. Peck[1]

An enduring research question and clinical problem is the impact of a disability in one family member on the larger family system. Equally elusive is an understanding of the effect of family dynamics on the rehabilitation process. Recent discussions (Framo, 1972) have amplified the need for an understanding of the relation between illness and the family. Unfortunately, this issue has received limited attention from researchers and practitioners (Glick & Haley, 1971).

The systems sciences, however, have provided a language and medium for expanding our awareness of the apparent reciprocal features of family living. To extend this understanding, a clinical-casework study of patient, family, and rehabilitation problems was conducted in three physical medicine settings over a two-year period. A primary purpose was to determine the role of family dynamics in the rehabilitation of a disabled family member and the effects of a rehabilitation intervention on the family.

In the course of this study, the reciprocal, interpersonal exchanges among the patient, his family, the physician, and rehabilitation personnel emerged as specific configurations—configurations that appeared to display separate and unique dynamics. Structurally, these reciprocal situations are similar to transactional games (Berne, 1961). Further, these recurrent configurations or model situations were relevant for geriatric, as well as for younger, acute patients.

To date, four primary configurations have been identified. This paper will consider these four interpersonal situations in terms of their core dynamics, the persons involved, the impact on rehabilitation outcomes, and the effects of interpersonal interventions.

Reprinted from *Family Process 13(4)*, pp. 469–479, ©1974, with permission.

The author wishes to thank Rollin Houle, Chief of Physical Medicine, United Hospitals Inc., St. Luke's Division, St. Paul, Minnesota, for including him as an active member of his rehabilitation family. Marilyn St. Martin, R.N., Referral Coordinator at St. Luke's Hospital, provided a number of valuable insights into the difficulties of working directly with rehabilitation families. Earl Pederson, Rehabilitation Coordinator, St. Cloud Hospital, St. Cloud, Minnesota, graciously allowed the author to be a foster child in his rehabilitation unit while this study was being conducted.

[1]From Emanuel Mental Health Center, Turlock, CA.

THE PHENOMENOLOGY OF DISABILITY

An early finding was that the phenomenology of disability is a common, key element in the four identified configurations. From the early days of a formal study of psychopathology down through Laing's (1959) *The Divided Self,* researchers have recognized a capacity in man to think of himself in parts, to "split" himself. Descartes' mind-body solution predates these studies and provides a philosophical base for looking at man in at least two parts. This two-sidedness is considered an integral feature of man such that psychotherapy procedures are frequently designed around this notion.

When viewed in a larger social context such as the family, a disability highlights and even amplifies this dual aspect in the disabled person. A disability in the physical medicine sense has the status of a natural entity. For example, a cerebro-vascular accident (CVA) is a something that someone has along with observable, concomitant *sequelae.* As a natural entity, a disability can be studied and treated in the natural science sense. This assumes that the object of study (CVA) forms no relationship in the personal sense. You cannot get chummy with a CVA unless you want to run the risk of being called *crazy* and treated accordingly. A CVA does not experience itself being studied nor experience the form and style of the scientist-object relationship.

However, a problem exists since the CVA is immanent in a person who, from a science of persons view, does have the capacity to reciprocate the personal relationship of the observer as a person, thereby confirming himself as a person and the observer as a person. A feeling of personhood breaks down if the observer and "object" do not reciprocate each other's awareness of the other's person. If the scientist responds to only one aspect—the disability—he simultaneously disconfirms the second side of this split—the person. This double-level potential is much more probable once an overt physical disability is introduced. At this point, the person is faced with a dilemma. Should he struggle to remain a person or give in to everyone else and become a non-personal disability.

The introduction of a disability in one family member frequently generates an unspoken, family-shared fantasy of death. Older persons are responded to "as if" they were dead. The socialized form of this fantasy is the family stance that the patient is not capable of caring for himself as in the past. Conversely, in younger disabled persons, the fantasy is played out between mother and child through the stylized, symbiotic dance of dependency. This gives mother and the family an opportunity to go back and re-raise their child with the idea of not making the same mistake twice. This "as if dead" or "as if re-born" fantasy gives rise to frequently occurring rehabilitation configurations.

The first configuration is an example of how the natural science approach to a disability infuses the relationship atmosphere of the family and affects the disabled person's progress.

Mr. Y., 65 years old, some two years prior had suffered a stroke. In the hospital he improved and was returned to his home. There his wife communicated with the doctors and generally assumed full responsibility for his living. She waited on him hand and foot. As a result of this inactivity, his leg atrophied to the point that it needed to be removed. During his second stay on the rehabilitation unit, the staff was worried about Mr. Y. because he was not involved with the activities around him. Some were even convinced that he had "lost contact with reality" and felt that a psychiatric consultation was needed. The rehabilitation team could not understand why Mr. Y. was not more energetic and eager to improve.

Finally, a psychologist was called in to see him; and his evaluation pointed in two directions. At a personal level, Mr. Y's self-concept was characterized by feelings of deterioration, decay, and lack of potency. He apparently had lost his sense of power as a separate person. Mr. Y. was communicating that all he could do was sit by and wait helplessly while his body slowly deteriorated. On the other side of the coin, Mr. Y. possessed a strong desire to reach out and be involved with other people.

Mr. Y. was in the untenable position of being invalidated as a person and being responded to as an organism incapable of reciprocating in any interpersonal context. As such, he was slowly and surely being driven mad.

It was decided that he was to be consulted directly concerning his rehabilitation progress. For example, Mr. Y. was given the job of scheduling his daily exercise regimen and OT appointments as well as choosing the specific PT skills that he wanted to develop. Once Mr. Y. was given an opportunity to be involved in *his own* rehabilitation, his spontaneity and sparkle reappeared. Rather than Mr. Y. being out of contact with reality, the larger rehabilitation team had been out of contact with Mr. Y., his power as a person, and his capacity to control his own future.

This is a common configuration and emerges when other family members assume an excessive amount of the patient's initiative once the disability has occurred. In these situations, rehabilitation is viewed as a *something* that happens in the absence of any personal involvement. This interpersonal style is also sustained by the sheer momentum of the rehabilitation team. The frenetic level of activity in a busy rehabilitation center creates an atmosphere in which the patient's initiative is taken over by the rehabilitation team's missionary zeal. Once all vestiges of his initiative are absorbed, the person of the patient is left in a strange land where his integration as a person is severely threatened.

A second configuration illustrates the difficulties involved during intervention into a heavily triangulated family situation. A triangle is a frequently encountered interpersonal configuration in the rehabilitation arena; it seems to emerge when a couple "decides" that the intensity of their prior conflicts is too great. The original dyad will then involve another person who becomes the third angle of the newly formed triangle and who absorbs or continually diverts the couple's struggles.

> Mrs. S., a 49-year-old mother of six, suffered a stroke. At onset, she entered a rehabilitation center for two months and returned home. There she assumed a helpless stance that forced her younger daughters to care for their mother as well as run the household. Father apparently was not involved either in his wife's problems or with helping his daughters. According to reports, he was gone from home often and "drank a little."
>
> Shortly after her return home and under pressure from the children, Mrs. S. returned to the hospital and was placed in the rehabilitation unit for intensive therapy. The expressed goal was for her to become generally independent so that she could return home to care for herself and her household with minimal assistance.
>
> While in the hospital, communication with the family was accomplished through the daughters. Mr. and Mrs. S. had limited meetings. When he did visit, it was noticed that they did not talk much. On the unit Mrs. S. was obstinate, passive, oppositional, and generally displayed no desire to cooperate in her rehabilitation. She seemed hell-bent on undoing any attempts to help her use the capacities for independence she possessed. Finally, the rehabilitation staff in a state of utter frustration asked that Mrs. S. be referred to the psychologist.
>
> This struggle with Mrs. S. continued throughout her stay in the hospital and seemed to reach its peak when discharge time approached. By then none of the family members seemed the least bit interested. The children had begun to be involved in other activities, while father was even more remote and unavailable. Mrs. S. was finally discharged to her home where she continued almost as before; except this time neither her children nor her husband were available to help her.

The two family interviews conducted prior to discharge identified a family that was in a state of progressive disruption, a disruption characterized by a migration of individuals away from the *family core*. The onset of mother's disability appeared to fracture the marriage to such an extent that Mr. S. made the first significant move away from his wife. The children who were living at home moved in to fill this void, thereby creating the initial triangle of mother-children-father. The children assumed the responsibility for mother's care, leaving father somewhat removed. This arrangement also generated the children's fantasy, "We'll have to stay home and care for mother the rest of our/her life, whichever comes first!" The agitation created in the children pushed them to have mother become more independent so they would be free to grow.

With the movement of mother into the hospital, a second triangle was created, i.e., rehabilitation team-mother-children. Within this new triangle, *mother* kept her position as before. The *rehabilitation team* assumed the children's former caring role. The *children* moved into father's previous spot of distant observer, while *father* moved into a fourth position outside of the new triangle. There he cultivated his disinterest in family matters and moved emotionally farther away from his wife and children. The children in father's old position quickly began to develop outside interests and had fun as young adults about to leave home.

As we learned, mother's fighting in the hospital was a struggle not to be abandoned. She felt the only way she could keep her family together was for her to remain helpless so the family would rally around to care for her. For Mrs. S., independence would ultimately mean the dissolution of her family. To the family, discharge meant the dissolution of the rehabilitation team-mother-children triangle and the resumption of the children-mother-father-triangle. It became painfully clear that it was almost impossible to resume a triangle when one of the angles has been on the outside (e.g., father) and lost his sense of involvement for even a short time. By discharge day, the children were living with the assumption that someone else would care for their mother. They would not give up their new-found sense of individual identity to take care of mother, and father would not regenerate his interest after having worked so hard to distance himself from the family.

Through the rehabilitation intervention, we destroyed the community effort and the capacity of the family to work out a democratic way to care for mother. Instead, the intervention set in motion a "hands-off" policy in which mother could potentially be passed from one rehabilitation unit to another. In retrospect, it seemed more useful for the rehabilitation team to remain as the outsiders and, thereby, sustain their power to move in and out of the family rather than extrude one critical family member (in this case, father) and risk further rupture of the family's unity.

Following is an additional configuration that is very difficult to treat without disrupting the core family. It is also a triangulated situation, yet is more subtle and vicious than the previous configuration.

Mrs. A., a 46-year-old woman, was severely disabled following an auto accident. She was thrown into the windshield and suffered considerable brain damage. During her outpatient rehabilitation, Mr. A. was her constant companion. He assumed almost primary responsibility for her speech and physical therapy. At one stage, Mr. A. reported that his wife was saying strange things. Apparently she felt that he was going to kill her in two weeks because he did not like her dogs and that he was selling some of their things. The rehabilitation staff referred Mrs. A. to the psychologist because of her "paranoid thinking and emotional problems."

A conjoint interview revealed a number of here-to-fore unnoticed aspects of the marital dyad. In addition to their stable, interlocking roles, Mr. and Mrs. A. evidenced a devastating communication style. A primary feature was his brand of help, which turned out to be a subtle, vicious attack, an attack that allowed him to express his resentment and foster her helplessness. Specifically, he would not acknowledge the content of her communications about her experiences. He would discount her feelings by translating them into what he felt she should be saying. At a symbolic level of communication, Mr. A. was truly kill-

ing his wife by invalidating her experiences, one of the most effective ways known to drive someone crazy (Peck, 1974).
Following this single interview, Mrs. A's "symptoms" disappeared. At the same time, Mr. A. turned his attention to members of the rehabilitation staff. He began to spread rumors about one staff person to another. These staff persons were all directly involved with Mrs. A's therapy.

The conjoint interview highlighted a subtle impasse and battle that had gone unnoticed. Mr. A. had seduced the rehabilitation experts into giving him advice on helping his wife. In the long run, he would not pay attention to them since he had his own secret agenda to drive his wife crazy.

The central impasse in this situation revolves around a phenomenology of disability issue. The family and the rehabilitation team "square off" over the issue of who will be allowed to respond to the disability as a natural entity. According to the rules of this interpersonal encounter, the loser must deal with the patient as a person while the winner assumes the expert status and responds to the disability as a scientific entity. The winner has the transactional right to be less involved and more distant from the person. The actual struggle consists of family members attempting to topple the rehabilitation experts by undercutting therapy progress.

A "squared-off" situation is generated by the working assumption that one family member can act as a primary therapist for his disabled relative. Typically, the rehabilitation team will teach a family member how to conduct a therapy regimen at home. Once this process is active, the rehabilitation team has unwittingly aligned itself with the resentment vector of the helper-disabled person relationship. As the helping family member increasingly becomes an out-patient therapy expert, he can more successfully mask his resentment under the guise of help. This live-in therapist is simultaneously related as a person, and as an expert, to a member of his own family. This leaves the disabled person in a painful, almost unassailable, double bind in the form: "Of course I still love you. I'm helping you, am I not?" The expert family member has absolute power over his relative, power so excessive that he can move the person toward psychiatric commitment.

Characteristically, the expert appears to be a truly saintly person who would go to the ends of the earth to help. Beneath this social appearance, the helper is locked into a vicious struggle to maintain control over the rehabilitation. This does not surface unless the rehabilitation team's efforts run counter to the "expert's" secret agenda for "rehabilitation." The painful reality is that the dynamics of this interpersonal mix ultimately hurt the very person the rehabilitation intervention was designed to help.

Often rehabilitation problems are complicated by the involvement of professionals who were previously concerned with providing care for the family. Current family therapy literature emphasizes the power a family unit possesses. For example, many therapists will not treat a family unless they have a co-therapist. The rationale is that the family system can easily absorb one person and render him powerless. One outsider can become enmeshed in the family's dynamics and unwittingly help continue the family's process. This is a particularly difficult problem for the physician who has known a family prior to a disability and who has truly come to care for them.

> Mr. M. suffered a stroke at age 70 and was moderately disabled with respect to his activities of daily living. He had some speech loss that returned shortly after onset. His demeanor on the rehabilitation unit was one of marked verbal activity and remarkable inconsistency during physical therapy. An initial battle emerged between the physical therapy department and Mr. M. over the issue of getting him to "walk rather than talk." In retrospect, Mrs. M. and Dr. H., the family physician, stayed on the very fringes of this struggle. The issue between Mr. M. and PT was resolved by the following strategy. The tactic was for the PT and OT staffs to be as, if not more, inconsistent than Mr. M. Therapists and schedules were altered randomly on a daily basis. The idea was that as long as Mr. M. could predict his therapy program he could maintain a sense of control over the situation and avoid working. Once this vector of unpredictability was introduced, he improved at a steady pace with only occasional plateaus.
> Once discharge was considered, Mrs. M. appeared and presented a durable core of ambivalence as to whether she could care for her husband at home. As the rehabilitation team mobilized trial experiences to help her decide, she became verbally more helpless. Finally, Dr. H. entered the dynamics by amplifying Mrs. M's ambivalence so that home care experiments never materialized. Even nursing home suggestions were ignored by both Mrs. M. and Dr. H. After their predictable unpredictability was introduced, Mr. M. reverted and failed to make any further progress. Following six weeks of this struggle, Mr. M. was discharged to a nursing home where he became increasingly inert.

After being absorbed into the family system, this "other" family member is a divided person in an unusual position with respect to the rest of the world. At one level, he is a symbolic family member who is emotionally and tactically aligned with the patient's family. At another level, he is a member of the medical community with a vested interest in the narcissism of the role and social concept, *physician*. In order to maintain a sense of identity as a separate person, the family physician will frequently flip-flop between these two levels.

This split in the person of the physician becomes more overt in the face of pressure from the rehabilitation team, on the one hand, and the family on the other. The family is pushing him to be a responsible family member, while the rehabilitation team is pushing him to be a responsible physician on their side *for the patient*. In the face of such pressure, the physician will simultaneously ally himself with the family's ambivalence and present himself to the rehabilitation unit as the physician-in-charge. In his desire to protect the family's overt sense of helplessness and his need to maintain his stance as a physician, he has double-bound the rehabilitation team, amplified the family's process, and stabilized its unwillingness to be useful to its disabled relative.

This fourth and final configuration is in full operation when the patient, by most criteria, is improving, while events in the family's world appear to be deteriorating. This configuration is also a classic example of how progress in one family member can be neutralized by other family members and by members of the social network surrounding the family.

DISCUSSION

The findings suggest that the family has a marked impact on the rehabilitation process, as well as on the rehabilitation team. Primarily, if the rehabilitation of one family member goes sour, it most frequently is a sign that other family members are involved in some uncooperative strategy. It is not safe to presume a blanket "good will" motivation on the family's part toward its disabled relative. The above configurations highlight the bilateral nature of this disruptive effect, i.e., the more disrupted the family is by the rehabilitation intervention, the less effective potentially will be the rehabilitation outcome.

Further, these model situations indicate that a disability and rehabilitation intervention will have at least a two-fold effect on the family. First, the growing family literature indicates that families have a capacity to care for their members in times of crises. However, the arrival of a disability seems to fracture the unity of the family with the result that the members lose this ability. A physical disability apparently leaves the family in a divided, chaotic condition.

Second, the four identified configurations highlight a primary dimension of family disruption. A disability and intervention disrupts the dependency vectors. A disruption of the family's dependency style makes it impossible for the younger members to complete their growth. The family then begins to depend upon the rehabilitation team to care for their relative. At the same time, the others begin to act as if the disability renders a person incapable of continuing his pre-disability family role. They seem to believe that they must find other things or persons to fill this presumed family void. Around these assumptions develops a core of resentment toward the disabled member that is often inverted and experienced as guilt by others in the family.

The results of this study point in two directions for further research. In terms of the potentially harmful aspects of rehabilitation intervention, a conjoint family interview prior to admission to the hospital would be useful for a number of reasons. First, an interview designed to give the family an opportunity to present itself as a unity reinforces its community capacity. This also evenly distributes the initiative for improvement so that rehabilitation is then a family affair.

Second, this interview would allow the rehabilitation team to learn how the family operates. Such information indicates what the potential is for the emergence of various configurations. With these data, the rehabilitation staff could structure its intervention so as not to rupture the family system.

Finally, it is certain that there are families with disabled members who make satisfactory adjustments. It would be useful to entreat these families to teach us how they arrive at this growthful balance. I think we will be severely limited in our usefulness to rehabilitation families until we learn how the "normal" disabled family works.

REFERENCES

Berne, E. *Principles of transactional analysis.* New York: Grove Press, 1961.
Framo, J. L. (Ed.). *Family interaction.* New York: Springer Publishing, 1972.
Glick, I. D., & Haley, J. *Family therapy and research.* New York: Grune & Stratton, 1971.
Laing, R. D. *The divided self.* London: Tavistock, 1959.
Peck, B. B. *A family therapy notebook.* New York: Libra Publishers, 1974.
Searles, H. F. The effort to drive the other person crazy—An element in the etiology and psychotherapy of schizophrenia. *British Journal of Medical Psychology,* 1959, *32,* 1-18.

CHAPTER 9

COUNSELOR SKILLS AND ROLES WITH FAMILIES EXPERIENCING VARIED DISABILITIES OR CONTINUED ADJUSTMENT PROBLEMS

Paul W. Power and Arthur E. Dell Orto

Different chronic illnesses can produce varied effects on families. In the introduction to Section III an approach is outlined that provides the reader with a general method to assist a family confronted by a disability situation. Such assistance includes showing the family members how they can help the patient lead a more satisfying life and teaching the family to live adaptively with the disability. Yet many disease conditions, because of the nature of the illnesses, can prevent a family from reaching a continued adaptive style. Multiple sclerosis, for example, with its uncertain periods of exacerbation and remission, can renew periods of family stress. For several months after the initial diagnosis the family members may be learning how to deal with the disease before finally reaching a stage of adaptation. Adaptation may be disrupted by a sudden worsening of the illness, however. A negative change in the patient's condition may revive anxieties, worries, role confusion, and anger. In his article in Chapter 6, Bray identifies the patient's own regression to an earlier, emotionally reactive stage as "reflux." This occurs because of a serious physical, emotional, or financial trauma. The family members can also experience a setback in their adaptation because of the traumas associated with an exacerbation of the disease or disability.

In another helping perspective, many families never really adapt to a disability. For many months or years after the initial illness or trauma family members may still be trying to find their coping resources. Communication patterns may have broken down. The children may show deviant forms of behavior, necessary home care for the patient may be neglected, and family life may be in a continually disorganized state. Unfortunately, the helping professional may not intervene until this critical time.

Such family situations require specific intervention skills, similar to those utilized when helping a family to assist a patient toward rehabilitation goals after the initial crisis for the family and patient has passed. The family is beginning to face the reality of the disability situation, namely, that the illness will probably be long-term and will affect the usual pattern of family life. The health professional perceives that the family members should become aware of their resources, that they need a sense of competence, and that they should become aware of their own strengths. These goals are also operative when the family is in a "reflux" experience or has never adjusted to the disability. Yet when the family is in a continued state of crisis or in a condition of lingering bereavement, particular intervention approaches are necessary; these are explained in Chapters 10 and 12. This chapter provides information to a helping professional who has the opportunity to work with families and patients experiencing reflux, continued maladaptation, or needed adjustment after the initial crisis. Specific roles for the helper to be used when assisting families and patients during a disability condition are also suggested.

A HELPING INTERVENTION

Health professionals need awareness, opportunity, and skills to intervene appropriately. Frequently, helpers are reluctant to get involved with a family that is "acting out" its anger about the disability. This hostility often occurs when the family members realize that the disability will not go away, but will instead intrude upon their daily lives. These feelings represent a threat to health professionals and diminish their motivation to utilize the family to help the patient. Also, working with the family usually requires some extension or flexibility of job demands. Often when attempting to include the patient's family helpers meet with much resistance from the agency, or work responsibilities are almost overwhelming to the extent that helpers have time only for the patient. Both instances require some preliminary work, e.g., advocating for the necessity of including the family in treatment efforts or reorganization of job tasks.

For organizational purposes, the intervention approach is viewed as the beginning phase, the middle phase, and the terminating phase. Each phase may represent many family meetings, and the delineation of these phases can only be determined by the helper.

Beginning Phase

After seeing the patient, the health professional determines whether a visit with the family could provide added information about the patient's rehabilitation-related problems. Consent from the patient to see the family should be obtained, and the family may be seen either in the helper's office or at their home. From their experience in working with families of the severely disabled the authors have found that family members initially share their thoughts more openly and more thoroughly in their own home environment. The helper should insist at some time upon seeing each family member living in the home in order to discover how each of them is involved with the adjustment problems.

During this beginning phase, the helper is concerned about establishing a positive relationship with the family and then stimulating the family members to talk about their own attitudes, feelings, and problems related to adjusting to the illness and its effects. Frequently the family is experiencing frustration, confusion, and feelings of inadequacy, guilt, and fear. They usually need to express these emotions and to be assured they are valid. This will demand patience from the helper and the suppression of any judgmental statements. Many beginning adjustment problems occur because the family members have not been given the chance to express and accept their disability-related emotions. Part of this expression will be a review of the past with the patient and family and a discussion of memories and shared experiences. The family often thinks about the past as it attempts to cope with the present, and past memories provoke resentment and disappointments.

During the family meetings it is also important that the helper: 1) attend to the family, namely, physically relate to family members in such a way that they believe the helper is sincerely interested in them. This may include the position of a chair and the way eye contact is established during the office or home visit (Anthony & Carkhuff, 1976). 2) Listen to the family members. This implies that the helper has not made any pre-judgments about the family and fully concentrates on what the family members are saying. 3) Respond. When questions are asked, only ask those that the family can handle emotionally at the time. Questions should be interspersed with frequent responses to the family members' feelings. Responding also includes attempting to label perceived family assets during the interview, giving information in a matter-of-fact, nonjudgmental manner, making "I value you" comments often, and responding to the feelings of the family members. 4) Observe. How are the family members dressed? How do they greet you? How are they sitting in relation to each other during the family visit? Who among the family members appears to dominate the conversation, and what family members are especially quiet? Family seating arrangements can be especially valuable for assessment purposes because they can provide clues to family member alliances, interfamily hostilities, or who is the family decision maker.

The objectives of the beginning phase also include:

Establishing a trusting relationship with the family. This is essential for intervention success and will demand much patience, endurance, and clarification of the helper's role. Active listening, especially during the first family meeting, can facilitate the building of this trust. Such listening shows an interest in the family members' feelings and opinions and expresses an active effort to learn and understand their conception of the disability or disease. It does not preclude, however, asking questions during the first family meeting.

Learning early in family intervention the meaning of the disability to the family members, their expectations for the patient and for each other, and family goals. Many adjustment problems have been created because the family had an inadequate knowledge of the disability, maintained negative expectations for the patient, and had lost the family goals in the struggle to survive as a family. The helper can discover how much the family members know about the disability and how much they really want to know. This information can be obtained as part of the family history, as discussed in Chapter 9.

Attempting to build self-esteem among the family members. Families who are witnessing an exacerbation of a child or adult disability often feel they have failed or have not responded in the best way to treatment demands. If inadequate feelings dominate, then family members should be helped to feel more confident in what they are doing, that they are likable, and have personal worth. This self-esteem can be developed by the worker through many "I value you"-type statements, labeling the family's assets, or providing reinforcement for the efforts the family has made toward the patient.

Observing the communication patterns among the family members. What goes on in the family (e.g., how family members relate to each other) is more important and of more concern than why it is going on. This observation focuses on process rather than content. Upon learning the family communication style the helper often can detect the source of the adjustment problems. A spouse, for example, resentful that the patient's disability has caused the family to drastically change its goals, might be deeply angry and show this by irritability, nagging, or long periods of silence. This person might need some individual attention before the rest of the family can hope to achieve any adaptation.

During these beginning family meetings the health professional is primarily a learner, assessing what is going on; discovering how family members are positively or negatively affecting the ill family member; identifying the values the family places on the roles, functions, and expectations that have been or may become disrupted by an illness; and understanding the meaning the illness has for the patient and family. Westin and Reiss (1979) believe that "the most important phase of the family's response to a problem is in how it defines and perceives the problem" (p. 27). Severe disability and chronic illness usually create a unique social difficulty. If the family perceives solutions to the problem, then it is likely that the family will become involved in the treatment program; if the family sees it as overwhelming and the treatment program as threatening, then it may withdraw from the patient's rehabilitation, and perhaps influence the patient to do likewise (Westin & Reiss, 1979). The helper is also a listener, providing support to others as they express their feelings. By being listened to family members slowly realize that their own feelings and convictions are respected, that the helper accepts them, and that the helper is not taking anyone's side. The helper's acceptance of and responsiveness to the concerns expressed by the family members can minimize feelings of helplessness and increase the likelihood of the family being able to recognize its circumstances. When family members talk about their loss, the fear and anxieties associated with threats to self-esteem, self-confidence, role functions, and plans for the future are lessened.

Middle Phase

The flow of time, the family members' realization that the disability is not going to disappear, and, perhaps, the facilitative presence of the helper cause the family to look at the reality of the disability situation. A denial of the implications of the illness may then occur, as well as depression, fatigue, and anger projected onto others, anxiety, and an attempt to begin to adjust to changing family roles. During this phase the family members are helped to understand their role in the family as a result of the illness trauma, the emotional needs of each other, the resources that are present in the family to cope with the disability, and their expectations for each other. This mutual awareness can be achieved by the helper's efforts in getting the family members to talk with each other about concerns related to the disability. Family communication can be considerably enhanced by the helper's encouragement of discussion, clarification of adjustment problems, and exploration of other's views in the family. Also, by responding to family members' requests and concerns, the health professional is likely to promote in them a feeling of being in control of the situation, rather than being helpless.

At this time it is important that the helper identify the problems that have intervention priority and with the family decide upon a plan to alleviate or eliminate these problems. It is necessary that all the family members understand the areas of adjustment difficulty and are willing to work together toward adaptation. Often this is the most difficult task of family intervention, because people are usually reluctant to change their behavior. However, imparting information like disease-related facts or positive expectations for the patient's daily living demands can pave the way for more effective adjustment attempts. The role of information, and especially facts that emphasize the more positive aspects of the patient's condition (i.e., remaining capabilities), cannot be underestimated; if the family believes differently about an illness, the family's way of acting can change. This is especially true with sexual difficulties. In adjusting to the disability limitations, as well as attempting to use the residual capabilities of the patient, the couple needs appropriate information. Yet many married persons are initially reluctant to obtain this knowledge and may only seek it after they have a trusting relationship with the helper and realize the critical need to improve this area of their relationship.

During this middle phase varied plans of action are suggested and then implemented to deal with the alleviation of the adaptive problems. These plans may revolve around information about the illness, the cultivation of mutual expectations between patient and family, the normalizing of family interactions, the suggestion of tasks to be performed that can help the family regain a sense of competency, the more effective utilization of community resources, and how family members can find constructive outlets for themselves without feeling guilty because of the patient's needs. In choosing these outlets the patient's needs are not neglected; rather, the family members' own needs are differentiated from those of the patient.

One of the assumptions for intervention is that the helper has understood the family influences on the patient, has assisted the family in acknowledging these influences, and, when necessary, has formulated a plan of action with the family that develops more constructive family behaviors affecting the patient. To generate this change family self-help groups may be utilized and/or the helper may meet regularly with the family for a selected time period to work on the designated problem. The health professional continues to be involved with the family until the family members realize that they are reaching out, trying to seek solutions, and are finding answers that satisfy them. Once the answers have been identified, the family can begin to progress toward reorganization.

Occasionally the family pathology may be so serious that it warrants extensive family therapy. The need for more prolonged family intervention may be explained to the family and referral sources may be suggested. Referring a family to another resource is a skill in itself, and should be done with tact, understanding, and a thorough knowledge of the community. If respect and trust have been established with the family, then the family members will be more receptive to the helper's directives.

Terminating Phase

The terminating phase occurs when, in the judgment of the helper, the family members have assumed some responsibility for tackling their problems and are following a course of action to achieve selective, adaptive goals. However, the health professional should never completely lose touch with the family. Some procedure for follow-up should be planned, such as periodic phone calls or family meetings. The family members will need the reassurance that they can turn to someone as a source of support or for additional information.

ROLES FOR THE HELPING PROFESSIONAL

When intervening with the family the helper assumes certain roles. These are functions that could be appropriately added to the helper's job responsibilities, but that should not pose a conflict to primary work demands. The initial assumption for the enactment of the roles is that the health professional is interested in helping the patient's family to assist the patient toward rehabilitation goals and wants to help the family itself meet adjustment goals. The authors have conceptualized three roles for the worker when working with the family with disabled member: assessor, resource person, and advocate.

Assessor

Chapter 8 provides an outline for family diagnosis. It is a suggested framework for the health professional to use when identifying the source of adjustment problems. The helper has to be able to understand what is going on within the family and know if the family has the necessary skills to adjust to the disability trauma and subsequent crisis. An effective intervention plan is built upon a sound family diagnosis.

Resource Person

As a resource person the emphasis for the helping professional is on having a fund of relevant information, including an understanding of what patients and their families are going through emotionally as a result of the illness, a knowledge of their social needs, and a knowledge of ongoing family behaviors that can be used by the professional to assist the patient to achieve optimal functioning. Severe disability constitutes a threat to family life and is a painful reminder to family members of satisfactions once enjoyed. Moreover, family roles must shift, even though the change may be only temporary. A husband may no longer be the primary breadwinner. A wife and mother may not be able to perform the customary household tasks. Any assumption of new roles may bring some form of anxiety or reluctance to accept or learn new tasks within the family. Also, there may be a genuine sadness, especially when children see a handicapped parent performing duties formerly handled with ease. Understanding how to cope with these feelings can be most beneficial to the family members. An opportunity to have someone to whom they can release their feelings of frustration and anxiety can become a beginning step to family equilibrium.

Advocate

In the role of advocate the health professional is functioning not only as a source of information but, more important, as one who can communicate this information to the family effectively. Often patients are unable to discuss with their families the emotional and adjustment considerations of an illness. A reactive depression and a lingering discouragement may be temporarily preventing the patient from discussing important facts of the illness with family members. In this helping context advocacy is "speaking up" and "speaking out" for the patient and the family members when it is appropriate. For example, because of a slow, degenerative disease in a family member many families experience drastic role changes and severe marital problems, especially sexual problems. Many of these problems can be alleviated if someone explains to the family members the dependency, emotional lability, and perhaps regressive behavior of the ill member.

An important element of advocacy is the early identification of emotional reactions and the resultant needs of the patient and the family. An early awareness of needs related to personality and motivational factors can encourage the health professional to speak for both the patient and the family when family interpersonal communication has faltered. In turn, such advocacy facilitates the family's cooperation because both the family and the helper assist the patient to move toward a way of life that accommodates the illness.

An advocacy role further presumes that health professionals examine their own feelings about illness and disability. It implies that they do not argue with the patient but rather perform their roles in a nonjudgmental fashion. Advocacy is not simply acting as a "go-between" but represents the efforts of an interested person who articulates the concerns of the patient and family, the emotional reactions of the family members, the mutual expectations related to performance in the sick role, and observed family behaviors that can influence the patient's adaptation.

CONCLUSION

The added perspective for the helper as an assessor, a resource person, and an advocate does not complicate the treatment situation, but eases the strain on the patient and the family, making it easier for the patient to develop and use his residual abilities. Implementation of these roles must be structured, focused, and problem-oriented, and must follow a trial-and-error approach. The authors have discovered that when health professionals enlarge their role so that they can respond to the emotional and social needs of patients and their families, their own treatment efforts are enhanced considerably. More important, productive living and continued comfort for the patient become more of a possibility.

The following articles illustrate the application of helping skills to families where different disability-related events have occurred. In focusing upon cancer and the effect it has on the family, Worby and Babineau emphasize the importance of the family interview. During the interview the helper can learn how certain feelings are handled by the family members, how families cope with a catastrophic life crisis, and how support can be given to the family. They believe that bringing the family together for discussion can be of great value in helping family members cope with a crisis, and explain how to conduct these discussions. Mary Romano examines how to prepare children to deal with a disabled parent. She views such a disability as a crisis, an event that demands that certain problem-solving tasks be accomplished by the children. She identifies the necessary tasks and outlines how a professional can help children perform these tasks. In contrast, Margaret Voysey explores the problems faced by the parents of disabled children and describes the necessary skills for parents to have when they and their children interact with others apart from the family. She believes that the arrangement of children in encounters with others is probably the most problematic area for parents, and the problem becomes more acute with disabled children. Voysey outlines the typical problems and strategies in "impression management," and says that parents of disabled children must acquire a special competence in managing interpersonal encounters. She also describes briefly how parents can develop this competence. All the articles identify specific helping suggestions for families in a disability situation. They contain valuable ideas for health professionals when family involvement is an integral part of rehabilitation.

REFERENCES

Anthony, W., & Carkhuff, R. *The art of health care.* Amherst, Mass.: Human Resource Development Press, 1976.

Westin, M., & Reiss, D. The family's role in rehabilitation: "Early warning system." *Journal of Rehabilitation,* 1979, January-February-March, 26–29.

THE FAMILY INTERVIEW:
Helping Patient and Family Cope with Metastatic Disease

Cyril M. Worby[1] *and Raymond Babineau*[2]

Studies of how families function in health and disease have become increasingly prominent within the last several decades (Liss & Sharma, 1970; McCollum & Gibson, 1970; Libo, Palmer, & Archibald, 1971). Psychiatry and its related disciplines of psychology and social work have been particularly active in exploring the relatedness of family processes to problems of mental health (Ackerman, Beatman, & Sherman, 1967). Working with the family as a group has yielded new theoretical insights, has provided a therapeutic method of considerable power, and has been used as an important research tool (Mishler & Waxler, 1968). The establishment of a specialty board in family medicine is further evidence of medicine's concern with the family as a unit (Worby, 1971).

Despite these developments, the direct application of the family perspective to everyday problems in medical practice still remains an opportunity unfulfilled. Most physicians avoid interviewing whole families together. Some do not see the necessity for it, ever. Others find the experience extremely taxing and perplexing and, perhaps most important, feel lacking in technics for interacting with the whole family as a group. These attitudes are understandable in view of the fact that physicians most often interact with one person, and it is tempting to maintain the status quo.

The family interview can be a useful technic in dealing with the difficult issues arising from the fairly common problem of metastatic disease.

Comprehensive care of the patient with metastatic disease and his family often presents conceptual, logistic and emotional paradoxes for the physician. The physician's domain of responsibility is one of multiple and continually shifting focus. At times, the physician's focus is on the individual patient; at other times, on the patient and family as a group. The family

Reprinted from *Geriatrics,* June, pp. 83–94, ©1974, Harcourt Brace Jovanovich, Inc., with permission.

The authors wish to acknowledge the valuable advice given by George Engel, M.D., and the helpful participation of Elta Green, M.S.S., A.C.S.W.

This work was partially supported by grants MH 11668 and MH 7521 from the National Institutes of Mental Health, Bethesda.

[1]Associate Professor and Vice-Chairman, Department of Psychiatry, Michigan State University, East Lansing, MI.

[2]Assistant Professor of Psychiatry and Chief, Mental Health Section, University of Rochester, Rochester, NY.

group is viewed here as a small social subsystem sharing a complex history, a unique way of defining and allocating roles among its members, and a distinctive style of coping with crises that threaten its integrity. The situation is complicated by the interactions of the patient and the total family unit with another social subsystem, the hospital, with its interlocking system of roles, services, rules and customs (Glaser & Strauss, 1969; Kubler-Ross, 1969; Christopherson & Lunde, 1971; Cokin, Colligan, & Ferrer, 1971; Korsch, Fine, Grushkin, et al., 1971; Salk, 1971; Simmons, Hickey, Kjellstrand, et al., 1971). In addition to paying attention to these discrete units—patient, patient and family as a group, and the hospital—the physician must deal in some way with his own feelings. How does he feel about the death of his patient as an inevitability, about the consequences to the family, about his own inability to reverse morbid processes? In short, he must face his own limitations.

BACKGROUND

In an effort to better understand these issues, we followed a 48 year old woman with terminal cancer for the last four months of her life. We were concerned with her as an individual, with how her past experiences influenced her manner of dying. We also were concerned with her and her family, with how they related to one another during the months preceding her death.

We first met the patient when she was admitted to the psychiatric service of a 700 bed university general hospital with symptoms of profound psychotic depression. She had been hospitalized on the medical service two months before, at which time metastatic carcinoma was found in the liver. This was traced to carcinoma of the breast treated two years before with radical mastectomy and bilateral oophorectomy.

While on the medical service, she was treated with antitumor drugs, and when the liver function tests returned to normal, she was sent home. In the ensuing weeks she became profoundly depressed and was admitted to the psychiatric service. Within a month, her psychotic ideation and depressive affect improved markedly in response to intensive support through individual interviews, sociotherapy on the ward, electroshock therapy, and a family interview.

The family interview took place on the day before the patient's discharge and included the patient, her husband, her 20 year old married daughter Mary, a psychiatric social worker, and a psychiatrist. The 23 year old son Tom was absent.

The goals of the interview were multiple. First, we wanted to learn something of the family's style of coping with the feelings generated by the fact that one of its members had cancer. Families often operate according to a set of rules designed to minimize emotional discomfort (Haley, 1959; Jackson, 1965). For example, some families have a rule against the open expression of feelings such as anger or affection. The rule is most often covertly stated and subtly enforced.

With the family under consideration, it was important to know how anger, disappointment, need for closeness, and other feeling states were characteristically handled. We thought that understanding this family's style of coping with feelings would allow us to be of greater help to them in the difficult days ahead.

A second and related goal was to provide an opportunity for the family to talk over with one another issues that they had assumed could not be openly discussed. Not infrequently, members of the family of a dying patient avoid one another to a degree detrimental to all of them (Norton, 1963). The presence of the physician may enable them to risk coming closer together.

A third goal was to provide a supportive climate to exchange information and correct misinformation. The experience with hospitalization and the contact with numerous members of the health care team often result in family members having highly idiosyncratic and at times distorted versions of what is wrong, what various procedures and tests mean, and what is to be expected in the future. A family interview may help achieve a common and realistic data base for the family as a whole.

THE INTERVIEW

The initial phase of the interview showed that the nuclear family is the crucial functional unit in this family; the extended family, which may be of enormous support in some situations, is not available. The children have not visited their mother often—the daughter once, the son not at all. At this point in the interview, the reasons for this are not clear. This family tends to deal with unpleasant emotions through denial or understatement. For example, the mother says they are a very close family, even though the son has not visited. The husband gives a superficial reason for the son's not visiting, as does the daughter in explaining her own behavior. Eventually, it is the mother who is able to be most direct: "He hasn't been up at all, to tell the truth."

The family justifies the son's preoccupation with his own family's affairs. The son's wife has had two miscarriages and waited six years for her first child, now overdue.

SOCIAL WORKER: Everything happened at once?
PATIENT: Yeah, so they had their own problems at that time. So it was kind of rough.

HUSBAND: And they felt, and I also felt, that with problems on both sides, it would be quite a clash if Tom and his wife were to try to see Mother, too, she having those problems at that time. As you say, everything just happened all at once.

DOCTOR: How do you see that as a clash?

HUSBAND: Well, their problems with the pregnancy and the trouble as Mary just said. And Mother having her problems, all at one time. Just wouldn't fit, that's all.

DOCTOR: Too overwhelming?

HUSBAND: Oh yes.

PATIENT: Especially at that stage of pregnancy. The waters broke, you know. That's pretty nerve-wracking, just to be waiting after that.

HUSBAND: What I really mean is that one should not burden the other. The way I felt, the two problems just didn't mix.

PATIENT: I think I was unaware of what was going on.

HUSBAND: Well, yes, you were, you were. But supposing you had been told about this. You see, Doctor, this could have had a very ill effect on my wife.

In this segment the husband protects his wife from the problems of their children. His use of the phrases "quite a clash," "the two problems just didn't mix," and "this could have had a very ill effect on my wife" suggests the extent of his distress over her illness and how fragile he perceives her to be. The patient feels isolated from her children, but she also experiences mixed feelings about their preoccupation with their own children. The excerpt shows the complexity of the relationships within and between the generations at this time of crisis, when death and birth must be dealt with simultaneously.

The physician's remarks "How do you see that as a clash?" and "Too overwhelming?" are aimed at clarifying and enlarging feelings and perceptions that not only are relevant to the past but might predict the family's behavior in the future.

In the next excerpt, the physician asks the patient directly about the onset of her illness. The husband and daughter seek to protect the patient by answering this painful question for her.

DOCTOR: When were the first signs you weren't feeling so well?

HUSBAND: I've been asked this question before, and I have found it rather hard to go back in my memory to the exact time.

DAUGHTER: It *is* hard. It was more or less—so gradual.

DOCTOR: Maybe your mother remembers.

PATIENT: I had my breast taken off, you know.

DOCTOR: That was when?

PATIENT: A couple years ago. And I lost my father with cancer of the esophagus. When he was only 47, he died. Well, I was 47 then. [laughs] I'm 48 now. I just turned 48. I had that awful feeling that I was going to die when I was 47 because he had and I had cancer. After all, this was malignant and they had performed the radical operation and all. And I had a morbid fear that they hadn't gotten it all, that I was going to die. I think that's what started it. I'd been told by the surgeon and my family doctor that they had gotten it all, that there was nothing to worry about. And they *finally* had convinced me before I went to the hospital this time that there was nothing to worry about. Well, then they did all these other tests and found I had it in my liver. Well, then that was it. After all, I had just gotten to the stage where I was beginning to believe I was going to live for awhile, you know, and then to have them tell me I had it in the liver. And they didn't pull any bones. They told me I had it. I mean, they took a biopsy. I was conscious, of course, while they took the biopsy. And I knew what they were looking for, and they told me what they had found.

DOCTOR: Did you know what your wife was feeling, was thinking about all this time? Did she let you in on it? Did she share her thoughts with you?

HUSBAND: Well, of course, I knew all this before she was told about it, you see. And naturally I suppressed all emotion when I was with my wife. I didn't let on that I knew any of these things, you know. It made it rather difficult for me. Well, after leaving the hospital, my emotions just broke, as my daughter will tell you.

First, the patient graphically describes her identification with her father's illness, her fear of a recurrence following initial surgery, and her despair over discovery of liver metastases. The physician asks the husband and daughter if they knew of the patient's turmoil in order to learn how receptive they had been to signals of distress by the mother. Often a conspiracy of silence develops in which the seriously ill person feels increasingly isolated from the rest of the family, all in the guise of not upsetting one another. The clinician attempts to reopen communication to whatever degree the family group may tolerate it.

The patient continues to talk of her feelings about the discovery of liver metastases.

PATIENT: Well, as I say, I had just gotten over feeling I was going to die. Of course, when they took the liver scan, they apparently found some signs of it. It was pretty frightening, you know, to think that you had something like this someplace. I didn't know where it was or how it was. I heard that you don't operate on a liver. You don't remove a liver like you can a breast or something, and you're just more or less stuck with it. Of course, at the time I didn't know they could treat it the way they are treating it [with chemotherapy].

DOCTOR: So it was hard for all of you to talk about this?

DAUGHTER: That I'll agree. I'll tell you something right now. This is the first time she has said anything in front of me, although I knew. But she never mentioned it when she was home. Never, never said anything about it at all.

The presence of a sympathetic physician and social worker enables the family to make explicit facts and feelings that they knew and experienced individually but were fearful to express among one another. These kinds of exchanges may facilitate the necessary grieving processes. Paul (1967) has drawn attention to the enduring destructive effects of intense, hidden and unresolved grief on family functioning.

The interview continues with the patient describing the impact that leaving the hospital had on her.

PATIENT: I came home from the hospital and I wasn't myself.

DAUGHTER: No. Well, I stayed with her. In fact, I think I handled her more than Dad did. So, she seemed to be pretty good when she was with me.

PATIENT: I was terribly depressed when I went home from the hospital. I didn't want to go home.

HUSBAND: No, she fought going home.

PATIENT: Oh, I didn't want to go home, Doctor. Why was that? When they told me I was going home, I just—I didn't think I was ready to go home.

DAUGHTER: That's all she'd say.

HUSBAND: I think it was the fear of leaving the hospital and the care she'd been receiving, knowing she wouldn't be able to get that same care at home. However, the doctors told me the care was not needed and there was *no* reason she couldn't go home.

PATIENT: I felt like I'd lost my last friend when they sent me home.

SOCIAL WORKER: The hospital being kind of a friend, so to speak?

PATIENT: Uh huh. Having what I have.

HUSBAND: That first night at home was like a nightmare. I sat up all night long with her. The next morning I called her doctor and explained the situation, and he immediately prescribed a sleeping capsule.

DOCTOR: You must have been scared.

PATIENT: I was.

DOCTOR: You must have been panicked.

HUSBAND: She was. She had some rather bad moments all night long.

PATIENT: I was just petrified. I was frightened, afraid of being alone. And, as I say, I got all that attention in the hospital. I had all that care and then to just be sent home on my own.

For the patient with a life-threatening illness, the transition between hospital and home can have ominous overtones. Such patients and their families often view the hospital as an institution with immense resources to sustain and prolong life, and in that sense the hospital represents a court of last resort.

The interview continues with an exploration of this theme.

DOCTOR: Did you think you were actually that bad off?

PATIENT: Yes, I thought I was going to die—soon. [laughs]

DOCTOR: What gave you that feeling?

PATIENT: Because they couldn't operate, and they couldn't operate on my father, either. Of course, he had it in the esophagus. I think they can do something for that now, but this was more than 20 years ago.

DOCTOR: Twenty years?

PATIENT: Uh hmmm. It was 23 years ago, because my son was born the same year he died. And they couldn't operate. They didn't say why, but they couldn't at that time. They discovered it at an early stage, and he just had to go on living. I saw him wasting away. Of course, it being in the esophagus, he couldn't swallow. He had weighed more than 170 lb, and when he died he only weighed 98. He was just skin and bones. An awful, tragic thing to see somebody you love waste away like that. Well, I had that memory, you see, and that's why I was so petrified. And that's why I was so petrified when I even got it in my breast. Of course, in the breast there is more hope because they've done wonderful things. I've heard of people who have lived 20 years after a breast operation. But then when I found out that I had it internal, I was just thrown for a loss. I was just petrified. And then when they said they were going to send me home... [laughs]

DOCTOR: You figured they gave up on you.

PATIENT: Yes, I just figured they would send me home to die, see? Now I can talk about it. I couldn't talk about it before. I was so scared, I couldn't even talk about it.

HUSBAND: This is the first I actually heard her talk about it.

DAUGHTER: Uh huh.

SOCIAL WORKER: Is this new to you, too, talking freely like this?

HUSBAND: Yes.

DOCTOR: You know, this inability to talk with each other must have made all of you feel very alone and separated.

HUSBAND: Well, of course, I was able to talk with my daughter.

DAUGHTER: We talked back and forth.

HUSBAND: Son, son-in-law, daughter-in-law.

PATIENT: But just that word "malignancy" is enough to scare me. If I hadn't experienced what I did with my father, it probably wouldn't have been so bad, but it was so tragic to see him. And he died at home and stayed at home most of the time, because there was nothing they could do for him. He was in a nursing home for awhile, and he knew he was going to die and he said, "Well, if I'm going to die, I want to be in my own home." So he was months at home wasting away. And he wouldn't go to bed until he was in a coma. He didn't stay in bed. He said, "As long as I'm alive and I can get up and around, I'm going to get up and walk," and he did. And he didn't go to bed until four days before he died. He was in a coma for four days.

A number of complex themes emerge in this segment. Each family member is faced with the task of integrating a terrifying fact: The patient has cancer that is inoperable. As they seek individually to cope with this fact, they tend to avoid being with one another. Before the family meeting, the quality of their relationship took on a stilted, superficial and formal character, so that forbidden topics and feelings would not come up and shatter the fragile equilibrium.

The patient once more returns to her experience with her father's malignancy as a source of her terror. She also poignantly illustrates the meaning she attaches to her discharge from the hospital. As she saw it, the hospital had the power of life and death. She had the magical belief that remaining in the hospital would prolong her life, perhaps preserve it. Going home implied a sentence of death. Had a family interview been held before the patient's discharge from the medical service, an opportunity would have been provided to clarify an important issue. The family could have been told that the patient had responded well to chemotherapy and that her liver tests had shown considerable improvement. Such clarification might have ameliorated the terror and abandonment that the patient experienced within hours of returning home. This terror was communicated to the whole family and seriously undermined their own capacity to cope. In turn, it compromised their ability to be supportive to the patient.

In the following excerpt, the husband is invited to share his perception of the events his wife has been describing.

DOCTOR: What was going on within you during this very difficult time?

HUSBAND: Well, I myself had never given up. I wouldn't. All this was working on my nerves, too, very much so.

PATIENT: It was terrible for the family. I know, from my own experience with my father and my mother.

DAUGHTER: I think the reason it didn't affect my brother and his wife so much is that they didn't *see* it. They didn't actually see anything that went on. So all they heard was what we tried to explain. And explaining like that, you don't actually get the whole picture. But being with someone is so much different.

HUSBAND: Eating concerned her at the time of going home. She mentioned that to me several times. "I'm not eating," "How'll I eat when I go home?" Things like that.

PATIENT: I just couldn't make myself chew and swallow solids. They just stuck.

DOCTOR: Kind of like with your father?

PATIENT: Yeah, I don't know. I wonder if that had something to do with it?

DOCTOR: What are your hunches about that, that you had symptoms similar to your father's?

PATIENT: Well, I don't know. Maybe I just associated malignancy with something like that. That I couldn't swallow. Because he couldn't swallow, see? They had to feed him intravenously and he just wasted away. Toward the end we had a nurse, private nurse, just to see that he got fed through the veins. Of course he was kept on dope, too.

The husband doesn't have much chance to elaborate on his feelings. The patient's fusion of her own situation with her father's is so prominent and insistent that the physician makes the connection explicit: "Kind of like with your father?" His purpose here is to suggest that her symptom of not being able to swallow may have less to do with her illness and more to do with her father's. The patient responds affirmatively to this and elaborates in her own words. In that sense, it becomes her own discovery. The suggestion may help her separate her situation from her father's, particularly the tortured nature of his death. Nevertheless, on the most fundamental level, she is right; they both had inoperable cancer.

Although hospital personnel acknowledge the frequency of terror, fear of aloneness, helplessness, and the concern over abandonment in the hospitalized child (Prugh, Staub, Sands et al., 1953), many do not sufficiently appreciate that adults may undergo similar experiences.

HUSBAND: Just before visiting hours she would worry for fear I wasn't going to come up.

PATIENT: Yeah, I was afraid he wouldn't come.

HUSBAND: We had perhaps about four nights this way. See, one night I found her crying.

PATIENT: I'd throw my arms around him and hug and kiss him. I was petrified he wouldn't come. I just feared he wouldn't.

HUSBAND: Some fear that I was *not* going to show up.

PATIENT: And then he was supposed to bring my daughter up, and I wouldn't let myself believe that she was coming because I was afraid she wouldn't come. And it wasn't until they both walked in that I was convinced.

DAUGHTER: Just before Easter I brought her a little Easter bunny, a little chocolate one, and she kept insisting it wouldn't be there when she got up the next morning.

PATIENT: Yeah, I was so afraid I was going to lose people and things.

DOCTOR: You were very afraid that you would lose people and things? What was that like, that feeling?

PATIENT: It was terrible, It was frightening. Just awful.

DOCTOR: Just thinking about it makes you tear, huh?

PATIENT: It even brings tears to my eyes, even now.

Another significant theme is the patient's fear that people important to her will disappear. Possibly this was both a metaphorical expression of her own fear of oblivion (dying) and an expression of her concern that those she depended upon most—her husband and her daughter—would abandon her. Such a fear is not uncommon among patients who have serious chronic illnesses, since they often must make extraordinary demands on other family members.

The situation between the patient and her daughter was complicated by yet another factor, illustrated in the next excerpt. Before her illness, the patient and her daughter had a very close relationship, with the daughter relying on the mother to be of help in many day-to-day decisions. Now the roles were reversed. In many ways, the daughter had to mother her own mother. The daughter describes these stresses while the mother was at home in the interval between discharge from the medical service and admission to the psychiatric service, a time when she had to attend to the competing needs of her mother and her own young child.

DAUGHTER: It threw everything at my house all out of kilter by going over there every morning. I was tired by the time I got home at night. I was ready just to go to bed. And we had a 14 month old baby. He had gotten a cold and started coughing really bad.

SOCIAL WORKER: Did you take him to your mother's?

DAUGHTER: Well, no, I had to shuffle him around. And my husband said, "It isn't fair to him." The baby had been shuffled around. He'd wake up in a different house. He didn't know what to make of anything; he was so confused. Near the end he got better, but it was just the idea of getting him up about 6:30 A.M. and taking him from the crib to the car. He was so confused. But at the end my mother started getting worse. I didn't come over as much. My doctor told me to "try to break away so she doesn't depend on you so much." When I'd go into the room, she'd start talking and be much better, but then when I'd leave she'd say, "I hate to see you go." Yet I *had* to go. I was stuck in the middle like she said she was, with my family and all.

Physicians often underestimate the importance of explanations to a family regarding changes in dosage or schedule of important drugs. The patient describes her reactions to the reduction in dosage of antitumor medication at the time of discharge from the medical service. She had been given a prescription for the drug, to be filled at her local pharmacy.

PATIENT: Oh, yeah, that prescription upset me, too.

DAUGHTER: Oh, she had a fit.

DOCTOR: You mean she was upset about the liver medicine?

DAUGHTER: Uh hmmm. And she said, "I can't see how somebody can get it from the drugstore." Then he cut her dosage down. He said, "She is doing so much better I am going to cut her down to 3 capsules instead of 5." And that upset her. She didn't like that at all.

DOCTOR: What did that mean, that you could get this stuff at a drugstore?

PATIENT: Well, you know, all you read about cancer and everything. I thought the only place you could get cancer medicine was through a clinic or something. I didn't think anybody could go to a drugstore and buy medicine for cancer. Because, the theory had always been that you can't cure cancer with medicine anyway. It had to be surgery, and then you were just fortunate if you cured it. To me cancer was hopeless. And that *word*. You were just a goner, that's all. And then, to be able to go into a drugstore and buy medicine for cancer. I had no faith in it.

Toward the end of the interview, a discussion ensues of practical arrangements for the patient's discharge and the immediate future. The patient then begins to cry.

PATIENT: I'm not depressed now, but the tears are still coming. I'm not depressed.

DOCTOR: What are you feeling right now?

PATIENT: Relief—just being able to talk about it.

DOCTOR: There *are* tears of relief.

PATIENT: I think that's what it is. I'm not depressed. I don't have that feeling. Just one of relief. Rolling down my cheeks.

DAUGHTER: Grandma, now you're going to get us all going. [laughs]

DOCTOR: It's all right to cry sometimes.

DAUGHTER: It helps a lot.

PATIENT: I couldn't cry, you know. I was so depressed, tears wouldn't come.

COMMENT

Knowledge of how families cope with typical and catastrophic life crises has been accumulating rapidly in recent decades. Application of such knowledge to diverse patient care situations by the nonpsychiatric physician too often is the exception rather than the rule. Metastatic disease is one example of health crises having profound effects on the family. We believe that bringing the patient and family together for one or several discussions may be of considerable value in helping all family members cope with a mutually shared crisis. Such discussions may enhance the intrinsic sources of strength often present within families.

The concerned and sympathetic physician who listens with care to the overt and covert communications can, by reflecting, clarifying and enlarging on difficult issues, encourage family members to risk dealing with previously unspoken subjects and experiencing feelings thought to be unacceptable. As a consequence, family members may be able to gain increasing cohesiveness as a group, even as they face the difficult task of losing one member.

REFERENCES

Ackerman, N. W., Beatman, F. L., & Sherman, S. N. (Eds.). *Expanding theory and practice in family therapy.* New York: Family Service Association of America, 1967.
Christopherson, L. K., & Lunde, D. T. Heart transplant donors and their families. *Seminars in Psychiatry,* 1971, *3,* 26–35.
Cokin, M., Colligan, E., & Ferrer, R. Helping parents in a pediatric clinic. *Child Welfare,* 1971, *1,* 504–509.
Glaser, B. G., & Strauss, A. L. *Awareness of dying.* Chicago: Aldine-Atherton, 1969.
Haley, J. Family of the schizophrenic: A model system. *Journal of Nervous and Mental Disease,* 1959, *129,* 357–374.
Jackson, D. Family rules: The marital quid pro quo. *Archives of General Psychiatry,* 1965, *12,* 589–594.
Korsch, B. M., Fine, R. N., Grushkin, C. M., et al. Experiences with children and their families during extended hemodialysis and kidney transplantation. *Pediatric Clinics of North America,* 1971, *18,* 625–637.
Kubler-Ross, E. *On death and dying.* New York: Macmillan Publishing Co., 1969.
Libo, S. S., Palmer, C., & Archibald, D. Family group therapy for children with self-induced seizures. *American Journal of Orthopsychiatry,* 1971, *41,* 506–509.
Liss, J., & Sharma, C. N. Multi-generational dynamics in a case of ulcerative colitis. *Psychiatry Quarterly,* 1970, *44,* 461–475.
McCollum, A. T., & Gibson, L. E. Family adaptation to the child with cystic fibrosis. *Journal of Pediatrics,* 1970, *77,* 571–578.
Mishler, E. G., & Waxler, N. E. *Interaction in families.* New York: John Wiley & Sons, 1968.
Norton, J. Treatment of the dying patient. *Psychoanalytic Study of the Child,* 1963, *18,* 541–560.
Paul, N. L. The role of mourning and empathy in conjoint marital therapy. In G. H. Zuk & I. Boszormenyi-Nagy (Eds.), *Family therapy and disturbed families,* pp. 186–203. Palo Alto, Cal.: Science and Behavior Books, 1967.

Prugh, D. G., Staub, E. M., Sands, H. H., et al. A study of the emotional reactions of children and families to hospitalization and illness. *American Journal of Orthopsychiatry,* 1953, *23,* 70–106.

Salk, L. Sudden infant death: Impact on family and physician. *Clinical Pediatrics,* 1971, *10,* 248–249.

Simmons, R. G., Hickey, K., Kjellstrand, C. M., et al. Donors and non-donors: The role of the family and the physician in kidney transplantation. *Seminars in Psychiatry,* 1971, *3,* 102–115.

Worby, C. M. The family life cycle: An orienting concept for the family practice specialist. *Journal of Medicine and Education,* 1971, *46,* 198–203.

PREPARING CHILDREN
FOR PARENTAL DISABILITY

Mary D. Romano[1]

The sudden acquisition of a physical handicap is a life event rarely desired by an individual. The very fact of the physical losses and changes that attend disability and that can resound through every aspect of a person's life represents a disruption of life-styles and life goals and expectations. Thus, to become disabled is a realistic crisis, whether it be in the lay terms of a disaster or in the technical sense of a disruption of a given homeostasis in which the individual's usual problem-solving means are inadequate to restore balance (Babcock, 1966; Rapoport, 1966).

Becoming disabled, then, may be seen as a personal crisis, but when the newly handicapped individual is a parent in a family, the fact of disability can present a crisis for the nondisabled members of the family as well as for the patient. The sudden presence of disability, with its attendant hospitalization and separation of a parent from his family, has an impact upon the family's, as well as the individual's, life-style; it may challenge the family value system, role patterns, and communication networks. It presents for the family a set of problems insoluble by their usual means, threatens the life goals of family members, causes acute psychological stress, and may mobilize anxieties and problems associated with past events (Parad & Caplan, 1966). In pragmatic terms, when a parent becomes disabled, there may be a dramatic cut in the family's income, a draining of the family's financial resources in order to provide for needed medical care and equipment, the necessity that the able-bodied parent assume new roles such as breadwinning or housekeeping, a forced change in the family's living environment to minimize architectural barriers, and so forth. Subjectively, both patient and able-bodied parent may feel lonely, abandoned, angry, guilty, or depressed over the situational reality. The adult's cognitive ability to perceive the problem and its ramifications in light of the family's value system and role patterns, while leading to anxiety, at the same time provides the basic tool for dealing with the crisis in an appropriate way.

A family's children, however, may not have developed the cognitive skills to understand realistically the events associated with becoming disabled. The young child cannot appreciate causality; he does not appreciate

Reprinted from *Social Work and Health Care* *1*(3), pp. 309–315, ©1976, The Haworth Press, Inc., with permission.

This paper was presented at the 52nd Annual Session of the American Congress of Rehabilitation Medicine.

[1]Supervisor, Social Service Department, Columbia Presbyterian Medical Center, 622 West 168th St., New York City, NY 10032.

contingency relationships. Pre-latency age thinking is primitive, magical thinking, and even into the latency years cognitive movement from magic to rational conceptualization is a gradual process (Fraiberg, 1959). Thus, "what," "why," and "how" become the questions of this period as the child tries to master the environment; abstract concepts, such as time, are mind boggling to the young child for whom an hour can seem an eternity.

With this in mind, it becomes easier to appreciate the staggering impact of a sudden parental disability upon a young child (Furman, 1974). A parent precipitously disappears from the child's life for a period of hospitalization the length of which may well be prolonged and unknown. The remaining parent is generally visibly distraught, which in itself is often frightening to children, and may spend long hours at the hospital with the spouse, or may be attending to reality problems. Such circumstances as these may deprive the children of both of their emotional anchors. Highly abstract medical and other reality problems may be discussed in the presence of the children; feelings about the disabled spouse and / or about the circumstances of the disability may be aired, such as, "He *had* to have that last drink! If only I'd been driving!" or "Why did this have to happen to us?" The inherent ambiguity of the medical situation heightens the anxiety of the able-bodied spouse, and this anxiety is communicated to the children (Bowlby, 1952; Freud, 1967; Kubler-Ross, 1969; Blacher, 1970).

The older child, while able to think in rational and conceptual terms, is not immune from experiencing the sudden disability of a parent as a crisis. He feels the same loneliness, the same apprehension, the same anger, and perhaps guilt; his identification with the disabled parent may be expressed in his trying to replace the hospitalized parent in the household ("I've got to be the man of the house now"), and since family value systems and communication networks are often such that adults' emotions are hidden from the children, the older child often expends vast amounts of emotional energy trying to suppress his feelings about the parental disability and its implications while at the same time pushing himself to fill parental shoes (Parad & Caplan, 1966).

In brief, then, a crisis is an event that causes disruption of a homeostasis in which the usual problem-solving tools are insufficient to resolve the feelings of tension, anger, despair, and guilt that follow the event. The sudden onset of disability of a parent is clearly a crisis for all family members including the children. In order to achieve effective resolution of this particular crisis, what problem-solving tasks must be accomplished by the children (Rapoport, 1970), and how can this problem-solving process be facilitated?

The first task is coming to terms with the absence of the disabled parent from the household in its most concrete implication, for example, the loneliness, the environmental changes, the possible situational deprivations, and the disappointments of failed expectations. The second task, related in some ways to the first, is for the child to master the threat of loss of himself; this fear of loss of self may be based on the absence of the parent on whom the child depends for emotional and physical survival, but it may also be based on identification with the parent which can produce in the child anxiety about his own frailty, anxiety about having caused the disability by angry wishes or inattention, anxiety about physical damage as punishment, or a need to try to replace the absent parent. The third necessary task is to reestablish contact with the disabled parent, and the fourth task is the reintegration of the changed parent into the family.

The means for facilitating the accomplishment of these tasks depends, to a great degree, upon the age and conceptual ability of the child. The older child or teenager can be helped to verbalize his concerns, questions, and feelings directly with the goal of working through them. In addition, because feeling helpless is part of the experience of crisis, older children and teenagers need opportunities for appropriate actions in understanding and dealing with the newly handicapped parent; it can be helpful for the child to meet with the parent's physical, occupational, and speech therapists to explore and learn about the adaptive equipment needed by the parent and to observe the parent as he learns to remaster task competence. Ordinarily, it is not helpful for children to be encouraged to do things for the disabled parent since this subverts the parental role and reinforces an inappropriate role reversal in which the child sees himself as having to parent the parent. Every effort should be made to encourage parent and child to interact with one another directly and in a reciprocal manner; for example, the child should be allowed to spend enough time in the rehabilitation setting in order to share thoughts, experiences, and feelings with the handicapped parent and vice versa, rather than simply to visit briefly and observe.

The young child also needs to spend time in the rehabilitation setting with the disabled parent, even if this involves changing hospital policy that prohibits visitors who are under 14. Young children, too, will want to explore the hospital environment and handle the parent's adaptive equipment, push wheelchairs, peer through prism glasses, and so on. The answers to their what-why-and-how questions, however, must be scaled to the child's level of understanding. For example, a question such as "Why can't mommy walk?" does not require an elaborate and fully scientific lecture of spinal cord lesions in response; instead, "Mommy hurt her back very badly, and that's why she can't walk" will suffice. The how questions—"How will she go to the store?" for instance—are answered equally simply and factually: "She will go in her wheelchair." Answers like these set the child's expectation that task competence and role maintenance will at least to some extent be resumed in the future; in other words, mommy will still be mommy. Similarly, one can assist the young child in establishing affective expectations as well, for example, "Now that mommy has a wheelchair, she will always have a lap for you."

Important as it is for the young child to understand parental disability, it is as important for the child to be able to share and deal with his feelings about these life events. Direct verbal acknowledgment of the feelings is one means of doing this: "It is very lonely for you, not having daddy at home. You miss him;" or "People feel mad and disappointed when they can't do something they wanted to do. I bet you feel that way when you think about daddy taking you to the ball game."

Another tool for reaching and expressing feelings is the use of creative play. The young child can use toys to play out events and express his feelings about them, thus distancing himself through the toys from a painful, immediate reality situation. Drawing materials, dolls, and hand puppets are used effectively to this end. Using readily available supplies and a little imagination, one can swathe a doll in bandages "like daddy's," splint a doll, place it in traction, and in so doing, use it to help prepare the child for the parent's appearance in the hospital and to help the child to start expressing his feelings about the situation. Projective drawing can be used in a similar way:

> Kathy, aged 7, was the second of three children whose father was quadriplegic. Asked to draw a picture of her family, she first drew a picture of three children standing on some grass; all the children were crying. Her second picture was of droopy flowers in the rain.

With the verbal child, mutual story telling with drawings or puppets can be used to elaborate further and resolve feelings. When asked, for example, to tell a story about a picture, the above child said, "The children are in their backyard; they're bored because their mother is at work, and their daddy is sick. They're kind of unhappy." Somewhat analogous stories are often told with hand puppets, especially animal puppets representing a range of animals from small and weak ones (rabbits, mice) to big and powerful ones (lions, elephants):

> Four-year-old Scott, whose mother had undergone below-knee amputation as a result of injuries sustained in an automobile accident, played out a number of stories in which a rabbit was angry at a "bad" lion who wouldn't play with him. With a mixture of excitement and fear, Scott's rabbit told the lion, "You're bad; you're terrible. I'm gonna beat you up. I'm gonna bite off your tail."

For the child with limited verbal skill or with constrained imagination, especially prepared stories can help the child deal with an overwhelming reality. Such a story might be about a family with a father who is hospitalized but who is preparing for his first visit home. The story might touch on the children's shyness of their father now that he is in a wheelchair, their loneliness for him, what his paralysis will mean to their lives, and so forth. The content of such stories should provide enough of a parallel to a given child's situation that the child can identify with it, yet the story should be sufficiently impersonal that the child can follow the story through to its conclusion and comprehend an ending in which the characters have achieved some peace with their situation and their feelings.

In order to master the task of reintegrating the changed parent into the family, it is important for the children in the family to have some preparation for the parent's first home visit, since this first home visit is often the model for subsequent reunification; if it is a successful experience, it will tend to lead to further reintegration. The child should have some understanding of what the parent will and will not be able to do, and, ideally, the children should have some choice in the schedule (e.g., perhaps in deciding what to have for dinner) with, if at all possible, time available for the family to be together without visitors. The special quality of that first visit can thus begin to be softened into a closer approximation of what it will be like to have the disabled parent at home, and this time together allows the family to resume their more typical patterns of communication and ritual (such as tucking the children into bed).

Methods such as these not only have the beneficial effect of helping children deal with the immediate crisis of having a newly disabled parent but also provide the child with models for dealing with the reactions of others to the parent's disability. Children are often the recipients of thoughtless or pitying remarks from peers, teachers, strangers, or neighbors; these remarks may initially mobilize a great deal of distress in the children of a newly handicapped parent, but as the children gain mastery over their feelings and life events, they can use their own growth to cope with this problem.

> Mike, 8 years old, was teased by children at school who told him that his father, paraplegic following a crush injury, would never come home from the hospital, and was a bad man whom God had punished. Instead of crying or fighting, Mike told the children that they were mean, that he was learning to help his father fix wheelchairs, and that his father loved him and could hardly wait to come home.

Children who do not have help in preparing for parental disability appear to have a much more difficult time in dealing with the handicapped parent, the rest of the family, and with outside relationships.

> Mrs. N., the mother of a 7-year-old son, could not bring herself to talk with her child about Mr. N.'s disability, nor could she allow anyone else to help the child understand more than that "daddy is in the hospital." The child became enuretic, withdrew from peer contact, and began to do failing work at school. Finally, with no preparation, Mrs. N. brought the child to the hospital to visit his father; at the entrance to the ward, she said, "Go find daddy." The child wandered from bed to bed, staring at each man, before returning to his mother and announcing "Daddy's not here!" in a panicky voice. Mrs. N. then brought the child to his father's bedside where the child said, "That's not my daddy" and began to sob. Following this event, the child's disturbance became so pronounced that the school insisted the child receive psychiatric help. Mr. N., the

patient, himself entered a severe depression as a result of this incident and soon elected to live permanently in a nursing home rather than return to his own household.

In summary, recognizing that the sudden disability of a parent is a crisis event in the lives of the parent's children, and responding to that recognition by preparing the children for parental disability, should be the key concern of helping professionals in acute medical and rehabilitation settings, whether the goal is to return the parent to the family in a maximally functional capacity or to work with the disabled parent and his family toward an intermediate or institutional continued care plan. Whether it be by working directly with patients' children or by training and assisting the able-bodied spouses in helping their children, a number of tools, including verbal recognition of feelings, creative play with special stories and mutual story telling, and involvement of the children in the total medical program, are feasible and rewarding means to this end.

REFERENCES

Babcock, C. G. Inner stress in illness and disability. In H. Parad & R. R. Miller (Eds.), *Ego-oriented casework*. New York: Family Service Association of America, 1966.
Blacher, R. S. Reaction to chronic illness. In B. Schoenberg, A. C. Carr, D. Peretz, & A. Kutscher (Eds.), *Loss and grief: Psychological management in medical practice*. New York: Columbia University Press, 1970.
Bowlby, J. *Maternal care and mental health*. Geneva: World Health Organization, 1952.
Fraiberg, S. H. *The magic years*. New York: Charles Scribner's Sons, 1959.
Freud, A. About losing and being lost. *Psychoanalytic Study of the Child,* 1967, *22,* 9–19.
Furman, E. *A child's parent dies*. New Haven, Conn.: Yale University Press, 1974.
Kubler-Ross, E. *On death and dying*. New York: Macmillan Publishing Co., 1969.
Parad, H. J., & Caplan, G. A framework for studying families in crisis. In H. J. Parad (Ed.), *Crisis intervention: Selected readings*. New York: Family Service Association of America, 1966.
Rapoport, L. The state of crisis: Some theoretical considerations. In H. J. Parad (Ed.), *Crisis intervention: Selected readings*. New York: Family Service Association of America, 1966.
Rapoport, L. Crisis intervention as a mode of brief treatment. In R. W. Roberts & R. H. Nee (Eds.), *Theories of social casework*. Chicago: University of Chicago Press, 1970.

IMPRESSION MANAGEMENT BY PARENTS WITH DISABLED CHILDREN

Margaret Voysey[1]

This paper is concerned with the interactional problems that parents face through having a disabled child and the strategies they adopt to manage them. It focuses specifically on encounters between parents and others outside the immediate family (including medical and other professional agents) where the child is either present or constitutes a potential constraint on interaction.

Other writers (Thomas, 1966; Haber and Smith, 1971) have analysed similar problems from the point of view of the disabled person himself and with a different theoretical perspective—that of more traditional "role theory." The approach adopted here is principally that developed by Goffman (see especially, 1959; 1961) but I am also indebted for many insights and comparative remarks to such writers as Davis (1961); Garfinkel (1967); Glaser and Strauss (1965); Sudnow (1967); and Weinstein (Weinstein & Deutschberger, 1964; Weinstein, 1969).

Goffman does consider parents of the disabled as an instance of his second type of "wise" person whose "relationship through the social structure to a stigmatized individual. . .leads the wider society to treat both individuals in some respects as one" (Goffman, 1968, p. 43), but he does not analyse the problems involved in this relationship in any detail. Birenbaum takes this as his main focus and finds that mothers of retarded children tend to adopt the adaptation designated as presenting a "normal-appearing round of life," upholding which claim requires that they avoid situations in which their obligations to the child are obtrusive. Thus, they discontinue relationships with those who do not show "consideration," i.e. who "indicate by their actions that the family (is) being re-evaluated as a result of having a retarded child" (Birenbaum, 1970, p. 199).

The argument in this paper differs from those of the two previous authors in respect to one most important point. Parents of the disabled are

Reprinted from *Journal of Health and Social Behavior* 13(1), pp. 80–89, ©1972, The American Sociological Association, with permission.

This project was supported by a grant from Nuffield Provincial Hospitals Trust. An earlier draft of the paper was read at the 5th National Deviancy Symposium held at York University, April, 1970. The author should like to express her thanks to Philip M. Strong for his help as the research and writing progressed. The author is grateful also to Gordon Horobin, Alan Davis, Anthony Elger, Norman Stockman, and Anthony Wootton for their comments on an earlier draft of this paper.

[1]From Aberdeen University.

crucially different from most members of the "wise" because they do not choose their position and, far from being expected to refuse, are encouraged to welcome its responsibilities (Voysey, 1970).[2] Hence, they are less likely to create embarrassment by "confronting everyone with too much morality" (Goffman, 1968, p. 44). Moreover, Birenbaum's (1970) findings appear to have limited applicability. Of the other two possible adaptations he considers, the first, "total disaffiliation" from the stigmatized, seems likely only in "extreme circumstances" and the second, "total acceptance," i.e. entailing the loss of one's own claims to a normal identity, may rather be widely legitimated. Evidently, it is necessary to discover the conditions under which parents adopt different methods of managing interaction with others. We may better do this if we examine why such encounters should be problematic for parents of the disabled.

THREATS OF A DISABLED CHILD TO PARENTS' COMPETENCE

The management of children in encounters with others is perhaps normally the most problematic area for parents. This for two main reasons. First, such encounters are places where definitions of parents' competence are constructed. The public appearance of any family member may be taken as evidence of the family's "private" state and, given their common identification, the behavior of any one member may reflect on the others. As "team-managers" it is the parents' responsibility to ensure that the proper impression of its individual and joint behavior is sustained. Children, however, are incompetent performers and untrustworthy participants in interaction (see Strong, 1971 for a more detailed analysis of the peculiar interactional status of young children) hence, secondly, such encounters are also places where parents' competence is most threatened. Nonetheless, their management can normally be largely routine and others routinely discount the impressions created by young children.

For parents of the disabled, however, all activities may become problematic. In general, the advent of a disabled child may be seen as breaching the institutionalized order of family life. The appropriateness of the old rules and recipes are called into question and parents may then be uncertain both as to how they should best perform their everyday tasks and what new

---

[2]That is, membership of the category "parent" imposes special constraints on their activities as the disabled child's "wise." Despite the great variation in child-rearing practices of different social groups in Britain (summarized and discussed by Wootton and Illsley, 1970) and the fact that parents normally enjoy great freedom in bringing up their children since the family is in many respects a "private" institution within which many "deviations" may remain secret, or known but tolerated by wider social groups, the actions of parents in our society are broadly constrained by what can be termed the "official ideology" of child-rearing. Whether or not individual parents believe in this, if they do become the concern of outsiders—friends, relations or professional agencies—they must accord with its prescriptions or make use of its rhetoric in "accounting" for their actions (Scott and Lyman, 1968a).

tasks may be necessary. For example, they may not know whether activities outside the home should be curtailed and visitors discouraged. The care and control of the disabled child may not only be physically more arduous but parents may not know whether routine methods are applicable or what special techniques are required. They may be uncertain as to what behavior it is appropriate to expect of the child both at home and in public and unsure as to how relationships outside the family may be affected.

SOME INTERPERSONAL TASKS OF PARENTS OF THE DISABLED

In any one encounter parents may thus have a variety of aims. As regards the proper upbringing of their child they may have to discover what is medically wrong with him and what action is therefore appropriate. Knowing this, they may be concerned with its implementation and getting help of various kinds from others. They have the conflicting responsibilities of teaching the child to define himself as essentially normal while guiding him in strategies for managing his stigma.

The performance of all these tasks is much aided by a knowledge of how the child appears to others, which may then, of course, inform parents' attempts to constrain alter's definition. Where parents are unsure of the child's real condition or their own general competence, they may be highly conscious of alter's opinion as implied by his treatment of parent and child.

These aims may conflict through time as well. The temporary relief of day-care may increase the likelihood of the permanent mortification of the special school. Concealing the true extent of the child's disability from over-anxious or over-sympathetic relatives may prevent their taking any part in his later management. Such conflicts may lead to changes in parents' aims, not only between, but within any one encounter. What starts off as an attempt to gain validation for a normal definition of the disabled child may become a plea for help.

Finally, one should note that, although parents' general aims may be those of covering up or coping with the child's abnormality and minimizing embarrassment, particular situations may require stressing or even exaggerating the stigma. Obtaining help often requires this strategy.

THE RESEARCH

This paper is based on interviews enacted by the author with parents[3] who had a child that had just been identified as suffering from one of a range of

---

[3]In fact, usually with the mothers as in many similar studies. Reference to "parents" throughout is justified on the grounds that mothers generally have more contact with professional agencies and it is at her that their efforts are mainly directed; the mother is the "center" of most families in our society and, moreover, principally responsible for the day-to-day care of the child. Hence it is her management of the experience of having a disabled child that is most important.

disabilities that were medically categorized as at least "relatively severe" and "probably permanent." Families were selected through frequent attendance at the various out-patient clinics and wards of local children's and maternity hospitals. Interviews were carried out in the family's home: one immediately after identification and three at equal intervals over the following twelve months. They lasted an average of one and one-half hours, were largely unstructured, tape-recorded, and transcribed in full. The priority given to recent identification plus the constraint that families live within one city excluded the possibility of holding other structural characteristics constant. Hence, the age of the children ranged from 0-9 years at first contact; their disabilities from obesity to spina bifida; the number of siblings from 0-7. Fewer than expected suitable cases became available in the contact period: 20 were initially interviewed and this decreased to 13 by the end of the 18 months of field-work. Two families could be called "middle class," the remainder "working class."[4]

TYPICAL PROBLEMS AND STRATEGIES IN IMPRESSION MANAGEMENT

Conveying the Desired Impression

For a variety of reasons, e.g. obtaining help or avoiding embarrassment, parents may wish to present a particular definition of their disabled child to others. However, they face problems in doing this. The child's disability may, of course, in fact discredit claims to a particular identity. But, even where this is not so, impression management is difficult because both the child's and the parents' actions are open to misinterpretation.

Like normal children, the disabled child may lack the social skills to cooperate with his parents' attempts and sustain their projected definition of him. Thus, the claim that a mongol child was "coming on as fast as his brother" was discredited when he made no attempt to hold the cup offered him by the paediatrician despite his previous ability in this skill. That is, the disabled child's "normal" disobedience and mistakes are more likely to be taken seriously and interpreted as symptomatic of his condition. All children let you down in front of visitors but the retarded child's tantrum was documentary evidence for his grandmother of the aggression typically associated with backward children. This is especially so since expressive behavior such as muscular reflexes and eye movements is generally seen as a spontaneous and therefore reliable indicator of underlying phenomena. Reliable, since young children are commonsensically held incapable of practicing artificial "spontaneity," they are as they appear (though, in fact, chil-

---

[4]According to the Registrar-General of England and Wales classification. The low number of middle-class families can be partly attributed to the greater "protection" they received from doctors whose opinions as to the suitability of families for study were sought. There was definite evidence of two or three instances of this.

dren do learn to produce "symptoms" that are rewarded by sympathetic adults).

Adults, of course, are assumed to possess such skills, hence parents may commonly be suspected of misrepresenting their child but this is often without basis. On the one hand, they may appear to overplay his normality but even in cases where this is in some sense true, what might normally be seen as the legitimate behavior of a proud parent is here more readily defined as "not facing up to reality"—a typical case in paediatrics. When, on the other hand, parents present the child as more disabled than he appears to others, their definition may be similarly discounted as "over-protectiveness." Parents of the disabled have more opportunities for being so misjudged because they engage in more encounters where the child's identity is in question. Moreover, the costs and rewards involved are likely to be higher. The dismissal of their pleas may delay the offering of necessary help.

Success in constraining alter to accept their interpretations of the child's behavior depends, first, on parents' own knowledge of the child's behavior, the recognition of its distinctively normal and abnormal characteristics. They may be uncertain as to what (if anything) is wrong with him or how severe it is, and where "expert" definitions are available these rarely provide an adequate guide to everyday management (even less where diagnosis and prognosis are unclear, cf. Horobin and Voysey, in press). Parents can only discover the extent to which the disability actually "obtrudes" in interaction through their experience with the child in different situations. A speech defect is not apparent to others when conversation does not include the child, while answering for him is a readily normalizable strategy. Secondly, success depends on a knowledge of how the child appears to others in what kinds of situations. When in doubt, parents may assume that what is evident to them is equally so to others. But some parents discovered that most people did not recognize their baby's features as peculiarly mongol, hence letting the child "pass" became a possibility. Parents may also find that others' perceptions of the "focus" of the disability vary and then attempt to control them. When others expressed their definition of diabetes as disqualifying a child from all effective interaction, his parents counter-asserted that "once he's had his injection he's just a normal little boy."

Given such knowledge, parents may discover the extent to which backstage work can produce a normal-appearing child. One mother concealed the "true" severity of her autistic child's condition from even the closest family by cleaning him and the house before they came home.

"Breaking-Through"

Interaction between parents and others is often problematic due to mutual ignorance of the other's definition of the situation. Even if the participants have attained what Scheff (1967) terms the "third-level of co-orientation" —that is, where ego knows that alter knows that ego knows that alter knows (that the child is disabled)—there remains the difficult problem of "breaking-through" and openly recognizing the fact.

Participants generally lack expertise in managing such situations. Further, the act of mentioning the child's disability redefines the situation and imposes a new set of rules upon action within it. Alter may have to express sympathy, the parents their grief, too great poise is inappropriate for either. Both may wish to avoid embarrassment and the possible reconstitution of their existing relationship. Even when the presence of disability has been acknowledged, similar problems may persist in the negotiation of its severity, visibility, and so on.

In each case, as Davis (1961) finds for the stigmatized adult, it is generally the task of the parents to indicate the appropriate definition of the situation. Of course, some complete strangers cannot restrain their curiosity, but more commonly it is only certain categories of others who, by virtue of their relationship with the parents can give unsolicited opinions. Grandparents suggest that the child should see a doctor since their motives must be assumed to be of the best. Even doctors, when they must break the news of the child's disability to parents, attempt to produce a context of growing awareness so that parents eventually ask what is wrong. Only when this and other indirect strategies (using the child's father as a "less-emotional" mediator) fail do they stage a showdown and insist that parents "face facts."

Information Control

Where parents know that their child is disabled, they have to decide who to tell what. Often they may wish to conceal their child's stigma. Where the disability is not very evident, parents may be able to control its "known-aboutness" so that they can act as if the child were normal, with all except the informed few. This is still problematic, however, since parents do not have objective knowledge of the meanings alter imputes to the disability. Thus, the doctor may only be fooled insofar as he is dependent on parents' admission of information (he need not know of the effects of the child on other members of the family). Moreover, parents often doubt the sincerity of, and therefore discount alter's expressed opinions. Close relatives are especially suspect of employing protective practices, tactfully appearing to concur with the parents' definition. Further, keeping secrets requires careful management. Parents must control the behavior of the whole family and themselves maintain a united front in order to sustain the desired impression of the disabled child. Young children may give the game away and are appropriately instructed even if they "don't really understand."

Sometimes, however, parents may wish to reveal rather than conceal. Letting others "in" may have definite advantages in terms of emotional support or practical help and such considerations may influence the parents' decision as to whom to tell. Thus, they can only appropriately express feelings of grief and resentment with close family and friends who can be expected to share in their sorrow; they may train certain others to manage the child in their own absence. But they are likely to weigh such advantages against the costs of involvement discussed in the previous section—too little help may be preferable to too much sympathy. Thus, parents conceal the true severity of the child's condition from grandparents who "will only get upset" and strangers (like the interviewer) are often the best confidants since both parties know that the involvement will go no further.

Such calculations are inappropriate in some cases since, whether or not they can help, certain people have a "right" to know. These persons are principally those relatives and friends who will share the parents' grief or who, like young siblings of the child, would themselves be hurt were they to hear it from another source. They should be informed quickly and by someone closely related to the parents—in fact, often by the child's father. Other than for this select group, given the complexity of information control, and the discovery that "bad news travels fast," parents may simply opt for the strategy "letting it get around." This removes some of the uncertainty in interaction, though it does not solve the problems of "breaking-through."

Obtaining Information

Often parents want to find out alter's real opinion of the child. This may be a central aim when they are themselves uncertain of the child's "true identity" or seek trustworthy advice on how best to help him. Others' definitions are also important in order to inform parents' activities as impression managers and suggest suitable strategies for different audiences and, finally, in order to teach the child the kinds of responses he will encounter should he become responsible for managing his own performance.

Given such intentions, there are two main categories of persons whose definitions of the child are important. First, those with desirable resources. Some people's opinions (e.g. doctors) are of intrinsic value; those of others may constrain their willingness to help. Friends may not babysit if they over-estimate the extent of the child's disability; employers may be unsympathetic to requests for time off work if they do not define the situation as serious. Second, it is important for parents to discover the definitions of those who have power over the child and can make important decisions about him whether now or in the future. If doctors and teachers between them largely control the child's entry into and progress through school, parents are in a better position to influence the child's future if they know to what extent he is "officially" disabled.

How can parents find out alter's real opinion of the child? Direct inquiry as an opening tactic is usually too threatening, both to the parents themselves—it may give the game away unnecessarily—and to alter from whom it may elicit only a vehement denial, which cannot be further pursued. A second tactic consists of checking alter's statements against his observable interaction with the child. Doctors may belie their assertions of the child's normality through their sustained testing of the child's reflexes. Parents may conclude that alter is himself uncertain or that "they never give you a straight answer" or "they don't want to hurt my feelings." A more subtle strategy is that of "testing" (cf. Edgerton, 1965 for the original use of this model). Parents proceed by "hinting" at the object of their concern whether it be the meaning of specific symptoms or general anxiety at the child's condition. One mother repeatedly presented her child at the clinic ostensibly for severe vomiting but "by the way" attempted to elicit an evaluation of the child's physical development.

Such tactics may be sustained over a number of encounters, but if they do not succeed in resolving the uncertainty, parents may then resort to "outrage," i.e. challenging alter with a definition of the situation that must be accepted or denied with at least a convincing show of sincerity if he is not to lose face, the parents' trust, or endanger his own and his profession's integrity. Thus, two parents confronted their doctors with the assertion that their children had leukemia; another said: "Are you trying to tell me my child is a mongol?" Such definitions may be seen by parents as "too awful to be true" but are used by them to define the boundaries of what is—unfortunately, sometimes such assertions prove correct.

RESPONSIBILITY AND POWER

These two factors are considered separately since they appear to produce fundamental differences in the styles that parents adopt to manage their interactional problems. "Responsibility" is defined as the degree to which parents or others define the parents as "responsible" for the child's disability, i.e. whether they have "caused" it either genetically or through negligence of their duties as parents. Inadequate care and control may result in the child falling victim to illness or injury, whether physical or psychological. One child was knocked down by a tractor and suffered permanent brain damage, another mother thought her son's epilepsy was partly a result of her inability to breastfeed him and consequent failure ever to feel "close" to him.

The second factor is the degree to which parents or others define parents as having power to "do something about" the disability. This depends on: a) the nature of the disability—e.g. the management of diabetes requires the parents' cooperation with doctors, b) the parents' knowledge of it— until they can recognize important symptoms they may feel helpless and doubt their competence should problems arise, and c) the parents' resources. Middle-class parents may suffer more from the "disgrace" of a mentally-handicapped child and be more isolated from kin and community help, but they are likely to make greater use of routinely available formal agency services, obtain preferential treatment through professional and informal "contacts," and possess more skills relevant to managing encounters with such agents.

It must be stressed that assessment of "responsibility" and "power" is based on actors' definitions. They are not objective facts to be "faced up to" but are always open to negotiation; parents and others may hold different definitions and each may influence the other. Doctors provide parents with "scientific" grounds for disavowing responsibility; parents may believe and convince others that their amateur physiotherapy is a help to the spina-bifida child. Such definitions are of central importance. They influence first the parents' management of the child and, second, the moral interpretation of parents' actions by themselves and others, which parents must take into account in managing interaction. The differences produced by the two factors are best shown if they are combined, since the ability to help partly mitigates the effect of responsibility and lack of power matters less where parents are not responsible for the disability.

If "power" and "responsibility" are treated as dichotomous then four logically possible types are produced. I want to suggest that for three of these situations there is a typical "line" or "style" which may be adopted by parents and proffered by others as an appropriate way of managing the situation and of establishing or maintaining the "good character" of the parents. In the fourth type, since such a line is not available, interaction concerning the child may be highly circumspect.

"Not Responsible/Have Power"

This is typical where the disability most approximates an "illness," i.e. it is known to be of "physical" and non-hereditary origin; treatment is possible, can alleviate and even control (though not cure) the condition—e.g. diabetes. Here parents have an important part to play if it is only to ensure that the child keep his appointments with the specialist. "Doing what the doctor says" is a ready defense against criticism and an excuse for rejecting advice. Others may even be impressed by, and express admiration of the parents' new competence in medical matters and incompetence is usually evident only to knowledgeable others, e.g. doctors. Hence, the predominant interpersonal style is "coping splendidly."[5]

---

[5]In fact this type of adaptation may well be the most common. It is often actively promoted and fully legitimated by others whether to decrease their own involvement or in admiration at the parents' competence. Parents are usually discouraged from thinking themselves responsible, at least by professionals, and encouraged to feel that they have some power since "thinking positively" and simply keeping the child happy can constitute "help" (see Voysey, 1970 for more discussion of these points).

"Responsible/Have Power"

Parents can feel guilt despite doctors' attempts to discourage them from "taking the blame." This seems to produce greater efforts on behalf of the child and an unwillingness to discuss him in routine encounters except when challenged. They may then dramatize their concern for his welfare and make evident their sacrifices on his behalf as the only way of neutralising threats to their identity as good parents. For example, the mother of the epileptic child cited earlier was extremely militant in her demands that the child be fully tested at the hospital and not discriminated against at school—if accused she could say with confidence: "I've done all I can." The typical line in this situation therefore is "making amends."

"Not Responsible/No Power"

This situation most resembles a bereavement and is most applicable to cases of "tragic" disabilities, e.g. congenital abnormalities. As with death, parents must learn to "face the (medical) facts." No one can offer any real consolation, neither can they accuse parents of negligence. Hence the parents' major problem may be the control of others' expressions of sympathy and ignorant advice. Since it is culturally assumed that most people are well-intentioned, parents must learn to listen patiently, however distressing this may be. The appropriate style here therefore is "stoic acceptance."

"Responsible/No Power"

These conditions typically apply in cases of "undifferentiated" mental subnormality. Since there is no known "physical" cause, parents may seek it in their own mismanagement of the child, but there are no "special" techniques that they can acquire to correct their mistakes, i.e. make amends. Hence, parents may try to keep the disability a guilty secret and restrict interaction to those who share in the responsibility or whose condemnation is mitigated by their knowledge of the parents' good character in other spheres. (This may therefore exclude even professional agents who might in fact be able to help.)

This seems to be the strategy described by Birenbaum (1970) but, as was indicated earlier, it is clearly the product of special factors. Moreover, though its adoption may be more common in cases of general retardation, it should perhaps be stressed that the child's disability alone does not determine definitions of parents' responsibility and power. This is demonstrated by changes in parents' strategies. If parents come to define themselves as less "responsible" for, or more able to influence the child's condition, then their interpersonal style may change accordingly. Thus, one mother avoided discussing her child's lack of growth with anyone but her husband. He finally persuaded her to see a specialist who diagnosed the cause as "something in the brain." Then, "She's got a growth deficiency," became her account to anyone who commented on the child's size. Another mother was asked by the child's nursery school teacher to cooperate with them using specific techniques to train him. She then showed a marked increase in willingness to discuss the child's present and future development with the interviewer.

To conclude: Parents who define themselves as responsible for, but powerless to change their child's condition, may avoid most encounters with others concerning him because there is no culturally acceptable line available to them. Even if they privately "accept" the child's condition, they may be unable to manage its public presentation. The alternative—carrying on as normal—can be sustained only in encounters where both parties are equally willing to honor its claims. Nonetheless, the fact that in the first three situations parents do have a legitimate way of managing encounters does not mean that any individual parents will never experience other problems of stigmatization, embarrassment, and so on. Interactional styles are related not to parents (or disabilities), but to particular definitions of the situation, which remain to some extent negotiable issues.

THE DEVELOPMENT OF COMPETENCE

It should be apparent that the management of interaction with others concerning a disabled child is highly complex. Embarrassment is inherent in many "normal" situations and parents may face many "strange" encounters with doctors, social workers, etc. Parents must usually indicate the appropriate definition of the situation. Hence if they are not to withdraw from all social relationships outside the family, they must acquire a special competence in managing encounters.

How do they develop this? We noted that middle-class parents are from the start more likely to possess relevant interpersonal skills. For all parents, specific sources of information are books and magazines written for and by the disabled or their parents, or other such parents met informally or through parent associations. The development from these of an ideology not only prescribes and legitimates, but provides a new basis for calculating costs entailed by particular actions. Personal experience is, of course, crucial and certain events may be particularly instructive. The first performance of "routine" activities such as taking the child out in a pram, on a bus, or to the clinic is often critical and may constitute a "turning point" after which it may "never be so bad again." Indeed, parents often expect such events to be the test of their acceptance. Areas of incompetence may still be revealed in atypical situations that are inherently unpredictable—e.g. the diabetic child who started to go into a coma in the street—or simply unpredicted. One mother only realised how disabled her spina-bifida child was when she took her to a party—"It was the first time it really hurt me." Events that cannot be managed within the parents' existing repertoire may occasion a drastic revision of tactics. Parents discover that "you have to be rude to some people" when more subtle cues fail to divert a stranger's inquiries. Some situations, however, may remain "un-manageable"—one cannot prevent people crossing the road to avoid an encounter. Parents may feel like shouting: "Look at him—he's not a monster," but never regard it as an appropriate strategy.

The skills that parents acquire enable them to typify embarrassing situations and predict alter's response, to define the actions of some categories of others as insignificant and distinguish true sympathy from mere curiosity. Thus, they are able to manage interaction such that they are not simply at the mercy of other's definitions. They may certainly continue to be influenced by and value such opinions but they need not just hope that alter will be considerate. This seems to be true only in the last situation discussed, where parents lack an appropriate line and their alternative "normal" interactional styles require alter's tactful acceptance. Parents' special skills may further be relevant to other situations. The frequent questioning of their actions by themselves and others may increase parents' awareness of the dynamics of interaction. Like others in marginal situations (cf. Scott and Lyman, 1968b), they may become generally more skilled as interactants. They often appear more able to "take the role of the other" and recognise that: "I'd be the same in their place."

CONSEQUENCES OF THE NEW COMPETENCE

Parents' competence may have fundamental effects on their identity and self-concept. Parents of the disabled learn to treat as routine occurrences which embarrass, distress, anger, or otherwise disorientate "normal" members of society. Such others may thus interpret parents' actions as evidence of special qualities of character—"kindness," "understanding," "self-sacrifice," and related skills—"they cope so wonderfully." These are the grounds for the "deep philosophy" that other persons with a stigma are often supposed to hold (Goffman, 1966, p. 147). Moreover, such definitions are likely to make sense of their conduct to parents. Several parents said: "I think I'm more mature now." However, such maturity may entail a degree of cynicism. We noted that parents may become more aware of the dynamics of interaction. This may include the recognition that one can manage even basic truths or natural emotions. It is fostered by such situations as: having to produce grief, projecting "false" definitions of the child, or having to prove themselves "good parents." Such an attitude is generally regarded as shameful but parents may still find that it has its rewards. Thus: "I feel I don't have to take anything from anyone now" or "I could never be so hurt again." Of course, to the extent that management of interaction again becomes routine, parents may be "taken in by their own game" and regain their natural sincerity.

The new competence can thus neutralize threats to parents' identity through effecting changes in that identity. Given the fact that they are parents of a disabled child, such changes are welcomed. They were anxious at the beginning to discover what new behavior was expected of persons in their situation and are glad to recognize in retrospect their unexpected capabilities. Of course, they retain "normal" parental responsibilities—many have normal children as well—and may continue to find difficult the performance of "unparental" actions such as restricting the child's freedom or administering painful treatment. But they may yet be different from normal parents. Since parents of the disabled may both be more concerned with and become more committed to fulfilling their responsibilities as parents, this identity may attain greater salience than normal. This may be one reason why they are often held to constitute a model for us all.

CONCLUSIONS

Much of the argument in this paper is, of course, tentative, given the constraints of the research design. Hopefully, it may further understanding of the problems and behavior of parents with disabled children. Its significance, however, can be extended beyond this substantive area. Like other events that question the basis of everyday action, the processes involved in learning to manage a disabled child provide the conditions of a natural experiment. It was pointed out that many of the problems discussed are not peculiar to parents of the disabled children. Hence, closer study of these processes may tell us more about normal parent-child interaction.

REFERENCES

Birenbaum, A. On managing a courtesy stigma. *Journal of Health and Social Behavior,* 1970, *11,* 196–206.
Davis, F. Deviance disavowal: The management of strained interaction by the visibly handicapped. *Social Problems,* 1961, *9,* 120–132.
Edgerton, R. B. Some dimensions of disillusionment in culture contact. *Southwestern Journal of Anthropology,* 1965, *21,* 231–243.
Garfinkel, H. *Studies in ethnomethodology.* Englewood Cliffs: Prentice-Hall, 1967.
General Register Office. *Classification of occupations.* London: Her Majesty's Stationery Office, 1961.
Glaser, B., & Strauss, A. *Awareness of dying.* Chicago: Aldine Publishing Co., 1965.
Goffman, E. *The presentation of self in everyday life.* New York: Doubleday & Co., 1959.
Goffman, E. *Encounters: Two studies in the sociology of interaction.* Indianapolis: Bobbs-Merrill Co., 1961.
Goffman, E. *Stigma: Notes on the management of spoiled identity.* London: Penguin Books, 1968.

Haber, L. D., & Smith, R. T. Disability and deviance: Normative adaptations of role behaviour. *American Sociological Review,* 1971, *36,* 87–97.

Horobin, G., & Voysey, M. Sociological perspectives on brain damage. In P. Black (Ed.), *Brain damage in children: Etiology, diagnosis, and management.* Baltimore: The Williams & Wilkins Co., in press.

Schatzman, L., & Strauss, A. Social class and modes of communication. *American Journal of Sociology,* 1955, *60,* 329–338.

Scheff, T. J. Toward a sociological model of consensus. *American Sociological Review,* 1967, *32,* 32–46.

Scott, M. B., & Lyman, S. M. Accounts. *American Sociological Review,* 1968a, *33,* 46–62.

Scott, M. B., & Lyman, S. M. Paranoia, homosexuality and game theory. *Journal of Health and Social Behavior,* 1968b, *9,* 179–187.

Strong, P. M. *Parent-child interaction.* Unpublished paper, Aberdeen University, 1971.

Sudnow, D. *Passing on: The social organization of dying.* Englewood Cliffs: Prentice-Hall, 1967.

Thomas, E. J. Problems of disability from the perspective of role theory. *Journal of Health and Human Behavior,* 1966, *7,* 2–14.

Voysey, M. *Ideologies of parents of the disabled.* Paper presented at the Fifth National Deviancy Symposium, 1970.

Weinstein, E. A. The development of interpersonal competence. In D. A. Goslin (Ed.), *Handbook of socialization theory and research,* pp. 753–775. Chicago: Rand-McNally, 1969.

Weinstein, E. A., & Deutschberger, P. Tasks, bargains and identities in social interaction. *Social Forces,* 1964, *42,* 457–465.

Wootton, A. J., & Illsley, R. Social influences on parents and their children. In R. G. Mitchell (Ed.), *Child life and health.* London: J. & A. Churchill, 1970.

CHAPTER 10

A FAMILY IN CRISIS
A Helping Approach

Paul W. Power and Arthur E. Dell Orto

When a family is in crisis the health professional is confronted by an event demanding the use of specific skills. Faced with a problem that appears to have no immediate solution, family members can become confused, extremely anxious, and can harbor feelings of intense helplessness. The crisis itself is perceived as a threat to the family's life goals (Rapoport, 1962). An event has disrupted the accustomed patterns of family living. If a crisis is responded to successfully, the family's life can be even more rewarding than it was before the trauma; if not, it can weaken the family and leave it more vulnerable to various everyday problems.

For the health professional who is available to assist a family in crisis, effective intervention requires knowledge of what family members are experiencing emotionally during the event and skills to implement appropriately certain helping methods. Both Chapters 4 and 5 identify many reactions of family members to a disability-related trauma. Chapter 9 outlines a general helping approach to families undergoing a disability. This chapter gives more of a specialized focus to the material explained in those chapters, since crisis intervention necessitates strategies that are somewhat different than the approaches already suggested in this section. These methods may be modified, or one aspect of intervention could be emphasized more than another for a continued period. The definition of the crisis problem may offer the helper a greater variety of possibilities for intervention. Before an intervention approach is explained, however, a brief review of the literature related to family crisis is presented. An understanding of the different reactive stages and crisis treatment methods provides a valuable resource of information for the development of the professional's helping perspective.

REVIEW OF THE LITERATURE

Many different events can cause a family disability-related crisis. A sudden trauma, e.g., heart attack, stroke, serious accident, the occurrence of a crippling, deteriorative, chronic condition or terminal illness, emergency hospitalization or a family member leaving the hospital after a long stay and returning home to recuperate, could be a precipitating cause to a family crisis state. After the initial crisis event the family usually goes through different stages. Caplan (1964) describes the first stage as the initial rise in tension that results from the crisis-provoking event, the second stage as one of increased tension because the family has not yet resolved the crisis, and the third stage as a period when the tension becomes so great that family members may experience acute depression because they feel so helpless and lost. In the final stage individuals will either experience a serious mental breakdown or they may resolve the crisis. These four stages are usually completed within 5 to 8 weeks. Hill (1958) has also developed stages of crisis reactions involving individuals and families. He believes that the course of an individual's or family's reaction to a crisis "follows a roller-coaster pattern." When the crisis occurs, the individual or family is "numbed" by the blow. As the family faces the reality of the crisis, it often becomes helpless and disoriented. The family then attempts to recover from the crisis after the brief period of disorganization by using "emergency coping mechanisms." Serious depression can occur if these devices fail, but some level of family balance is established by these emergency procedures.

Just as the family's reactive pattern has been viewed as occurring in stages, so treatment with individuals or families in crisis has been conceived as taking place in different phases. Rapoport (1962) believes that the health professional needs to have rapid access to clients during the initial stage of a crisis. Smith (1978) states that crisis therapists should complete six tasks in the initial contact with the patient: 1) identify the precipitating event with the patient, 2) learn how the patient feels about the crisis, 3) discover how the patient has tried to cope with the crisis, 4) assess how and where the patient should be helped, 5) explain to patient why they are still in a state of crisis, and 6) discuss with the patient tasks that could be accomplished to resolve the crisis successfully.

In their work at the Family Treatment Unit of the Colorado Psychiatric Hospital in Denver, Langsley and Kaplan (1968) help the family to focus, during the initial meeting, on the precipitating event that led to the crisis. They encourage the family members to share their experiences and feelings about the crisis, and a return interview is usually scheduled the morning after the first visit. Home visits and daily family contacts are held for 3 or 4 days and then become less frequent as family balance is slowly restored.

Oppenheimer (1967) has also performed most of her crisis intervention work in hospital settings. She believes that with the hospitalized cancer patient and the family the techniques of intervention should include: 1) assisting the family and patient to develop an awareness of their problem, 2) diagnosing accurately and quickly the total situation for the patient and family, and 3) helping the patient and family to develop new and more effective problem-solving skills.

In a crisis different approaches may have to be adopted according to the particular crisis and the unique needs of the family. The general goals of intervention emphasize the here and now and include both helping the family to restore itself to a state of equilibrium and to assist the family in giving support to the patient. In contrast to other goals of family treatment, helping a family in crisis assumes that after a brief period of effective helping the family will regain its ability to meet its own needs as it adjusts to the new reality of disability.

A HELPING APPROACH

Intervention with the family occurs in three phases: beginning, middle, and terminating. Each phase varies in length, and it is important that as many significant family members as possible be involved in the intervention. This enables the helper to evaluate family intervention, to encourage communication, and to discuss the nature of the crisis problem openly with the family. Crisis also involves a sense of urgency and immediacy, and an active approach must be used in order to relieve tension and counteract feelings of helplessness and hopelessness (Parad, 1965). Families in crisis are "not interested in long-term treatment, and should be helped to find solutions in a few meaningful sessions" (Kirschner, 1979, p. 211).

Beginning Phase

When the family is in crisis because of a traumatic event, the family members initially express fear, guilt, confusion, shock, and feelings of inadequacy. At this time the family primarily needs emotional support. Health professionals often feel that they have to ask many questions upon first meeting a family in crisis. What the family initially needs is just someone to be with them to attend, to listen, and to respond to their feelings. Gradually the family members will want to talk about the trauma and the patient, and are more willing to do so when they perceive that the helper wishes to listen and to share their grief, anger, and disappointment.

During their initial reaction to the event family members usually want to ventilate their feelings and need empathy and warmth. When helpers listen and stimulate this verbalization of feelings they can begin to learn how the family is expressing the precipitating event. A health professional wants to hear information that will be helpful in identifying the stresses within the family's life, as well as understand the particular needs resulting from the trauma of the family members. Such needs may be continued emotional support, help in confronting the reality of the situation, more information about the trauma, help in responding to the patient, or community resources that can be utilized during this crisis. By listening the helper is attempting to create an atmosphere of acceptance and to let the family know that someone cares (Anthony & Carkhuff, 1976). Once this is established, the family can become more receptive to the worker's helping efforts. The helper will also need to understand what adaptive mechanisms are already operating in the family and how the family members have coped with past crises. Appropriate questions can be asked following the expression of feelings. Gradually, intervention goals are formulated as the helper begins to understand the meaning the crisis has to the family.

The health professional needs to make contact with the family at the family's level of reality. Some families may be too overwhelmed with the realistic problems caused by the crisis, e.g., housing, money, employment, or child care, to have any energy immediately available for expressing grief. The expression of feelings may follow the temporary resolution of these practical difficulties.

On the helper's part, however, this stage is characterized by giving support, identifying immediate adjustment problems, and understanding how the family can assist, if and when possible, the patient's recovery. Often the family is not emotionally ready soon after the trauma to provide this help. They may need assistance in reorganizing family roles before they can be contributors to the patient's rehabilitation.

Middle Phase

As the family members gradually face the reality of what has happened, they will begin to ask such questions as, "Why has this happened to us? What can we do to help the patient?" Their search for answers may demand a specific response, but many questions will have no answer. There may be no discernible reason why the traumatic event has occurred.

In questioning the family members health professionals need to recognize that the family's emotions may take many forms. For example, anger may be expressed as passive resistance, sarcasm, or blame of persons on whom the patient or family depends. Frequently the health professional will become the target of anger, and when this happens he should assist the family members in learning the origin of these feelings and how they are being expressed.

During this intervention stage the helper continues to listen, but encourages the family members to understand the possible problem areas for adjustment. The helper may also have to assist the family to acknowledge the possible life-threatening situation of the patient. The family might even have to be prepared for the loss of the family member. Interpreting the meaning of the traumatic event, providing and utilizing support during the crisis, and establishing an accepting relationship and communicating with empathy and respect can, singly or together, help the family face unpleasant alternatives.

It is important for the helper to respond to the family with concreteness, to focus on the present, on the current crisis, and not give false reassurances. The family members may deny what has happened, but denial may be necessary in order to give them time to gather their resources. As the family begins to understand more fully the meaning of the crisis, the health professional may assign the family members certain tasks related to family reorganization. These duties may involve contacting, when possible, the extended family, performing other chores in the home, or using designated community supports. The helper should be aware of the separate needs of each family member and what each person is struggling with most. These may vary from the mother who wants to spend more time in the hospital with the ill child to children who may wonder how they are going to be cared for if one parent is away from home so much of the time. When the health professional helps family members to communicate with each other about disability-related concerns, family reorganization is handled more easily. As the family makes the adaptive changes, reinforcement and encouragement from the health professional help family members to regain self-confidence and feelings of adequacy.

Of course, the type of specific intervention depends upon the main problem areas identified. The main goal of this phase is to assist the family to begin to adapt to the disability occurrence. Included in this goal is helping the family move from a state of disorganization to one of balance, or from a family atmosphere where anger, confusion, and feelings of helplessness dominate to a family life where these emotions may at least be controlled, if not removed. The latter may be the only feasible solution so that family life can continue to function.

A further aid to family members in crisis is a regular opportunity to express their feelings to someone outside of the family. As time passes there may still be much unresolved grief or guilt. If the family can be seen at the helper's office at regular intervals for a prescribed period of time, they can be helped to vent and understand their own emotions and reach a stage where they can live with the loss, disappointment, or even sense of failure. These meetings can also provide the chance for the helper to inform the family of how a particular loss can be compensated for, or what activities will help alleviate feelings of grief.

After understanding the main adjustment problems, health professionals should determine whether these problems can be handled in their job function or whether a referral should be made. Referrals may have to be made when helpers believe that extended, intensive family counseling is necessary that is beyond their own skills and helping opportunity. Often such counseling is needed because the precipitating event of the trauma was just one in a long series of traumatic occurrences that culminated in a state of family crisis.

Terminating Phase

When the health professional realizes that family equilibrium is being restored, adjustment problems are being tackled, and the family is involved, to the extent they are capable, in the patient's rehabilitation, then contact with the family may diminish. Many families may only need someone immediately after the initial crisis to provide information or serve as a listener. Other persons, after family life has been reorganized to the best extent possible, may not desire any further contact with the health professional who aided them in family adjustment. To the family this helper may represent a time of sadness, and they do not want to be reminded of that period. However, whether the family members have assumed adequate responsibility to control the implications of the crisis or whether they request that helping services no longer be provided, it is often reassuring if the health professional lets them know that he will be available if they need him. An occasional phone call to assess the family's progress is also generally welcomed. Follow-up often prevents a recurrence of the severe adjustment problems.

CONCLUSION

During crisis intervention the health professional has multiple functions. As an assessor he tries to determine how the crisis affects the entire family and considers the possibility that emotional symptoms may be related to a previous family crisis (Ruben, 1975). The situation is evaluated as adequately and thoroughly as is possible, and the helper learns the total situation of the patient and family and how they can develop, when necessary, effective problem-solving skills. The health professional is also a resource person, providing information about: a) the disability or illness and its implications for family life, b) the financial resources available in the community for the family, c) how family roles can be readjusted to accommodate the new, caring needs of the patient, and d) how the extended family or kin network can be temporarily utilized. Because the family members should recognize their feelings and attitudes related to the crisis, the helper is a facilitator for the expression of these feelings, as well as a source of support by listening and reinforcing the collective strengths of the family. This support may help the family to make the necessary decisions to get through the crisis (Kirschner, 1979).

In helping a family to alleviate their crisis situation the worker is indirectly assisting in the patient's possible rehabilitation. A family in confusion and a high state of anxiety will have difficulty in attending to the needs of the disabled family member, even if one of those needs is simply emotional support. When it is possible the patient should participate in crisis treatment intervention. Family members need to know, for example, the patient's own understanding of what has happened and come to realize that patient and family influence one another. If the family is going to reorganize its life after a traumatic event, the patient should be included in reorganization plans.

The two articles that follow in this chapter highlight the reactive family process to a sudden crisis. Margaret Epperson identifies six family stages that are experienced before family members regain their balance. With each stage there are particular intervention approaches, and her explanation of the stages and intervention contains valuable insights. Barbara Giacquinta's article discusses one particular disease, cancer, and illustrates how it can provoke family crisis. She explains family reactive stages, and her explanation of the family hurdles and intervention goals associated with each stage is particularly helpful. Both articles contain a wealth of material on intervention strategies in crisis.

REFERENCES

Anthony, W., & Carkhuff, R. *The art of health care.* Amherst, Mass.: Human Resource Development Press, 1976.

Caplan, G. *Principles of preventive psychiatry.* New York: Basic Books, 1964.

Hill, R. Generic features of families under stress. *Social Casework,* 1958, *39,* 139-149.

Kirschner, C. The aging family in crisis: A problem in living. *Social Casework,* 1979, April, 209-216.

Langsley, D., & Kaplan, D. *The treatment of families in crisis.* New York: Grune & Stratton, 1968.

Oppenheimer, J. Use of crisis intervention in casework with the cancer patient and his family. *Social Work,* 1967, *12,* 44-52.

Parad, H. *Crisis intervention: Selected readings.* New York: Family Service Association of America, 1965.

Rapoport, L. Working with families in crisis: An exploration in preventive intervention. *Social Work,* 1962, *7,* 48-56.

Ruben, H. Family Crises. *American Family Physician,* 1975, *11,* 132-136.

Smith, L. A review of crisis intervention theory. *Social Casework,* 1978, July, 396-405.

FAMILIES IN SUDDEN CRISIS:
Process and Intervention
in a Critical Care Center

Margaret M. Epperson[1]

Mr. and Mrs. Smith (fictitious name), the middle-aged parents of two teen-agers, were awakened by an early-morning phone call from the Maryland State Police. John, their nineteen-year-old son, had been in a serious car accident and was being flown by helicopter from the accident scene to the Maryland Institute for Emergency Medicine (MIEM). One of the car's occupants had been killed. By police estimate, John appeared to be in critical condition.

The Smiths and their seventeen-year-old daughter, Lisa, drove from their home in western Maryland to the Institute in Baltimore, a two-hour trip. They were met in the family waiting area by a social worker trained in family process. The way they spoke, their body language, and agitated behavior indicated that these family members were under severe stress.

Mr. Smith began pacing the floor, shouting, "Where's my son?" and "Can't someone do something?" Mrs. Smith sat on the edge of a chair with her hands clasped between her thighs, repeating over and over, "My God, what happened? I hope he's all right!" Lisa, with red eyes and nose, quietly wove a torn facial tissue around her fingers as she sat tensely in the corner of the couch.

The Maryland Institute for Emergency Medicine is a special critical care center equipped to give intensive, comprehensive treatment to multiple-trauma victims. In the mid-1950s, Dr. R. Adams Cowley, the Institute's director, began his war against the second greatest killer in the United States —death due to serious accidents. By using rapid air transportation, advanced technology, an interdisciplinary medical and nursing team approach, and special treatment techniques, the MIEM offers many critically injured persons a better chance of survival. The mortality rate is 20%. (For statistical reasons, this figure also includes those patients who are pronounced dead on arrival.)

PURPOSE OF STUDY

Current literature discussing critical care patients and ICUs emphasizes the need to give special consideration to families of severely ill patients (Brodland & Andreasen, 1974; West, 1975). Effective treatment for such families

---

Reprinted from *Social Work in Health Care* 2(3), pp. 265–273, ©1977, The Haworth Press, with permission.

[1]Chief, Family Service Division, Maryland Institute for Emergency Medicine, 22 South Greene St., Baltimore, MD 21201.

needs to be developed. The purpose of this study was to determine the needs of families under sudden, severe stress due to life-threatening injuries of a family member, and to develop appropriate treatment methods.

Because many of those families studied were "fragmented" families (i.e., families with one or more members temporarily or permanently absent), and because of the currently differing views of the sociological composition of the so-called modern family grouping, the definition of "family" used in this paper is based on that of the philosopher-theologian, Thomas Aquinas: family as the community of one's household—the person or persons one is living with.

The phrase "sudden, severe stress due to life-threatening situations of family members" describes the state of acute crisis the family experiences when a family member is in critical physical condition due to multiple injuries as a result of a catastrophic event. The families in this study had to deal with the reality that one of their members was suddenly in danger of death because of a road accident, violent criminal assault, industrial mishap, recreational miscalculation, or some domestic tragedy.

The Smiths are typical of the 230 families of MIEM patients studied over a period of twelve months. Charting the behavior of these families and noting their verbal responses allowed similar, repeating patterns to emerge. The investigator was able to identify a process of recovery from the crisis state, and to develop treatment modalities to help families through the various phases. Each family's treatment time averaged two and one-half interviews, or approximately five hours of intervention.

The theoretical framework used for this study was the crisis model as developed by Dr. Erich Lindemann and Dr. Gerald Caplan. Crisis intervention is a brief treatment modality having the current crisis as its only focus. Its goal is to reestablish the equilibrium that is disrupted by the crisis situation (Parad & Caplan, 1960).

"Crisis" in its simplest terms is defined by Caplan as "an upset in a steady state" (Caplan, 1959–1960). This definition rests on the systems-theory concept that an individual, a family, or any social system strives to maintain a state of equilibrium through a constant series of adaptive maneuvers and characteristic problem-solving activities that allow for basic need fulfillment to take place. Whether a situation or event becomes a "crisis" depends greatly on how the family defines or interprets the event in light of its own cultural and historical experiences. What may be a crisis for one family may not be so for another.

Throughout a system's life span, many situations or events occur which can lead to sudden breakdowns in the system's functioning. One event that can disrupt the usual homeostatic state of a family system is the sudden, catastrophic illness of one of its members. The Smith family is typical of a family thrown into a sudden crisis state.

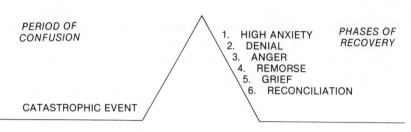

Figure 1.   Families under sudden, severe stress in life-threatening situations undergo a six-phase recovery process.

It is postulated that in a state of crisis the system's usual problem-solving mechanisms are insufficient and do not rapidly lead the system back to a state of equilibrium. Often, a family must find new solutions to deal with that which, up to the current crisis state, had been outside the realm of their family system's life experience (Spiegel, 1957). The Smiths needed external help in coping with their situation until they could mobilize their own adaptive capacities and activate their inner resources which would eventually help reestablish the family's pre-crisis "steady state."

DESCRIPTION OF PROCESS

Families under sudden, severe stress appear to go through, or at least touch on, six distinct phases before the family system is able to reorganize, reintegrate, and regain its homeostatic state. It is to be understood that families differ both in regard to the sequence of phases and in the rate by which family members pass through the various stages. Also, it is to be noted that some families skip over stages and eliminate them altogether in the adaptive process. Furthermore, all family members do not go through the phases at the same time, and each member is unique in his or her completion of the process. Each family member, like each family group, is individualistic in his pattern of the adapting process. However, despite this diversity, there remains a distinct, identifiable method of recovery to a "steady state" (see Figure 1).

High Anxiety

A period of high anxiety is most often the phase families go through first, and it is usually experienced by most family members at the same time. The high-anxiety phase is characterized by great physical agitation, high-pitched voice, tight neck and shoulder muscles, and other body reactions, such as fainting, nausea, and diarrhea, found to be typical of persons under severe stress. On their arrival at the Institute, Mr. and Mrs. Smith overtly demonstrated many of these physical signs of stress. Lisa sat quietly to the side;

only her body language revealed her stressful state. Sometimes anxiety is manifested by withdrawal and body tenseness as if one were using all his energies in body containment. This acute anxiety can last anywhere from a few minutes to several hours.

Three things are done to help diminish the family's anxiety:

1. Brief, accurate information is given about the patient. The family is told where the patient is at the moment—the admitting area, operating room, or the critical care area. They are also told the general condition of the patient, e.g., "His condition at the moment appears to be serious." The family is assured that a physician and nurse will be in to give a complete medical report as soon as the physician team has done a thorough examination and x-rays have been read—usually within an hour.
2. The life saving methods and advanced technology of the Institute are explained. This seems to reassure the family that the patient has every advantage modern medicine can offer.
3. The family members are encouraged to ventilate about the initial impact of the news of this sudden catastrophe, e.g., where they were, what they were doing, and what they were told about the accident.

These three steps, coupled with definite information from the physician's report, are most often sufficient to relieve the anxiety to a level at which the family members can begin to consider other issues, e.g., what this means, what they should do now, and other pragmatic considerations which lead to another phase, usually that of denial.

Denial

John was severely damaged in the car accident. He had multiple fractures and several lacerations that would heal over time. But a spinal-cord injury would leave him permanently paralyzed from the waist down. After a lengthy discussion with the family, the doctor left and Mrs. Smith began to cry. Her husband tried to comfort her, saying, "Everything will be all right. You know John; he's a tough kid. He'll be walking again, you'll see." He repeated this statement to Lisa and to the therapist. Later he told the nurse of spinal cord-injured army buddies who had learned to walk again and that there was no reason why John couldn't do the same. Mr. Smith's denial of the situation was real.

The denial phase is important because it seems to act as a psychological preparation for any further bad news the family may receive about the patient. It also seems to have in it the essential element of hope needed to carry on. Further, denial is a regression to a comfortable childhood stage of "magical thinking" that says "in spite of what happened everything will be all right."

It is important for the therapist to maintain a balance in this situation by recognizing the need for denial as well as the need for the family to deal with the reality of what has happened and what now is. Statements such as "Mr. Smith, John was such a healthy boy, it must be difficult for you to believe that he is now paralyzed" are often helpful. Appropriate reiterating of like statements to the family conveys to them that the therapist understands and accepts their struggle with reality. These statements also act as a reminder of what is, without removing the denial defense.

Often, the denial phase lasts until the family is able to speak to the patient, usually after a 48-hour stabilization period. Some family members hold on to their denial for long periods of time and special efforts must be made through follow-up sessions to help these persons deal with the reality of the situation.

Anger

Anger expressed by families under sudden, severe stress seems to be amoeboid, taking many different shapes and directions. During this phase, anger can be directed toward oneself or another family member in an apparent attempt to place the blame, or part of the blame, for what has happened. It can be directed toward the physician and nursing staffs, the state police, emergency medical technicians, the therapist, and others. Often, it is a diffuse kind of anger that lashes out at society or at life in general for allowing to exist circumstances such as high speeds, lack of gun controls, or lenient drunk-driving laws, that may have contributed to the tragedy.

Often families unite in their expressions of anger. In the Smiths' case:

> Lisa was the first to articulate her angry feelings. In response to her father's statements of denial, she began to accuse him of always having to be in control, of telling everyone what they could or could not do: "You're always telling everyone what they're going to do. Just because you say he is going to walk again doesn't mean he is going to." She began to blame him for the accident: "You're the one who told him to 'get out.' This wouldn't have happened if he was at home." (John was living outside the parental home.) Mrs. Smith lashed out at Lisa for being disrespectful to her father. After siding with her husband, Mrs. Smith began to express angry feelings about the inefficiency of the state police. Her husband joined her in her accusations. Lisa began to criticize society in general.

During this phase, the therapist encourages ventilation of angry feelings. It is the therapist's task to help the family focus on the real cause of their anger. When families have a chance to really listen to their accusations, they often see the illegitimacy of their charges. Eventually, the family comes to realize that they are really angry at the patient himself for disrupting the family routine and causing great stress and disorganization within the family system. It must be noted, however, that there are times when outside agents are legimately responsible, at least in part, for the accident.

It was of interest to the investigator that in families which appeared to have good, open patterns of communication, the expressed anger was often immediately directed toward the patient for being so "careless," "dumb," or "stupid" in putting himself in the dangerous situation which was now causing the family such stress. But these same families often expressed feelings of guilt for blaming the sick person for what had happened.

All families who express anger toward the injured member, whether immediately or through a circuitous route, need reassurance that they are not "bad" persons for feeling angry. Often, individual members need repeated "permission" from the therapist to say their angry words. Our society says that it is not nice to be mad at sick, helpless individuals. Consequently, some members experience a sense of uneasiness for blaming the injured member. It is the experience of this writer that, unless the anger family members feel toward the patient is expressed and dealt with, it can cause further destruction to the family system by being later expressed in passive-aggressive behavior toward the patient during his rehabilitation.

Remorse

The sense of guilt families feel for blaming the patient for the current crisis is different from what is considered to be a period or phase of remorse. Guilt feelings say "somehow I have done wrong; I am culpable." Remorse, on the other hand, includes the elements of both guilt and sorrow. Remorse seems to describe best what family members feel about the part they may have played in contributing to the accident. They regret not only that the incident occurred, but that they did not, or could not, do more to prevent it. It is the "if only..." stage.

> With great sorrow, the Smith family expressed their remorse with such statements as "If only I had not bought him that car, this would never have happened"; "If only he had still been living at home, he would not have been out so late"; and "If only I had given him the money to get that car fixed, this might not have happened."

It is important to listen to these expressions of remorse and to try to inject some reality as to how much blame the family members can take for the accident. What is it that the family members actually could have done to prevent his tragedy from happening? Usually, there is little, if anything, they could have done to prevent it, but the family can come to this reality only by open discussion.

What family members seem to need and want most during this phase is a reassurance that they are "okay" people in spite of what has happened. Often, the news media compound this problem by giving inaccurate reports that appear to show negligence on the part of the family. Families find it very difficult to cope with the public censure as well as that of other systems with which they must interact, such as in their job situations, school, clubs, and church groups. It is the task of the therapist to help the family relieve themselves of the burden of taking responsibility for the accident, as, in the judgment of the investigator, it was a rare case that a family member could or should have taken legitimate blame for what had happened.

Grief

During the second interview with the Smith family, Mrs. Smith began to express the meaning of her loss. As is characteristic of family members beginning to deal with their grief, Mrs. Smith began by talking about how others would miss her son. "He's such a good boy, the other kids really depend on him to help them out. If anything happens to him, I don't know what they'll do." Eventually, after much discussion about how others would feel about John's temporary absence from his social groups and how they would be affected by his paralysis, both Mrs. Smith and Lisa were able to internalize their feelings of loss. Through her tears Mrs. Smith was able to say "I love him so much—he's my oldest baby; he's always been such a comfort to me. Why did this have to happen?" Lisa's statement showed a recognition of at least temporary loss of old, familiar family patterns and the need for role reversal: "He has always taken care of me. I guess now I'll have to take care of him."

The grief phase usually follows the period of remorse, but not always. It is to be remembered that each family system and each family member differs when going through the phases. The family, at one time or another, experiences an intense period of sadness, a grieving time when their sense of loss, even temporary loss, becomes almost overwhelming. At this time, tears and deep sobbing are frequent. Some family members withdraw into privacy. Tears shed during this phase are different from those that offer a cathartic release of tension in the anxiety phase. This stage is the beginning of a grieving process, the duration and intensity of which depend on such factors as the medical condition of the patient, length of hospitalization, the family solidarity, and the degree of remorse experienced by the family.

During the grief phase, the therapist remains with the family. Grief cannot be taken away, nor should there be any attempt to do so. Grief is a very natural, human response to the loss, or threatened loss, of a love object. Most often, the therapist just sits quietly with the family members, offering a silent support. Many times physical closeness, holding a trembling hand or embracing limp shoulders, conveys an empathy for and an understanding of what the family members are experiencing. These empathic gestures are often all that are needed to begin the flow of copious tears that give some release to the deep emotional feelings of loss.

Reconciliation

Reconciliation usually occurs last, and it seems to be a culmination point in the therapist's intervention during the acute family crisis. At this time the high state of anxiety is diminished, the reality of the situation is clear, or is becoming clearer to the family, anger and remorse have usually been expressed, and the grieving process has begun.

Choosing an accurate word to describe what transpires during this phase is a problem of semantics. The word "reconciliation" is used because it differs from "acceptance" or "acquiescence" in that it connotes a "bringing together" or "bringing into harmony" all that has taken place. Reconciliation is not acceptance of what has happened; most families cannot accept the tragedy, especially if it appeared to be a senseless occurrence. This is a phase of putting things in place, of being reconciled to the fact that something terrible has happened that deeply affects, and will continue to affect, the total family unit. Included in this period of reconciliation is a realistic sense of hope that, whatever hardship this tragedy may impose, the family can and will survive.

This is the time when mobilization of the family system's resources begins, if it hasn't already, to enable the family to adapt to the current situation and cope with whatever is to come. During this phase, a family solidarity seems to emerge and concretize through a concerted effort on the part of the family to plan for the future.

> The Smiths gave evidence that they were becoming reconciled to the tragic reality of John's injuries by such statements as "We've been through hard times before and we've made it"; "There's no reason we can't ride this storm out"; "Tragedy is nothing new to us"; and "We'll have to pull together and take each day as it comes."

During this phase, the social worker helps the family to start thinking about and begin to develop a feasible plan of action: what needs to be done now? who will be able to do these things? what are the available resources that can be utilized? who and what helped the family pull through previous crises? For a variety of reasons, either current or long standing, some families appear unable to activate adequate coping mechanisms and must rely heavily on outside resources. Other families are better able to cope, but require minimal outside support. In both cases, appropriate referrals to community agencies must be made.

DISCUSSION

No attempt was made in this paper to consider the long-term effects of life-threatening situations on the family system. Others have made observations in this area (Mueller, 1962; Fahy, Irving, & Millac, 1967). The purpose of this presentation has been to discuss the process that families in the acute crisis stage undergo when the family unit has been disrupted because of the traumatic, life-threatening injuries to one of its members. Also, treatment techniques utilized within the crisis-theory framework are presented as methods of intervention that have been effective in treating families of critical patients brought to MIEM.

Trauma centers such as MIEM are the wave of the future. There is increasing interest in the medical field of traumatology and trauma nursing. As more critical care centers are established across the country, there will be a great need for social workers to work with the families of multiple-trauma patients as well as with the patients themselves.

This paper offers a method of family intervention for these workers to adapt to their own critical care situations. It presents the therapist with some important insights as to what the family experiences when a member is suddenly in critical condition because of a serious accident secondary to our highly technical society.

REFERENCES

Brodland, G. A., & Andreasen, N. J. Adjustment problems of the family of the burn patient. *Social Casework*, 1974, *55*, 13.

Caplan, G. Formulated in seminars at the Harvard School of Public Health, 1959–1960.

Fahy, T. J., Irving, M. H., & Millac, P. Severe head injuries—A six-year follow-up. *Lancet*, 1967, *2*(7509), 475.

Mueller, A. D. Psychologic factors in rehabilitation of paraplegic patients. *Archives of Physical Medicine*, 1962, *43*(4), 151.

Parad, H., & Caplan, G. A framework for studying families in crisis. *Social Work*, 1960, *5*(3), 34.

Spiegel, J. P. The resolution of role conflict within the family. *Psychiatry*, 1957, *20*(1), 15.

West, N. D. Stresses associated with ICU's affect patients, families, staff. *Journal of American Hospital Association*, 1975, *49*(49), 63.

HELPING FAMILIES FACE THE CRISIS OF CANCER

Barbara Giacquinta[1]

Traditionally, the family is viewed as the first line of defense to support one of its members who faces a crisis. But an entire family may be in crisis because one of its members is diagnosed as having cancer. In this perspective, the nuclear family is not viewed solely as the principal refuge for the sick, but rather as the unit facing crisis and, therefore, the target of nursing care.

The diagnosis of cancer for any family member is experienced as a personal tragedy and an assault on the integrity of the family system. Many families fail to cope successfully with either the tragedy or the threat to family stability. Furthermore, it is becoming more evident that the treatments of cancer place additional strain on the family, strain that must be fully understood and alleviated.

In working with families facing cancer, I have attempted to find a model of stages and phases for the systematic description of the functioning of family members. Kübler-Ross (1969) proposed a model of five stages through which the dying person proceeds emotionally in the living-dying continuum. Kavanaugh (1974) described a model of seven phases in an individual's bereavement process after the death of a loved one. My model, in contrast, focuses on 10 phases of family functioning within four stages— living with cancer, the living-dying interval, bereavement, and reestablishment. This model, based on analysis of 100 families, describes hurdles for the family to overcome and goals of nursing intervention at each phase.

There is always an inherent danger in proposing such a model. A model can be misused to stereotype and reduce the complexity of human behavior and to distance health professionals from the uniqueness of their clients. I hope, rather, that nurses will use this model as a starting point and will further elaborate it by identifying resonating themes of behavior within families and to incorporate these themes into the model.

STAGE I: LIVING WITH CANCER

During this stage, an individual in a family receives an initial diagnosis of cancer and continues to carry out familiar obligations by functioning in var-

Reprinted from *American Journal of Nursing* 77(10), pp. 1585–1588, © 1977, The American Journal of Nursing Company, with permission.

[1]Assistant Professor of Nursing, New York University, New York City; and co-practitioner in oncology with a private family practice for those dealing with such issues as living with cancer, dying, death, and bereavement.

411

ious ways as a family member. Within this first stage, a family may undergo five phases: impact, functional disruption, search for meaning, informing others, and engaging emotions.

Impact is the phase in which the family learns that one of its members has been diagnosed as having cancer. Shock and strain, evident in this first phase, can conceivably lead to a high rate of such nonproductive behavior as withdrawal, anxiety, and agitation. The entire family group may be disorganized or key members may come forth to help the others cope. Having strongly motivated, clearly defined role responsibilities within a family tends to reduce nonproductive behavior. Those who are with the individual at the time he or she receives the diagnosis of cancer are found to be less shocked, dazed, or highly agitated if the person communicating the diagnosis does so with candor and confidence.

The hurdle for the family to overcome in this phase is despair. Nursing intervention must be geared toward fostering hope. "Hope comes close to being the very heart and center of a human being" (Lynch, 1965). But hope cannot be sustained without the support of significant others; it must be generated in the family.

Hope is the feeling that the family can live with cancer and that each family member can use this experience for growth. It offers a sense of security that approaches like surgery, radiation, immunotherapy, or the newest drugs are available and may help. Hope allows the patient and the family to imagine a future.

Family members at this time, although in shock, are able to perceive the attitudes of hopefulness or hopelessness in the health professionals around them. The nurse with hope helps the family members explore and combat feelings of despair, separation from their thoughts and feelings, and withdrawal from one another.

Functional disruption may follow as the second phase. Shock experienced by family members in the first phase may weaken their commitment to mutual role obligation. The hospital vigil may supersede former responsibilities. Role dilemmas may occur. Initiative and leadership in the family may be lacking, household management may need adjustment, and even the daily needs of children may be difficult to meet. The stability and autonomy of the family may weaken as members are pulled in various directions of daily living. As stability and autonomy decrease, the family becomes less able to reach out to other systems of support.

The hurdle for the family to overcome in the second phase is isolation. Isolation arises when family members are separated from one another or from other systems of support in their interaction, communication, cooperation, and social and emotional involvement (Theodorson & Theodorson, 1969).

Nursing intervention that fosters cohesion of the family and that strengthens interaction, communication, cooperation, and social and emo-

Points of Transition in Individual With Cancer	Family Stage	Family Phase	Family Hurdle	Goal of Nursing Intervention
Individual receives initial diagnosis of cancer, continues to carry out role obligations with the family, and functions in varying ways as a family member.	Living with Cancer	impact	despair	fostering hope
		functional disruption	isolation	fostering cohesion
		search for meaning	vulnerability	fostering security
		informing others	retreat	fostering courage
		engaging emotions	helplessness	fostering problem solving
Individual with cancer ceases to perform familiar roles and is cared for either at home or in the hospital.	Restructuring in the Living-Dying Interval	reorganization	competition	fostering cooperation
		framing memories	anonymity	fostering identity
Individual with cancer dies.	Bereavement	separation	self absorption	fostering intimacy
		mourning	guilt	fostering relief
	Reestablishment	expansion of the social network	alienation	fostering relatedness

413

tional involvement will combat isolation and will enable the family to increase its autonomy and decrease its instability. Stability and autonomy are requisite to the ability to sustain relationships within the family and with other support units. Delineation of needs and priorities, addition of resources both material and social, and full engagements of each family member in family life will further reduce the isolation that might be experienced.

A search for meaning may occur as the third family phase. There appears to be an attempt to gain intellectual mastery over the cancer process. A family member may go to the library to read about cancer. Others may ransack their memories for evidence of the patient's prior vulnerability. There is a need not only to find meaning for the present occurrence of cancer in the family, but also a need to ensure that this could *not* happen to another member. Family members may harp on the ill person's never having eaten properly, having drunk too much alcohol, coffee, or diet soda, or having smoked too much. This behavior can be particularly difficult for the seriously ill member because what is implied is that he or she is at fault in causing the cancer.

The hurdle for the family to overcome is vulnerability. As each family member comes in touch with his or her own mortality, fusion and identification with the patient can occur. The focus of nursing intervention, therefore, is toward security and toward supporting the family system to maintain the identity, integrity, and continuity of each member under the pressure of changing life conditions. Security for each member of the family is enhanced if each makes a commitment to experiencing his or her changing identity.

The fourth family phase, *informing others,* may occur before the family has overcome the hurdles of despair, isolation, and vulnerability. Family members may not have fully dissipated the impact of the patient's diagnosis nor assimilated the information concerning the course of treatment and expected outcomes. The response of those whom they inform can cause the family to retreat, the next hurdle to overcome.

Some families face regret in having shared the news prematurely. They may be faced with questions that they cannot answer, with pressure to seek additional opinions regarding diagnosis and methods of treatment, with what seems to be intrusiveness of friends and relatives, and with the necessity to support others outside the family.

Nursing intervention that fosters courage will help the family sort out and share feelings within the immediate circle. Strengthening the communication and the cohesion of the family will override their search for outside sources of primary support.

Once the family has increased internal open lines of communication and support and has knowledge, direction, and commitment concerning priorities of action, it is more likely to experience courage rather than to retreat in relationship to others.

The fifth and final family phase in the first stage is *engaging emotions.* When a family member has cancer, there are profound changes for the entire family. Volatile emotions come to the surface as former family values, goals, satisfactions, and positions of security are changed. Family members greatly fear losing control by displaying bursts of strong emotion. Loss of control, however, does not occur when people acknowledge and express their emotions. Rather, loss of control occurs if feelings are suppressed and individuals lose touch with themselves and with each other.

Helplessness is the fifth family hurdle to overcome. Helplessness evolves from the belief that everything that can be done has been done (Shea & Hurley, 1970).

When the individual with cancer progresses to recovery, the feeling of helplessness, as well as the flow of volatile emotions, gradually ebb away. But if the condition of the ill family member progresses gradually toward death, family members slowly get in touch with what is happening. They begin to recognize the defeat and loss they feel, the strain of carrying additional role obligations, and their need to change sights, to find satisfactions with life as it is evolving, and to plan more realistically for their life together. Grieving usually begins at this phase.

Family members will usually evidence a fluctuating desire at this time for someone to set a final date. They believe if they have a time limit they will be able to cope better. Often, when families are given a specific number of months, they direct their energies toward postponing death or toward bearing up to that day. The family as a whole may survive the date, but in coping in this way, they are robbed of valuable life together.

Directing nursing intervention toward daily problem solving will decrease the helplessness that families feel. It will also crystalize their realization that the life of the family will be changed but ongoing after the death of their loved one.

STAGE II: RESTRUCTURING IN THE LIVING-DYING INTERVAL

During this stage, the individual with cancer ceases to perform familiar roles and is cared for either at home or in the hospital. Within this stage, a family may undergo the sixth and seventh phases—reorganization and framing memories.

Reorganization is the sixth family phase. Role obligations must be redistributed among family members to lessen strain and overcompensation by some members. The performance of these new roles must be rewarded by others. True reorganization necessitates open and honest exploration, compromise, and consolidation.

The sixth hurdle for the family to overcome is competition. The nurse attempts to foster a sense of cooperation so that family goals are met more effectively. Some of these goals may include helping the family feel a greater sense of wholeness, facilitating relationships of mutual support among family members, and enhancing their lives with the individual having cancer. The nurse supports their movement toward acceptance of the eventual death and fosters continued grief work by encouraging a cooperative system that will support the continued growth of the survivors.

Framing memories is the seventh and final phase in the second stage. Just as the family needs time to form a clear picture of the impending death of their loved one, they need time for remembering the individual's life history. They may spend hours gazing at scrapbooks and pictures of the loved one and recalling the person in all of his or her individuality.

The threat of anonymity of the dying person is the hurdle for the family to overcome at this phase. Family members may not be able to recall their loved one prior to the diagnosis of cancer. Their focus may be fixed on a seriously ill and dying person.

Because of the emotional pain involved in such a visualization, family members attempt to block out recollection of their loved one. Through utilization of pictures, scrapbooks, and family storytelling, nurses may foster the family's recall, help to crystalize the person's relationships through time with significant others, and promote the identity of the person through the entire continuum of his or her living-dying. Identity rather than anonymity will be the outcome of such nursing interventions. As the family's image of their loved one strengthens, they can relinquish their dependence on his or her physical presence, and remember their loved one without pain.

STAGE III: BEREAVEMENT

This stage coincides with the imminent dying and death of the individual with cancer. Separation and mourning are the two phases within this stage.

Separation, the eighth family phase, occurs when the loved one's consciousness diminishes and awareness of the environment vanishes. At this time, the family fully experiences their loss and the loneliness of separation. Self-absorption is the hurdle for the family to overcome now. Nursing intervention must be directed toward promoting intimacy if family members are to be supported in their ability to grieve within their family network.

Mourning is the ninth family phase, and the obstacle for the family to overcome here is guilt. Human grief is as strong and as unique as the relationship that has been severed. Grief is a personal experience, different for each member of a family who is grieving over the loss of the same person.

Nursing intervention is geared toward fostering relief expressed through mourning. The family members may have reached the limits of their own endurance and may initially confess relief that their loved one has died and that they remained with the person through that time. Echoes from previous losses may then surface, and these mournings, if uncompleted, may hinder relief. The mourning process is relieved only when the deceased person becomes internalized and enriches the continued family life.

STAGE IV: REESTABLISHMENT

This final stage of family functioning occurs after the completion of mourning and encompasses the tenth and final family phase, *expansion of the social network*. Only after successful resolution of grief will the family fully reenter their social environment that extends beyond the family.

The final hurdle for the family to overcome is alienation. Alienation occurs when involvement with one's society and culture is estranged or lacks meaning. The goal of nursing intervention is to foster relatedness so that self and family estrangement and meaninglessness may be overcome. Individuals in the family may be helped to look back on their family life with acceptance and self respect. Their lives may have taken on dimensions of new growth and self-actualization.

In overcoming feelings of alienation, each person must be open to experiencing his or her changing identity. As families become closer and expand their social network, they begin to accept that the death in the family was inevitable, but not insurmountable.

REFERENCES

Kavanaugh, R. E. *Facing death,* p. 107. Baltimore: Penguin Books, 1974.
Kubler-Ross, E. *On death and dying,* pp. 38–137. New York: Macmillan, 1969.
Lynch, W. F. *Images of hope,* p. 31. Baltimore: Helicon Press, 1965.
Theodorson, G. A., & Theodorson, A. C. *Modern dictionary of sociology,* p. 216. New York: Thomas Y. Crowell, 1969.
Shea, F., & Hurley, E. Hopelessness and helplessness. *Perspectives in Psychiatric Nursing,* 1970, *2*(1), 32–38.

CHAPTER 11

PHYSICAL DISABILITIES AND GROUP COUNSELING:
A Proactive Alternative for Families of the Disabled

Arthur E. Dell Orto and Paul W. Power

PERSPECTIVE

The impact of physical disability or chronic illness creates new roles, expectations, challenges, and demands for the disabled as well as for their families (De Lamata, Gingas, & Weitkower, 1960; Deutsch & Goldstein, 1960; Vincent, 1963; Nagi & Clark, 1964; Gordon & Kutner, 1965; Currier, 1966; Ludwig & Colette, 1969; Olsen, 1970; Pless, Roghmann, & Aaggery, 1972; Shellhase & Shellhase, 1972; Power, 1974; Krupp, 1976; MacVicar & Archbold, 1976; Bray, 1977; Bruhn, 1977; Parks, 1977; Foster & Thomas, 1978; Peterson, 1979). Health professionals need to understand the encompassing nature of disability in order to design adaptable and relevant intervention strategies. Group counseling is one approach that has been documented to respond to selected needs of the disabled.

GROUP COUNSELING OF THE DISABLED

As reflected in the literature, group counseling has applied to a variety of populations and disabilities: arthritis (Henkle, 1975), cancer (Blandford, 1968), coronary disease (Adsett & Bruhn, 1968; Mone, 1970; Bilodeau & Hackett, 1971; Rahe, Tuffli, Suchor, & Arthur, 1973), the elderly (Isaacs, 1967; Burnside, 1970, 1971), myasthenia gravis (Schwartz & Cahill, 1971), multiple sclerosis (Day, Day, & Hermann, 1953; Mally & Strehl, 1963; Schwartz, 1974; Hartings, Pavlou, & Davis, 1976; Power & Rogers, 1979), pediatric illnesses (Milman, 1952; Luzzatti & Dittmann, 1954; Cofer & Ner, 1976), renal disease (Shambaugh & Kanter, 1969; Wijsenbeek & Munitz,

1970; Hollon, 1972; McClellan, 1972; Buchanan, 1975), spinal cord injury (Roessler, Milligan, & Ohlson, 1976; Banik & Mendelson, 1978), stroke (Piskor & Paleos, 1968; Oradei & Waite, 1974), the terminally ill (Yalom & Greaves, 1977), and visual limitations (Herman, 1966; Avery, 1968; Kubler-Ross & Anderson, 1968; Manaster, 1971; Keegan, 1974; Lipp & Malone, 1976; Roessler, 1978).

All of these group counseling interventions emphasize developing a support system that would create a buffer zone between the patient and the ravages of illness and disability. Group counseling, therefore, can be a counter-force to helplessness, isolation, and desperation because it brings people together to share their individual concerns as well as their common resources.

The uniqueness of group counseling is that it provides an opportunity for people to explore the dimensions of their disability and develop the skills to maximize their rehabilitation potential through a peer-oriented support system.

GROUP COUNSELING AND THE FAMILY

Interventions that focus solely upon the disabled person apart from the family system are often limited in their scope as well as their effect, because disability affects the total family.

In discussing the impact of long-term and fatal illness upon the family, Gordon and Kutner (1965) point out the following to indicate the multitude of problems faced by such a family:

1. There may be an initial traumatic reaction when the diagnosis is revealed to the parents.
2. The parents' self-attitudes as well as their relationships with other members of their families, friends, and neighbors may be seriously altered.
3. There may be difficulty in adjusting to the medical needs of the sick child.
4. A variety of relationships with physicians and other medical personnel in clinics and hospitals must be established.
5. A long-term readjustment of life-style, depending upon the nature of the illness and the economic, biological, and social consequences following in its wake, may be required.
6. Latent emotional problems may be brought to the surface by the demands of the situation.

These concerns focus upon the demands made upon the family, but they also allude to the consequences if a family is unable to bind its resources and to obtain assistance during traumatic periods. Family group counseling is one alternative that can help put disability into perspective and result in the development of responses that help the family meet the challenge facing them. Family group counseling has the potential of: a) supporting both the client and the family during hospitalization, rehabilitation, and community re-entry, b) exposing the family unit as well as family members to role models, and c) teaching the necessary skills to effectively respond to past, present, and future problems.

This proactive response is essential for families of the disabled, because the impact of a disability is often the beginning of a long, isolating journey that may deplete family resources and erode the foundation of the family system. Owen (1972) indicates the value of a group process for the family of the disabled:

> Most people know nothing about severe disability. When a serious accident occurs to one of their family group it may seem like the end of the world. Fear may be so gripping that their overriding response is to run away. The doctor needs to spend some unhurried time with the spouse as soon after the accident as possible. He cannot, of course, make promises that may not come true, but he can give support to a person in dire psychological need. If he will take the time to acquaint himself with the many successful handicapped persons who are leading active, rewarding lives he will be in a better position to be constructive in these discussions. At this time, he can point out the great value of the group discussions to the family (pp. 13).

As a result of the demonstrated value of groups as a response to the demands of disability, group counseling with families of the disabled is becoming an integral part of the health care delivery system (Linder, 1970; Wilson, 1971; Mattsson & Agle, 1972; D'Afflitti & Weitz, 1974; Heisler, 1974; Huberty, 1974; Abramson, 1975; Wellisch, Mosher, & Van Scoy, 1978). A major emphasis of family group counseling is providing families of the disabled and chronically ill with the support and skills needed to meet the unique demands of various disabilities.

Although there are many commonalities among the use of family group counseling with various disability groups, there are also unique features relative to the specific disability. For example, there may be variation in the format, size of group, length of time, and role of the leader as well as the content, intensity of emotion, and the nature of the crises (see Table 1).

CRITICAL ISSUES RELATED TO GROUP
COUNSELING WITH FAMILIES OF THE DISABLED

Often the major goal of family counseling groups is the resolution of critical problems related to illness, disability, and rehabilitation. However, there are many other potential consequences of disability that can intensify the trauma and further deplete personal and family resources, which can surface in the following ways:

Table 1. Perspective on family group counseling with the disabled

Author	Population	Size of Group	Setting	Time	Goals	Leadership
Huberty (1974)	Stroke, oncology, diabetic, tumor, cardiac	Not specified	Hospital	Variable	Adaptation to illness	Co-lead; social worker, occupational therapist, nurses, chaplains
Wilson (1971)	Children, cerebral palsy, blindness, deafness, spina bifida, mental retardation, muscular dystrophy	12	Outpatient	1 hr	Provide information, support	Professional who is parent of disabled child
Linder (1970)	Mothers of disabled children	5	Hospital	Once per week	Support and alternatives	Psychologist
Mattsson and Agle (1972)	Parents of hemophiliacs	10	Hospital	25 weeks; 1½ hr	Cognitive awareness and adaptation	Psychiatrists
Abramson (1975)	Families of burn patients	Varied	Hospital	12 sessions	Orientation, support	Social worker and nurse
D'Afflitti and Weitz (1974)	Stroke patient and families	Four groups of three to five patients plus family	VA Hospital	12 weeks; 1½ hr	Encourage communication	Nurse and social worker
Heisler (1974)	Parents of cerebral palsy children	Not specified	Outpatient	66 sessions; 1 week; 2 hr	Actualization of parents	Psychologists
Wellisch et al. (1978)	Families of cancer patients	Four to 16, average of six	Outpatient, private medical practice	11 months; 1 week; 2 hr	Maximal utilization of life	Psychologist, nurse/oncologist

1. Marital relationships can begin to deteriorate, and parents or spouses may see separation or divorce as the only way to save and remove themselves from a situation they cannot handle.
2. Children may act out at home and in school as a result of loss of attention and lack of understanding regarding their needs, especially when no alternatives are perceived.
3. Excessive alcohol or drug abuse can occur.
4. Work performance of family members can deteriorate, reflecting the strain of the home situation and resulting in financial uncertainty.
5. Individual family members as well as the total family can neglect themselves both physically and emotionally by not tending to individual or mutual needs.
6. Financial pressures can be seen as a cause of disharmony when, in fact, they may be symptomatic of underlying stress that is more difficult to concretize.
7. Traditional support systems, such as friends and relatives, may remove themselves from supporting roles because of their inability to respond to the emotional demands upon them.

The challenge of the family group counseling is not only to prevent these and other realities from occurring but to provide families with the opportunity to more clearly understand their reactions and develop their resources.

One of the most powerful insights that can take place in a family counseling group is the awareness that the individual is not alone in the situation and that there are others who can help families to resolve what has happened as well as help prepare them for what will occur. This is poignantly illustrated in groups focusing on terminal illness. In such groups, members are able to participate in an unfolding process that gradually prepares them to face their own individual loss. In a sense, it is an opportunity to see some people faced with intense loss, tragedy, and suffering who still can cope. On the other hand, there is the opportunity to share what cannot easily be shared with others. As Yalom and Greaves (1977) state:

> First and most important, the group offers an arena in which all concerns can be aired and thoroughly discussed. There are no issues too deep or morbid to be discussed openly in the group. These issues include physical concerns (e.g., loss of hair from chemotherapy, disfigurement from mutilating surgery), fear for the actual act of dying, fear of pain, the possibility of afterlife, the fear of becoming a "vegetable," the desire to have decision-making power concerning the time of death, euthanasia, the "living will," funeral arrangements, etc. These concerns are foremost in the minds of many patients, but they are unable to discuss them with any living person. The group affords considerable relief by simply allowing patients to share these thoughts (p. 398).

This statement reflects the intensity of the emotions surrounding disability as well as the complexity of the issues involved in medical care and rehabilitation. A significant factor in this process is the family group leader's skills, sensitivity, and perspective on the process, procedures, and problems relative to family group counseling.

GROUP LEADERSHIP AND DISABILITY

Leaders of groups that deal with intense physical and emotional realities must be highly skilled; they must have medical knowledge, leadership skills, be personally integrated, and have the ability to cognitively and experientially appreciate the impact of disability.

Medical knowledge is critical in working with the disabled because of the complexity of the procedures involved in the initial steps of hospitalization and throughout the rehabilitation process. In addition, comprehension of how a disability or illness affects the client is critical in being able to respond to both physical and emotional change.

Leadership skills must be based upon a sound theoretical base, combined with extensive supervision and experience in working with generic as well as specific populations. In addition to group work, group leaders must have extensive background experience and supervision in working with families. Wellisch et al. (1978) emphasize a model that includes a specifically trained clinician with involvement of medical specialists and support personnel. This model indicates the power of a co-leadership approach that utilizes the skills of a variety of professionals.

Personal integration refers to the life-style of the group leader. Basically it can be summed up as whether leaders practice what they preach and can demand of themselves what they ask of the client.

The following is a list of some of the characteristics of an effective group leader with the disabled or their families:

1. Humanness—an appreciation of the plight and struggle of clients and their families, which manifests itself in a caring response that can approximate the intensity of the problem.
2. Compassion—the ability to feel in a constructive way.
3. Resiliency—the ability to continue with the tasks of one's role in spite of personal emotional drain, which often accompanies a repetition of "failure" experiences or personal loss.
4. Intervention skills—ability to design and implement programs and responses that are timely and relevant to the changing needs of clients, family, and group.
5. Medical knowledge—the ability to understand aspects of disability, such as the specific manifestations of various disabilities and illnesses and how they affect the patient and the group process.
6. Communication skills—the ability to relate to patient, family, and medical staff.

7. Ability to differentiate between individual and family problems.

8. Awareness of the synergistic effect a combination of problems and crisis situations can have on the group process, the individual, and the family system.

9. Ability to orchestrate group process.

10. Awareness of the independent and conjoint functioning of family subsystems.

11. Ability to implement a variety of intervention techniques, e.g., role-playing, didactic material, structured experiences.

12. Ability to work with a co-leader, which is helpful with large groups and provides a feedback and support system for leaders.

13. Ability to resolve personal prejudices as they relate to roles of group members, e.g., traditional male/female roles, stereotypes regarding the potential of the disabled.

14. Cognitive and experiential awareness of the impact of the disabilities represented in the group. Traditionally, group leaders have had the advantage of only verbally reflecting on understanding of disability; only in selected cases have health professionals experienced in a training format what disability means, what its impact is on others, what it would mean to them and their families, and whether they could handle it. Lasky and Dell Orto (1979) have developed a variety of experiential group procedures that explore the impact of disability on the nondisabled, which are helpful in training professionals who work with the disabled.

15. Comprehensive understanding of a theoretical model that is relevant, applicable, and useful to the disabled and their families.

MULTIDIMENSIONAL GROUP: A THEORETICAL MODEL

A viable family group counseling model in health care settings must go beyond a token response to the needs of the disabled. It must be accepted and supported by administration, the staff, the patients, and their families. This can occur only when the family group counseling program addresses critical issues encountered during rehabilitation.

A model of group counseling for the disabled and their families must be designed to be comprehensive and proactive rather than limited and reactive. A comprehensive proactive group model is one that:

1. Is available throughout the rehabilitation process

2. Has the potential to be adapted to a variety of settings, populations, and issues

3. Is flexible to meet the evolving and changing needs of the disabled and their families

4. Can be fully integrated into a hospital or rehabilitation setting

5. Is capable of transcending the hospital environment and meeting the demands faced in the community
6. Has didactic components to teach the skills needed to respond to a range of medical and nonmedical problems and issues
7. Can respond to the various subsystems that may have an important role in client treatment and rehabilitation
8. Is proactive in anticipating problems rather than only reacting to them

With a multidimensional model, the needs of the families of disabled and ill persons can be more effectively met by providing a system of alternatives as well as a system of supplementary groups. The following is a list of subgroup descriptions:

Core family group   Perceived as a critical factor in rehabilitation, the family group is the central, core group. It is from this group that the other groups evolve.

Client/patient group   A peer group. Some needs of the client are best responded to by peers.

Parent group   Focuses upon needs of parents in their personal adjustment to a disability as well as developing behaviors that will support their relationship.

Sibling group   Enables siblings to express and resolve their feelings, such as anger or disfranchisement.

Male group   Addresses role issues that are relative to male problems and concerns.

Female group   Addresses role issues that are relative to female problems and concerns.

Theme group   Permits the addressing of various issues, such as medical, financial, or vocational issues.

Children's group   Opportunity for disabled children to share feelings and learn how to respond to their unique situations, e.g., the loss of a parent.

Didactic group   Provides information and teaches relevant skills.

Spouse/marital group   Concerned with nurturing and maintaining the marital relationship.

Medical staff group   Opportunity for physicians, nurses, and other rehabilitation workers to discuss issues relative to their individual functioning and provide a professional support system.

Significant others   An opportunity to involve those persons who are a part of the families' or clients' interactional system.

Multiple family group   Several families sharing common processes, which can put problems and resources into perspective.

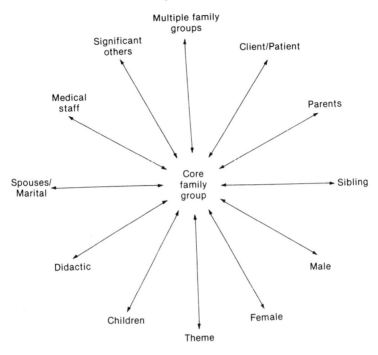

Figure 1.   Theoretical multidimensional group model.

The theoretical model in Figure 1 is presented to create a perspective of the potential of the group process and to show the possible relationship of subgroups to the Core family group.

CONCLUSION

The message of this chapter has been that group counseling is a valuable resource in working with the disabled and, therefore, family group counseling is an alternative that can:

1. Expose families in crisis to role models, that is, other individuals in similar situations who were able to meet the challenges posed by a personal disability or the disability of a family member.

2. Provide a system that will respond to long-term needs over the total process of rehabilitation rather than be limited to the concerns associated with acute care.

3. Create a structure within which family members can respond to their individual as well as collective needs and receive feedback from persons in similar situations.

4. Introduce family members to community resources based upon the knowledge and expertise of group members to avoid the unnecessary strain and stress of individual families having to struggle for information that is already available.
5. Teach families how to cope by developing a proactive rather than a reactive response to problems that are common to individual disabilities.
6. Provide a structure for the introduction of medical knowledge that is relevant to group members, e.g., effects of chemotherapy, procedures emphasized in burn injuries.
7. Establish a consumer point of view in a professional world and facilitate dialogue with medical and human service workers (the development of self-help groups is one manifestation of this).
8. Establish an additional level of accountability for all who are involved in treatment and rehabilitation. A collective of consumers is often more aware of what should be happening compared with an individual family in a state of crisis.
9. Diffuse problems before they become overwhelming to the family or its individual members. This can be accomplished by exposing families to the problems and solutions employed by other group members.
10. Enable families to share a common burden rather than be fragmented by the desperation that is often a by-product of isolation.
11. Personalize the treatment process by processing information in a caring, structured manner rather than in an impersonal, random, unstructured manner, as is often the case in busy hospital environments.
12. Develop the group as an evolving resource that can result in social contacts, which are essential in coping with disability over an extended period of time during and after hospitalization.

The existence of a family group counseling program does not mean that all problems will be eradicated, but it can mean that critical elements in the rehabilitation of a disabled or ill person will have a better chance of being attended to.

Based on the principals of mutual support and understanding of unique needs, the group process for families of the disabled can be a significant factor in the adjustment to disability as well as facilitation of the rehabilitation process. However, there is a need to expand the range of supportive services that are available to the consumers of health care.

The following articles in this chapter have been selected to provide the reader with an overview of group counseling with the disabled and their families as well as to illustrate group counseling with specific populations. Huberty explores family group work with stroke, oncology, diabetic, tumor, and cardiac populations. The value of the family counseling group program is the awareness created for the hospital community regarding the emotional, social, and family components of adjusting to illness and hospitalization. The goals groups are described by Huberty as "assisting the patient with his family in working through the stages heading toward the acceptance of disability of illness and adjusting to it as a family unit." The needs of parents of leukemic children are the focus of a group program discussed in the article by Heffron, Brommelaere, and Masters. The focus of this group counseling program was to provide information regarding leukemia as well as to offer support to family members in their attempt to cope with its many peripheral issues. Abramson describes a group counseling approach employed to attempt to minimize the trauma and reduce the crisis surrounding burn-injured patients and their families. This approach emphasizes the need for group support from acute care through rehabilitation, thus stressing the need for a developmental support system that can respond to changing needs of family and patient.

Group counseling programs are a major resource in personalizing the health care system and providing patients and families with the support, skills, sensitivity, honesty, caring, and consistency that can facilitate rehabilitation.

REFERENCES

Abramson, M. Group treatment of families of burn-injured patients. *Social Casework,* 1975, April, 235–241.

Adsett, C. A., & Bruhn, J. G. Short-term group psychotherapy for post-myocardial infarction patients. *Canadian Medical Association Journal,* 1968, *99, 577*–584.

Avery, C. Para-analytic group therapy with adolescent multi-handicapped blind. *New Outlook for the Blind,* 1968, *68*(3), 65–72.

Banik, S. N., & Mendelson, M. A. Group psychotherapy with a paraplegic group, with an emphasis on specific problems of sexuality. *International Journal of Group Psychotherapy,* 1978, *28*(1), 123–128.

Bilodeau, C. B., & Hackett, T. P. Issues raised in a group setting by patients recovering from myocardial infarction. *American Journal of Psychiatry,* 1971, *128,* 37–38.

Blandford, B. R. Peer group membership of young women with cancer. *Journal of Chronic Disease,* 1968, *21,* 315–322.

Bray, G. P. Reactive patterns in families of the severely disabled. *Rehabilitation Counseling Bulletin,* 1977, March, 236–239.

Bruhn, J. G. The effects of chronic illness on the family. *The Journal of Family Practice,* 1977, *4*(6), 1057–1060.

Buchanan, D. C. Group therapy for kidney transplant patients. *International Journal of Psychiatry in Medicine,* 1975, *6*(4), 523–531.

Burnside, I. M. Loss: A constant theme in group work with the aged. *Hospital Community Psychiatry,* 1970, *21,* 121–173.

Burnside, I. M. Long-term group work with hospitalized aged. *Gerontologist,* 1971, *11,* 213.

Cofer, D. H., & Nir, Y. Theme focused group therapy on a pediatric ward. *International Journal of Psychiatry in Medicine,* 1976, *6*(4), 541–550.

Currier, L. The psychological impact of cancer on the cancer patient and his family. *Rocky Mountain Medical Journal,* 1966, February, 43–48.

D'Afflitti, J. G., & Weitz, G. Rehabilitating the stroke patient through patient family groups. *International Journal Group Psychotherapy,* 1974, *24,* 323–332.

Day, M., Day, E., & Hermann, R. Group therapy of patients with multiple sclerosis. *Archives of Neurology and Psychiatry,* 1953, *69,* 193–196.

De Lamata, R., Gingas, G., and Weitkower, E. D. Impact of sudden, severe disablement of the father upon the family. *Canadian Medical Association Journal,* 1960, *82,* 1015–1020.

Deutsch, C. P., & Goldstein, J. A. Family factors in home adjustment of the severely disabled. *Marriage and Family Living,* 1960, *22,* 312–316.

Foster, R. M., & Thomas, D. F. Anger, disability and demands in the family. *American Journal of Orthopsychiatry,* 1978, *48*(2), 228–236.

Gordon, N. B., & Kutner, B. Long term and fatal illness and the family. *Journal of Health and Human Behavior,* 1965, *6,* 190–196.

Hartings, M. F., Pavlou, M. M., & Davis, F. A. Group counseling of multiple sclerosis patients in a program of comprehensive care. *Journal of Chronic Disease,* 1976, *29,* 65–73.

Heffron, W. A., Brommelaere, K., and Master, R. Group discussions with parents of leukemic children. *Pediatrics,* 1973, *52*(6).

Heisler, V. Dynamic group psychotherapy with parents of cerebral palsied children. *Rehabilitation Literature,* 1974, *35*(11), 329–330.

Henkle, C. Social group work as a treatment modality for hospitalized people with rheumatoid arthritis. *Rehabilitation Literature,* 1975, *36*(11), 334–341.

Herman, S. Some observations on group therapy with the blind. *International Journal of Group Psychotherapy,* 1966, *16*(3), 367–372.

Hollon, T. H. Modified group therapy in the treatment of patients on chronic hemodialysis. *American Journal of Psychotherapy,* 1972, *36*(4), 501–510.

Huberty, D. J. Adapting to illness through family groups. *International Journal of Psychiatry in Medicine,* 1974, *5*(3), 231–242.

Isaacs, B. Group therapy in the geriatric unit. *Gerontologist,* 1967, December, 9.

Keegan, D. L. Adaptation to visual handicap: Short-term group approach. *Psychomatics,* 1974, *15*(2), 76–78.

Krupp, N. E. Adaptation to chronic illness. *Post Graduate Medicine,* 1976, *60*(5), 122–125.

Kubler-Ross, E., & Anderson, J. R. Psychotherapy with the least expected: Modified group therapy with blind clients. *Rehabilitation Literature,* 1968, *29*(3), 73–76.

Lasky, R. G., & Dell Orto, N. E. *Group counseling and physical disability.* North Scituate, Mass.: Duxbury Press, 1979.

Linder, R. Mothers of disabled children—The value of weekly group meetings. *Developmental Medicine and Child Neurology,* 1970, *12,* 202–206.

Lipp, M. R., & Malone, S. T. Group rehabilitation of vascular surgery patients. *Archives of Physical Medicine and Rehabilitation,* 1976, *57,* 180–183.

Ludwig, E. G., & Colette, J. Disability, dependency and conjugal roles. *Journal of Marriage and the Family,* 1969, *31,* 736–739.

Luzzatti, L., & Dittmann, B. Group discussions with parents of ill children. *Pediatrics,* 1954, *13,* 269–273.

McClellan, M. S. Crisis groups in special care areas. *Nursing Clinics of North America,* 1972, *7*(2), 363–371.

MacVicar, M. G., & Archbold, P. A framework for family assessment in chronic illness. *Nursing Forum,* 1976, *15*(2), 180–194.

Mally, M., & Strehl, C. B. Evaluation of a three years group therapy program for multiple sclerosis patients. *International Journal of Group Psychotherapy,* 1963, *13,* 328–334.

Manaster, A. The theragnostic group in a rehabilitation center for visually handicapped persons. *New Outlook for the Blind,* 1971, *65*(8), 261–264.

Mattsson, A., & Agle, D. O. Group therapy with parents of hemophiliacs. *Journal of Child Psychiatry,* 1972, *11*(3), 558–571.

Milman, D. H. Group therapy with parents: An approach to the rehabilitation of physically disabled children. *Journal of Pediatrics,* 1952, *41,* 113–116.

Mone, L. C. Short-term group psychotherapy with postcardiac patients. *International Journal of Group Psychotherapy,* 1970, *20*(1), 98–108.

Naji, S. Z., & Clark, D. L. Factors in mental adjustment after disability. *Journal of Marriage and the Family,* 1964, *26,* 215–216.

Nir, Y. Theme-focused group therapy on a pediatric ward. *International Journal of Psychiatry in Medicine,* 1976, *6*(4), 541–550.

Olsen, E. H. The impact of serious illness on the family system. *Post Graduate Medicine,* 1970, February, 169–174.

Oradei, D., & Waite, N. Group psychotherapy with stroke patients during the immediate recovery phase. *American Journal of Orthopsychiatry,* 1974, *44*(3), 386–395.

Owen, S. Is group counseling neglected. *Journal of Rehabilitation,* 1972, *38*(6), 12–15.

Parks, R. M. Parents reaction to the birth of a handicapped child. *Health and Social Work,* 1977, *2*(3), 52–65.

Peterson, Y. The impact of physical disability on marital adjustment: A literature review. *The Family Coordinator,* 1979, January, 47–51.

Piskor, B. K., & Paleos, S. The group way to banish after-stroke blues. *American Journal of Nursing,* 1968, *68,* 1500–1503.

Pless, D. B., Roghmann, K. J., & Aaggery, R. J. Chronic illness, family functioning and psychological adjustment: A model for the allocation of preventive mental health services. *International Journal of Epidemiology,* 1972, *1,* 271–277.

Power, P. W. *Family behaviors in chronic illness: A perspective for rehabilitation.* Unpublished doctoral dissertation, Boston University, 1974.

Power, P. W., & Rogers, S. Group counseling for multiple sclerosis patients: A preferred mode of treatment for unique adaptive problems. In R. G. Lasky and A. E. Dell Orto (Eds.), *Group counseling and physical disability,* pp. 115–127. North Scituate, Mass.: Duxbury Press, 1979.

Rahe, R. H., Tuffli, C. F., Jr., Suchor, R. J., Jr., & Arthur, R. J. Group therapy in the outpatient management of post-myocardial infarction patients. *International Journal of Psychiatry in medicine,* 1973, *4*(1), 77–78.

Roessler, N. T. An evaluation of personal achievement skills training with the visually handicapped. *Rehabilitation Counseling Bulletin,* 1978, *21*(4), 300–305.

Roessler, R., Milligan, T., & Ohlson, A. Personal adjustment training for the spinal cord injured. *Rehabilitation Counseling Bulletin,* 1976, *19*(4), 544–550.

Schwartz, M. Group psychotherapy with multiple sclerosis patients and their spouses. *Proceedings American Psychological Association,* New Orleans, 1974.

Schwartz, M. L., & Cahill, R. Psychopathology associated with myasthenia gravis and its treatment by psychotherapeutically oriented group counseling. *Journal of Chronic Disease,* 1971, *24,* 543–552.

Shambaugh, P. W., & Kanter, S. S. Spouses under stress: Group meetings with spouses of patients on hemodialysis. *American Journal of Psychiatry*, 1969, *125*, 928–936.

Shellhase, L. J., & Shellhase, F. E. Role of the family in rehabilitation. *Social Casework*, 1972, *539*, 544–550.

Sorenson, E. R. Group therapy in a community hospital dialysis unit. *Journal of the American Medical Association*, 1972, *221*, 899–901.

Sussman, A. E. Group therapy with severely handicapped. *Journal of Rehabilitation of the Deaf*, 1974, *8*, 122–126.

Vincent, C. E. The family in health and illness. Some neglected areas. *Annals of the American Academy of Political and Social Science*, 1963, *346*, 109–116.

Waite, N. S. Group psychotherapy with stroke patients during the immediate recovery phase. *American Journal of Orthopsychiatry*, 1974, *44*(3), 386–395.

Wellisch, D. K., Mosher, M. B., & Van Scoy, C. Management of family emotion stress: Family group therapy in a private oncology practice. *International Journal of Group Psychotherapy*, 1978, *28*(2), 225–231.

Wijsenbeek, H., & Munitz, H. Group treatment in a hemodialysis center. *Psychiatric, Neurologia, Neurochirurgia*, 1970, *73*, 213–220.

Wilson, A. L. Group therapy for parents of handicapped children. *Rehabilitation Literature*, 1971, *32*, 332–335.

Yalom, I. D., & Greaves, C. Group therapy with the terminally ill. *American Journal of Psychiatry*, 1977, *134*, 396–400.

ADAPTING TO ILLNESS THROUGH FAMILY GROUPS

David J. Huberty[1]

Group work for behavioral problems, psychiatric disorders or family pathology is readily accepted in most social agencies or settings where a social model of treatment is the primary modality. In hospital work, however, social work is properly described as an ancillary or supportive profession which provides supportive services to the primary professions of medicine and nursing. In this secondary setting, the role of the social worker is frequently limited to those functions assigned by the medical staff or by the hospital administration. While group treatment or group therapy is an accepted function on hospital psychiatric units, the suggestion that group counseling be done on general medical floors is often met with suspicion by the nursing staff and with reluctance, apprehension, and at times refusal of permission to see the patient from the strictly medically-oriented physicians.

Prior to 1971, medical social work at St. Mary's Hospital and St. Mary's Extended Care Center was recognized as a supportive service, the primary function of which was to assist in the more traditional medical casework problems of patients, such as making referrals to nursing homes, arranging financial assistance through local welfare departments, and facilitating other referrals, such as finding a babysitter for a patient's children, arranging remedial reading for a patient's husband or helping patients with job problems.

The counseling potential of social casework was, in fact, accomplished indirectly through counseling that necessarily related to the specifics of the referral. However, referrals by physicians rarely, if ever, were made specifically to provide psychological support or assist a family in working through the difficult emotional changes that always accompany disability and lengthy hospitalization.

During the last three years at St. Mary's, major efforts have been made to develop and implement social group work within a variety of medical diagnostic categories. This paper describes the evolution and development of five such groups: Stroke, Oncology, Diabetes, Out-Patient Tumor Clinic and Cardiac Surgery.

Reprinted from *International Journal of Psychiatry in Medicine* 5(3), pp. 231–242, © 1974, Baywood Publishing Co., Inc., with permission.

[1]Formerly Director of Social Services, St. Mary's Hospital, Minneapolis, MN; currently Coordinator of Detoxification and Halfway House Services, The Central Minnesota Mental Health Center, 1321 North 13th St., St. Cloud, MN 56301.

PURVIEW OF SOCIAL WORK

First, it was quite natural for group work to develop out of the Social Service Department as there are three areas of expertise relevant to group work to which social workers may lay claim. While these areas of expertise are in no way limited to social work, they are distinct areas of professional training in a master's degree curriculum in accredited schools of social work.

1. *Group work*   Social group work is one of five specialized methods in the field of social work. Schools of social work provide both academic and experiential training in group dynamics and group therapy under the supervision of experienced group workers and group therapists. Therefore, the social worker does bring specialized training and developed skills to the group method of counseling.

2. *Family dynamics*   The process of adapting to illness is not one that takes place within each patient in isolation but rather is an interactional process of adjustment between the patient and his spouse, his children, his parents, as well as among those significant others as they form a network of emotional and social supports. It is the family system that encounters major adjustments as a result of one member's hospitalization. Changes in employment and income, decision-making roles, and responsibility are just a few of the non-medical components that affect and complicate the patient's adaptation to his medical diagnosis and very possibly impinge upon his rehabilitation. As a result of specific training in family dynamics and family therapy along with a theoretical framework of a "systems" approach to counseling, social workers tend to view the family as a necessary component in any individual's healthy response to change.

3. *Emotional and social components of illness*   As a profession with its training orientation balanced between sociology and psychology, social workers are oriented by training and experience to the emotional and social components of the vicissitudes of life, including illness, disability and dying.

With these three areas of focus within the purview of social work, the Social Service Department at St. Mary's Medical Complex was available to be of broader service to the patient by working with him and his family in group counseling sessions. Also, social workers had demonstrated their group work skills on the psychiatric unit and on an adolescent drug unit. Therefore, development of the medical groups was essentially an extension and combination of two approved areas of social work practice within the hospital—psychiatric *group work* (and family counseling) and *medical* casework. While the five medical groups discussed in this paper did not begin meeting at the same time, they do have a number of elements in common, discussed here in a generic way, followed by a more specific description of each medical group with examples illustrating the development of the program and the success of a particular group session in a patient's life or that of his family.

ADAPTING TO ILLNESS

There are similarities among the broad diagnoses of cancer, stroke, heart attack and diabetes and the group formations in these areas. First, in adapting to a major change in one's life, it is universally true that the person goes through a *process* moving towards acceptance or an adjustment to his new status in life. Accompanying long-term hospitalization, physical limitations from a chronic illness or disability may be perceived as a loss of freedom and the beginning of unwanted dependency. Whether a patient uses his illness and feelings for self-pity or for motivation for recovery will largely depend on how successfully he works through various emotional stages leading to assigning some significance of his illness to his life's goals.

Kübler-Ross (1969) identifies five stages of grief in the dying process. Similar stages, which may manifest considerable overlap, may also be applied to a patient and his family who are adapting to a major medical change in their lives. There is initially some *denial* of the limitations of the disability followed by *anger* over "why me?" This is frequently followed by *bargaining* with medical personnel, family members or just within one's own mind: "If I am a good patient, I will get well quicker," or "If my surgery is successful, I'll start going to church again regularly." This phase is likely to be followed by *depression* as one realizes that the disability is permanent or that the limitations imposed by the disability are, in fact, real. The final stage in the adjustment process is an *acceptance* of the *realistic* limitations of the disability with perhaps an alteration of life goals or an incorporation of the illness into the meaning of life resulting in a calm optimism. Thus, the *process* of adapting to the illness and disability is a working premise in medical group work with the patient.

A second *common* characteristic, if not completely universal, is that families will also go through a similar kind of process. Although this is perhaps more dramatic and therefore more apparent with the family of the dying patient, it is nevertheless just as real in any serious illness. For both the patient and his family there is a great degree of psychological uncertainty. This, of necessity, results in anxiety, frustration, anger and depression. In terms of family dynamics, it is of note that in one study where the patients were recovering from myocardial infarction, 100 per cent of the families interviewed evidenced "steady eroding conflict" and disruptive family relationships (Cassem & Hackett, 1973). It is not unreasonable to anticipate that similar family disruption may occur in an equally high percentage of families where the patient has some other serious disability. Even the most stable marriage and family relationships are challenged if not marred by the disability. Of course, couples and families frequently will respond to the crisis of hospitalization and disability with increased sensitivity and understanding. In these cases the result is closer interpersonal ties and a deeper emotional strength. Every major crisis provides the dual opportunity for destruction or growth. It is not crisis that destroys families, marriages or individuals, but how they choose to negotiate that crisis and deal with it.

Throughout these universal processes of adaptation to illness, it is appropriate that even very normal and emotionally healthy families experiencing such crises be assisted in this adjustment and grieving by the use of group work. Over and over again families remark on how helpful it is to talk with others experiencing similar circumstances. Sharing and comparing unfamiliar challenges and pain draw a strength previously untapped, partly achieved through giving emotional support to other patients or families who are hurting more. Families are specifically invited and encouraged to attend each of the group sessions. Although attendance by family members varied, family involvement did increase as the groups became more universally understood and accepted by the medical and nursing staff as well as the families themselves.

The group setting is unique in providing the opportunity for development of a mutual support system. Also, more advanced or experienced group members may provide assurances from their broader perspective on the disability and the adjustment process to the newer members. No other counseling context provides for this mutual support.

DEVELOPMENT OF MEDICAL COUNSELING GROUPS

All medical group work at St. Mary's follows the multidisciplinary team approach, each group co-led in some combination by a social group worker, a nurse, an occupational therapist and chaplain. Each group evolved out of a different area within the hospital and required different administrative procedures for implementation. Each of the groups was initiated after a hospital staff member identified a need for some level of counseling for a patient and/or his family in order to help them adjust to the particular disease.

Goals of the Group

Each group has the general goal of assisting the patient, preferably with his family, in working through the stages leading toward acceptance of disability or illness and adjusting to it as a family unit. Working with patients and their families requires sensitivity to a wide range of emotions which may interfere with a healthy adjustment and to the various ways a health crisis will be interpreted by family members. A family's interpretation of a crisis will have a great effect on how the patient responds to treatment and rehabilitation. If interpreted as a threat, the crisis will produce anxiety; if interpreted as a loss, it will produce depression; if interpreted as a challenge, both anxiety and hope will create problem-solving energy and promote motivation and individual growth as well as emotional growth within the family unit (Rapoport, 1965). Certainly if different family members interpret the crisis in different ways, the initial goal is to help the members identify and clarify to each other the various subjective meanings of the crisis. Thus, while we may describe some specific goals for each group, the goals for an individual patient and his family within a group session may become very individualized to fit their needs at that moment.

CASE EXAMPLES

While the specific cases below are not uncommon, they have, nonetheless, been chosen to illustrate some of the more dramatic positive results of the group work process. The support of other persons in the same situation is a powerful tool in helping families cope with a difficult change in their lives. There are also case examples of people who have stayed away from the groups because they were not yet ready to face the crisis or who preferred to adapt through their own family supports or directly with the help of their physician. The groups were consciously designed to permit people the option of not attending or of freely leaving a group session if they felt uncomfortable for any reason.

Stroke Group

This first medical counseling group evolved out of the need for families to obtain more information about strokes in general and the rehabilitative progress of their family member in particular. After an afternoon lecture approach failed to meet these needs, a family group discussion format was initiated during evening hours. Since the stroke rehabilitation program ranges between two weeks and three months, patients and families could be expected to attend between two and twelve group sessions. In addition to helping them adapt to communication problems and the physical limitations imposed by a recent stroke, the "Family Involvement Evening," as the group was called, enabled the staff to get a better picture of the patient's family and therefore begin discharge planning earlier and more completely. The groups enabled the social worker to work with the family earlier in the rehabilitation process in an effort to help them and the patient work through the guilt, anger, and stigma (Hyman, 1972), always present to some degree. Since these three feelings tend to get in the way of *expecting* and *allowing* maximum independence from the patient, it is extremely important that they be openly discussed and confronted.

Case Example   The patient was a women in her late 60's. She and her husband had been very close most of their forty years of marriage. Their daughter lived out of town and was therefore unable to attend the group; one son, age 35, the patient's favorite, sided with his mother on most issues; another son, age 29, appeared to be favored by his father and, although quiet, supported his father's point of view.

The patient's husband was completely overwhelmed by her stroke and debilitated condition. Because of his deep feelings of love and concern, he immediately made it clear to the doctors and the staff that he would spend whatever was necessary to give her the best of care: "She deserves the excellent care that she is getting here. She can stay here for the rest of her life!" The thought of ever taking his wife home with the responsibility for her care was more than he could face.

The staff soon realized that despite the patient's good potential to return home, the husband's attitude was a major rehabilitation barrier. His level of coping with the crisis was to "pay for the best of care." Counseling also needed to be done with the older son who, through his denial of the real limitations imposed by his mother's stroke, maintained that she could be *completely* independent again. The younger son's blind acceptance of his father's view of the stroke and plan for institutional care needed to be tempered too.

Each new step in rehabilitation was interpreted by the patient's husband as a set-back. When the patient was scheduled to receive a leg brace, he interpreted this as a crisis and "proof" for his belief that she would never recover. In the group setting, however, another patient who had recently received a brace announced, "This is what your wife's brace is going to do," and he stood up and began walking around the group. This well-timed demonstration helped the husband realize that a brace was progress. Within a few weeks, however, the husband had moved to the other extreme: "I look forward to the day when I can dance with Joan again." At that point a non-patient in the group strongly confronted: "You're putting your goals on her and she probably won't be able to reach them and do you know what that's going to do to her?" The husband's gradual realization that he was projecting his own unrealistic hopes was followed by depression. Because he had not really faced her disability realistically, he was still hesitant to take his wife home and only did so reluctantly on a "trial weekend." That weekend his wife proved that, although limited, she could generally function well at home *with his help*. He *experienced* that she *needed* him and that he could, in fact, assist her and provide good care. Her affect improved markedly over that weekend and only then did he begin to understand how important it was for her to return home.

Over a period of twelve weeks and twelve group sessions the patient's husband moved from a denial of rehabilitation and his role in that process, through anger and depression, and finally on to an acceptance of the realities of the stroke, including both its *limitations* and *potential*. Without this rather lengthy process in group, the patient would most likely have been institutionalized because her husband simply wanted "the best possible care," which he was convinced was expensive, long-term institutional care.

Oncology Family Group

Patients who are either weakened by the disease itself or by treatments for their cancer are hospitalized in the Extended Care Center's specialized Oncology Unit for two weeks to several months. These are patients with disseminated cancer in advanced stages. Therefore, the goals of this specialized unit are totally directed towards helping the patient increase his physical strength and achieve optimum health and independence within the confines of his disease.

The Oncology Family Group was more specifically directed towards helping the family and patient to assess on a physical, social and psychological level what would be the best placement upon discharge; frequently this was back home, but at times nursing homes or other placements are more appropriate for all concerned. While the group's primary function is to help the patient, one of the most effective and efficient ways of helping and supporting a patient is to deal with the whole system of people involved with that patient (Brennan, 1970). This means a process of adjustment working its way down from the spouse, children, perhaps extended family members and also staff members who may get very involved and feel very close to the patient (Carey, 1974). These are all people who *directly* affect the patient. The following case illustrates the impact of dying on other members in the family network.

Case Example   The patient, a woman age 56, with stomach cancer and metastasis to her lungs and breasts, had been in the Extended Care Center nine weeks. She was failing rapidly at the time of the group session recounted here and was too ill to attend. It was the sixth group for her husband, her two sons and the wife of the younger son.

The younger son told the group how he had always felt left out of the family process. He frequently did things contrary to his parents' preference, including marrying against their wishes. He felt guilty about having to stand by what he felt was right and yet watch his parents grieve and hurt. Now with his mother dying he felt he wanted to be forgiven for some of his decisions. He wanted to have the opportunity to express to his mother how he really had made some mistakes and how she was right in many ways. The group accepted what he said and suggested his going to her and telling her how he felt. One nurse added her support by telling this son how his mother had expressed her desire to forgive her children of some things; the mother had said she felt bad that they had been reaching out to her for so many years and yet never really touched despite their being a close family; that because of the dying process, things had fallen into a different perspective for her and what really mattered was that they were together.

For the family this process provided a new perspective and new ways of relating: The husband of the patient really heard what his son had said and responded with the brief comment that "I've always had a hard time expressing my emotions in a physical or verbal way too." At this point, his daughter-in-law looked towards him and told him she never realized he could not express his feelings: "I've always been afraid of you, but now I feel like hugging you." Her father-in-law said nothing, but other group members encouraged her to do just that.

A death in a family is still a death and a loss but also a "rebirth" for many family members, depending on how they choose to negotiate the crisis. This family's searching into themselves allowed the patient to die a relatively peaceful and happy death and enabled the living members to become closer. As one nurse observed after the group: "He lost a wife but gained a daughter-in-law and a new kind of son he never knew existed before." This patient died four hours after the group session ended.

Diabetic Group

The Diabetic Group developed from a need identified by a nurse parent-teaching coordinator who felt that the five classes which offered factual information to in-hospital diabetic patients simply did not deal with some of the emotional components of diabetes. She noted that inaccurate information about diabetes within the family network was not getting clarified because of the families' apparent emotional blocking of clarifications. On her request a social worker sat in on one of the classes each week and attempted to take the last twenty minutes of the class to discuss how patients felt about being diabetic. After a number of relatively unsuccessful weeks using this structure, a sixth hour within the diabetic class schedule was added and geared towards the feeling level of the patients.

The goals in this group were three-fold: 1) to give the patient an opportunity to share his feelings regarding his diabetes, 2) to clarify misinformation, and 3) to evaluate the patient's level of adjustment to his diabetes. This evaluation was then communicated to the attending physician by charting in the Physician's Progress Notes any concern about the progress of the patient's adjustment.

Case Example   Mr. Stevens, a 37-year-old laborer, had, a year prior to the hospitalization, been doing a great deal of heavy lifting at his job. At that time he was promoted to foreman, which meant his work time was spent supervising rather than lifting. Despite clearly explained etiology of diabetes, Mr. Stevens in the group setting continued to blame his job promotion for his "catching diabetes." "If I had kept working hard I wouldn't have this [weakling's] disease." He further described that the disease meant a real *loss of freedom:* "Instead of being able to eat a twelve ounce steak I am now limited to a three ounce steak." Severe depression was the most accurate way to describe Mr. Stevens' reaction to his diabetes. The threat to his masculinity was hinted at in his reference to his job. With his high level of anxiety and the way in which he was interpreting his diabetes, it would not be unlikely for this patient to return home and experience temporary sexual impotence along with other manifestations of depreciated self-esteem.

Since the physician's major concern in the effective management of diabetes is the *reaction* of the individual (Kimball, 1971), this information was relayed to the attending physician for follow-up with the patient after discharge from the hospital. It should be added that Mr. Stevens' obvious depression was not only ignored but chastised by some well-meaning nursing personnel. Since they understood the disease process of diabetes, they were quick to try to cheer up that patient by telling him just how lucky he was not to have a more serious disease and that he "should not feel depressed." Not accepting his depression meant that he was not accepted as a person, which further confirmed his interpretation that "it is not okay to be a diabetic."

Tumor Clinic Group

In June 1973, a new chaplain joined St. Mary's staff. He questioned many hospital personnel on what they thought he might bring to hospital programming. A nurse in the emergency room mentioned that a group of outpatient cancer patients came to the hospital every Tuesday for blood analysis, medication and an examination by their physician. Since they usually had a long wait in the clinic, she thought that perhaps he could "visit" with them and therefore help their time go faster. The result was informal group discussions initiated by the chaplain and a social worker for a period of about two months during which time the group became more formalized and structured. Since the discussions repeatedly returned to the side effects of radiation and chemotherapy and the terminal possibilities of cancer, this group provided an opportunity for an exchange of experiences, thoughts and feelings that are often avoided by relatives and friends of cancer patients. Weekly memorandums provided feedback to the attending physicians of a patient's social and psychological developments.

Since the patients in the tumor clinic have cancer in an advanced stage, many of them will be returning to the hospital as inpatients sometime in the foreseeable future (six months to three years). Usually family contact with hospital personnel ceases during periods of outpatient cancer treatment. At the very time they need support the most they frequently have no one to talk with (Hertzberg, 1972). One result of the weekly group sessions has been the development of a close relationship with the chaplain who has assisted some of the patients and their families through the dying process many months later.

Case Example   One member of the group was a 17-year-old girl with a primary tumor (fibrosarcoma) on her wrist with metastasis to the brain. She and her family and hospital personnel knew that her life expectancy was short. Also in the group that day was a 65-year-old man whose wife was being discharged from inpatient care to a "cancer home" where she would, with all certainty, soon die. He had just received that news and came to the group somewhat lost, emotionally numb, fearful of the future, and near to tears.

The young girl was able to leave that group with some hope for herself and a thanksgiving over still having a number of weeks, or months, or perhaps a few years, ahead of her in contrast to the man's wife who had a limited number of days or, at most, weeks to live. Although saddened, the older man was also able to leave the group having shared his grief with some people who could relate closely with his loss. He left feeling somewhat better that he had had many good years with his wife. There was no way of making the situation better for either of them and there was no attempt on the part of the group to do that. But it was clear that he was supported by the group and the group members were able to give of themselves and to share in his pain. He was not alone!

Cardiac Family Group

The Cardiac Group was the only one that grew directly out of the social workers' assumption that cardiac patients and their families likely experience emotional reactions similar to that of other chronic disease patients. Based on that assumption a review of the literature was made and a proposal written to the hospital Coronary Patient Education Committee. After several rewritings and assurances to the physicians and nursing staff, the group began under co-leadership of a head nurse, chaplain, occupational therapist and social group worker.

A specific goal was to provide families an opportunity to discuss with staff their concerns regarding the unexpected current hospitalization of their cardiac patient and what might be expected when he returned home. Prior to the group effort, families were seeking out busy nurses on a one-to-one basis. The group setting allowed time for such questions as well as an opportunity to discuss possible changes in family life that might result from the illness.

Case Example   At the time of this writing, the Cardiac Group has been in existence only four weeks. While no specific case is cited here, we have noticed with this group an extension of the mutual support system that builds in all of the groups. Families have quickly gotten to know each other on a personal level surrounding the crisis of cardiac surgery.

Having met and shared their fears, guilt and uncertainty, they continue supporting one another outside of the group sessions throughout the hospital stay. Group members help alleviate the loneliness experienced during hospitalization. They spend time together in waiting rooms, at meal time and during evening hours, visiting one another's hospitalized family member and often continuing this concern and support after discharge.

CONCLUSION

In developing a number of medical groups, the Social Service Department has attained greater visibility and consequently increased casework referrals. More importantly, the existence of the medical family counseling groups has called widespread attention within the hospital to the emotional, social and family components of adjusting to illness and hospitalization. As a result, the groups have served as a tool for inservice education for nursing staff, physicians, and other ancillary hospital personnel. Social group work skills have been learned well by non-social workers and leadership for some of the groups has been assumed by non social work personnel. Nurses, occupational therapists and chaplains co-lead in all the groups with the assistance of the social worker. This interdisciplinary approach has facilitated staff relationships.

It should be emphasized that all of the groups have worked mainly with emotionally healthy patients and families experiencing acute stress related to hospitalization. As a result, family pathology and underlying family problems have not been the focus of the groups; the groups have, however, consistently helped reduce the anxiety of patients and their families about the particular disease and prepared them for more full and independent lives while living with the disease or disability.

REFERENCES

Brennan, M. J. The cancer gestalt. *Geriatrics,* 1970, *25,* 96–101.
Carey, R. G. Living until death. *Hospital Programs,* 1974, *55,* 82–87.
Cassem, N. H., & Hackett, T. P. Psychological rehabilitation of myocardial infarction patients in the acute phase. *Heart and Lung,* 1973, *2,* 382–388.
Hertzberg, L. J. Cancer and the dying patient. *American Journal of Psychiatry,* 1972, *128,* 40–44.
Hyman, M. Social psychological determinants of patients' performance in stroke rehabilitation. *Archives of Physical Medicine,* 1972, *53,* 217–225.
Kimball, C. P. Emotional and psychosocial aspects of diabetes mellitus. *Medical Clinics of North America,* 1971, *55,* 1007–1018.
Rapoport, L. The state of crisis: Some theoretical considerations. In H. Parad (Ed.), *Crisis intervention: Selected readings,* pp. 129–139. New York: Family Services Association of America, 1965.

GROUP DISCUSSIONS WITH THE PARENTS OF LEUKEMIC CHILDREN

Warren A. Heffron, Karen Bommelaere, and Ruth Masters[1]

Group therapy as part of medical treatment may well have been started by Anton Mesmer in the early 1700s with mass hypnosis. In the early years of this century, some therapeutic groups were formed to help with the management of tuberculosis, stammers, neurotic conditions, alcoholism, and sexual disturbances. In midcentury, the greatest group therapy impetus was furnished by psychiatry, as large numbers of groups were formed to aid in the management of a variety of psychiatric problems (Graham, no date).

More recently, expansion into other areas of medicine has occurred, including rheumatology, hemodialysis units, pulmonary disease, diabetes, myocardial infarction, blindness, deafness, and obesity control. Groups are also being used in programs for underachieving or disabled children, drug abusers, unwed mothers, gamblers, and smokers, as well as in prison and other rehabilitation programs. In these areas, group therapy sessions have been shown to make a significant contribution to medical management (Annual review of the group psychotherapy literature, 1969, 1970, 1971; Linder, 1970; Siegel, 1970; Sorenson, 1972).

While group interaction has proven to be a meaningful and effective means of sharing and communication in many diverse areas, our search of the literature revealed few reports of groups being used in a comprehensive approach as an ancillary modality in the treatment of childhood acute leukemia.

Ablin et al. (Binger, Ablin, Feuerstein, Kushner, Zoger, & Mikkelsen, 1969; Ablin, Binger, Stein, Kushner, Zoger, & Mikkelsen, 1971) have reported a step in this direction by utilizing a family conference as part of the total management of the family involved with leukemia. They used a single conference session as a means of identifying and solving emotional as well as physical problems. They felt that the initial discussion set the stage for a trusting relationship between physician and family.

Vernick and Karon (1965) and Friedman, Chodoff, Mason, and Hamburg (1963) utilized the group concept to include families of hospitalized

Reproduced from *Pediatrics 52*(6), © 1973, with permission.

This paper was partially supported by National Cancer Institute Grant HEWCA 12213-02.

[1] All from the Departments of Family and Community Medicine and Internal Medicine, Albuquerque, NM.

leukemic patients. They reported "highly gratifying results" (Vernick & Karon, 1965).

Bozeman, Orbach, and Sutherland (1955) discovered that parents of hospitalized leukemic children sought one another in lounge areas. In so doing, they formed spontaneous groups since they regarded other parents "as the most important source of emotional support."

METHOD

Our group sessions provide a conference setting on a continuing basis for parents of inpatient and outpatient children. The setting is a part of the clinic of the University of New Mexico School of Medicine where children with acute leukemia are treated in a comprehensive manner.

Most of the chemotherapy is done on a research protocol basis as a part of the Southwest Cancer Chemotherapy Group. Treatment involves chemotherapy and radiation, as well as management of the intercurrent acute problems encountered by these children.

The group meets weekly for an hour and a half prior to the pediatric hematology clinic. The staff have included a medical social worker, a physician, and a registered nurse on a continuing basis. Initially, a psychiatrist was present for the sessions. There have been physicians, nurses, and medical students participating for shorter periods of time.

All parents who have children being treated for acute leukemia are invited to attend the sessions. A total of 18 parents attended at least some of the sessions during the initial year when we followed 24 children with acute leukemia. Occasionally a father attended, but participation was almost exclusively by mothers.

The format of the meetings was informal with no definite ground rules. Each meeting was allowed to go wherever the needs of the group dictated. The time was spent in dealing with questions of a purely medical nature, lighthearted discussions seeking advice, or sharing deep and personal feelings.

Attendance was variable. In general, it tended to be up when one or more children were in relapse and down when all children were in remission. Attendance ranged from one to seven parents, but most meetings involved four or five.

This report defines some of our findings after the first year of group meetings during the calendar year 1972.

DISCUSSION

Much of the discussion was oriented toward identification and solution or problems related to medical and emotional aspects of leukemia.

Problems of the Patient

If the child was old enough to have heard of, or have some understanding (or misunderstanding) of leukemia, it was important how he was told that he had it. Most of the children were too young for the name to have any significance. The older children seemed to better handle their reaction to diagnosis if they were told by their parents or a physician whom they knew. A kind and supportive attitude by the physician may have been as important as anything he said.

Leukemic children at a very early age realized the possibility of death even when not told directly. Recognition of this eventuality was contributed to by numerous clinic visits, painful procedures, and parental anxiety, as well as exposure to accidental comments by siblings, playmates, and even unthinking adults. Parents expressed considerable difficulty in discussing death with their leukemic or normal children. However, children kept bringing the matter up, albeit obliquely at times. When parents were aware that the child needed to talk about death and then discussed it meaningfully, all felt better.

Initially, parents had difficulty answering such questions as: "Will my sister get my radio when I die?" Frequently they avoided responding. In one instance, the child developed severe behavior problems and was unmanageable on the ward during a hospitalization for relapse and reinduction. About this time the parents became able to discuss fears of death with the child. The parents and child felt relief, and in the ensuing months the child verbalized many questions and thoughts on death. The whole family was comforted when the parents expressed to her that they certainly didn't want her to die, but that whatever happened, they would be there, stand by her, and do all that was possible. She no longer had a behavior problem, and her eventual death was peaceful.

Other children presented different openings to the parents for discussions of death. Some children would ask point-blank questions about death, embalming, and graveyards. One child developed quite an interest in cemeteries. Another child, who had seen a movie in which the hero died, presented a comfortable opening by commenting: "That's the way I would like to do it." Children seemed better able to face death as an eventuality if their parents were aware of the significance of these comments and did not block a natural discussion. One child even wanted to discuss such things as: "What happens to your body after you die?" She became interested in caskets and gained some reassurance from these discussions.

Some of the children expressed overt suicidal thoughts, although none of them made any attempts. This usually surprised, and was distressing to, the parents. However, if the parents accepted such an expression as honest and provided loving support of the child, suicidal thoughts were kept from becoming increasingly important. One mother even told her son, "In your position I would feel exactly the same way; however, we will all face this illness together." This helped him sufficiently so that suicide did not become a problem. Suicidal thoughts generally were not anticipated by the parents, and discussion of this topic in the group helped to prepare them to give their child the needed support.

Frequently, the children were admitted to the hospital for infections, drug therapy, diagnostic procedures, platelet or blood transfusions, granulocytopenia, bleeding, or evaluation of other problems. These admissions were often quickly arranged after an abnormal blood test was reported or a fever was discovered. Usually these hospitalizations were for conditions which were not immediately life threatening. However, the children reported later that they were fearful of dying, but did not admit this to staff or parents. The medical staff realized the improbability of death and therefore failed to reassure the children that there was no danger at this time.

Manipulativeness on the part of the sick child was present in every case. Most children learned that at times their disease could be used to get extra favors or advantages. Considerable variation in the ability of parents to discipline their children was noted. Some parents would think, "She is going to die one of these days," and would be incapable of administering discipline. In general, however, those parents who disciplined as they had before had fewer behavioral problems with their children. One mother commented that she felt guilty whenever she disciplined the child because she feared the eventual loss or that punishment would precipitate an untoward effect on the youngster. The child's behavior became more uncontrollable, and this mother found herself punishing the child even more than the other children. She then felt guilty about overpunishing.

Loss of hair due to radiation and chemotherapy was a much more traumatic aspect of treatment to both child and parent than was initially realized by the staff. During periods of baldness, the child wanted to stay home and socialize less, even with close friends. It was particularly distressing when playmates at school would pull off a wig to tease the patient. Embarrassment was much less if the child made no attempt to hide that he was wearing a wig. One girl periodically went to school without it. Another boy would take off his wig and start a game of "catch" with it when he saw a teasing session developing. Such openness negated the fun other children derived from ridicule and made the burden of baldness much easier to bear. No matter how well it was handled, alopecia at some time in the course of illness was an emotional problem for children and parents. Some parents could cope with bone marrow aspirations, repeated IVs, and radiotherapy but were greatly distressed to see their child's hair fall out by the handful.

Children responded differently to the variety of procedures which were a part of their management. Intravenous injections, lumbar punctures, and bone marrow aspirations were painful. Many of the medicines were toxic and caused several days of sickness. Many parents were embarrassed when their children expressed fear, violence, hatred, or contempt toward the physician or nurse during painful procedures. Some parents tended to instill guilt in the children when they reacted unfavorably. However, it was helpful when children were allowed to vent their true feelings. In general, parents and staff reported that children were easier to handle in clinic when they were not denied this freedom of expression.

Problems of the Parents

Kübler-Ross (1970) has identified five stages that the dying patient experiences: denial, anger, bargaining, depression, and acceptance. The parents in this group underwent adaptive behavior similarly. Unprovoked anger, threats, and uncooperativeness were all manifestations of early parental nonadaptive behavior. These behaviors were precipitated when more stress was introduced. For instance, parents became upset if medications were given even a few minutes late. They became greatly concerned with the speed of IVs and counting pills. Minor problems were occasionally magnified, and many parents became overprotective.

The attitude and knowledge of the physician who first told the family that the child had leukemia were stressed as being very important by all parents. One family had an unfortunate experience at the time of diagnosis which interfered with their acceptance of the disease and its management during the entire course of treatment. They were never really able to discuss leukemia or death with their child. The father walked away when his daughter tried to bring up the possibility of dying. He said, "To discuss it with her would make my ulcer bleed again for sure." Another family was greatly incensed when their physician telephoned saying, "Your child has leukemia; I'll get with you later," and then hung up.

The initial shock of the diagnosis of leukemia is great for all parents. Perhaps their greatest need from the physician is compassion, understanding, and the assurance that he will be there and do all he can. At that point, they need hope and are not ready for all the "facts, figures, and protocol information." They will be back in a few hours or days with lots of questions, and that is the best time to start the educational process. The first diagnosis confirmation is best handled with decorum and concern.

Parents appreciated hearing others discuss their experiences of telling their children that they have leukemia and how it should be done. Some parents initially tried to avoid the use of the word leukemia and would not discuss it with their children. However, the children invariably heard the word from people in the waiting room or lab, physicians, siblings, or playmates at school. Being frank and letting them know that their parents would be with them for support was especially important.

Parents discussed concepts of life and death in the group; in some instances, for the first time in their lives. This led to increased ease in similar discussions within the family and tended to be supportive.

At times there was a cathartic effect in just being able to come to the group and say things that could not be said at home. One mother reported a feeling for the past few days of extreme weakness and helplessness. She had been bothered with a persistent realization of "how can I stand it if my child dies?" The severe impact of the realization of possible impending loss was ameliorated considerably simply by talking about it.

Some families tended to divide their lives into a "sick" world and a "well" world and behaved differently in each situation as the disease process changed. During "well" periods, they tended to repress thoughts of leukemia, and there was little discussion of the disease and only minimal contact with the hospital. However, when relapse or other complications arose, the "sick" phase occurred, and of necessity, the family was faced intimately with leukemia and the hospital. Stress, worry, and verbalization regarding the illness increased. The stress was considerably relieved among those families which were able to integrate the "sick" world into their normal living.

In addition to sadness and stress, parents reported almost a constant state of frustration and futility. One mother said, "It is just as if I am paralyzed." Another added, "At times I just wish it were somebody else's problem."

Religious beliefs were a source of strength for some families. In the adjustment to handling the leukemic state, all parents expressed depression, and asked repeated questions, such as, "Why me?" and "Why my child?" Some of those with a deep religious faith believed that there were reasons even though they could not be understood at that time. One mother's religious faith led her to the belief that her son was an exceptional person who had been given to them for 12 years. Faith was expressed and accepted readily within group discussion even though there were significant differences of belief within the group.

In the bargaining and guilt phases of some families' adaptation to leukemia, God was accepted as long as all went well. However, when the child's condition became worse or he died, frequently God was blamed for the suffering or death, and then religious beliefs offered no source of strength. When parents felt that God was punishing them, they also rejected religion as a means of emotional sustenance. One family which had no religious beliefs expressed feelings of "nothingness."

When a child died, some parents attended the memorial services and felt that their presence helped the bereaved parents. Others, however, felt that the situation would be too stressful and chose not to attend.

The group had been meeting for several months when it was discovered that the parents were quite interested in how the child dies but had never asked. This had not been discussed with any of them, and they all expressed considerable relief to learn that terminal stages are usually quite peaceful and almost always painless.

The group presented a forum for sharing concerns, strengths, problems, and solutions among families. Attendance generally increased when someone's child was in relapse and the mothers wanted to share whatever might be possible. Parents reported that their contacts with other parents were the best source of comfort. As one mother said, "No matter how hard the staff tries to understand our needs, they are unable because they haven't walked where we walk." This close sharing of feelings led to the deepening of interpersonal relationships between the family members and staff members.

Discussions about the disease or death were difficult within families. The ease with which open discussion could be carried out varied greatly from family to family and tended to correlate with predisease ability to communicate. Some families never discussed death within the family circle. One mother felt encouraged by techniques of discussion she had learned in the group. When a series of problems started causing explosions and lack of communication within the family, she and her husband found that setting aside time for dialogue about family stress and behavior was quite helpful.

Parents used the group for help in solving family interaction problems. They discussed how doting grandparents and other relatives who showed preferential treatment to the leukemic child could best be handled. In general, the consensus was that parents should be firm if necessary to see that leukemic children did not get preferential treatment as compared with siblings. Also, some parents were excessively permissive, tending to lead to behavioral problems. This was helped if at least one parent recognized excessive permissiveness and tried to prevent it.

Some parents noted that they felt responsible for some of the various moods and attitudes of their children. Many times the children appeared to adopt the mood of the mother on any given day. Mothers realized that they could be responsible for hope, cheer, and happiness, on the one hand, or depression, gloom, and little productivity, on the other. It seemed best to some mothers to make a conscious effort to accentuate what they felt were positive values.

Mothers especially were frustrated when faced with excessive dependency and depression on the part of their children. At times, the children were so dependent that they literally would cling to their mothers all day long with constant and excessive demands. This led to recognition of a need for the parents to be away from their children at times—a need which was stressful when related to fear and guilt, but not if recognized as an actual need.

Problems arose with husband-wife relationships. Husbands could disappear at work and frequently "had" to work long overtime hours. Wives were left to handle the trips to the clinic and the constant exposure to a sick and often unreasonable child. Wives felt that they were subjected to more than their share of the emotional involvement of chronic illness and frequently resented this role. Some could verbalize this and some could not. Wives generally wanted their husbands to participate to a greater degree in the emotional support of the child. One wife suggested that each parent work half-time so that the emotional trauma could be shared and each would have some time away from the stressful situation.

Considerable stress was placed on the family when another member became sick. The mother usually had all she could do getting the leukemic child to the lab, doctor, etc. When someone else had even a relatively insignificant illness, the anxiety level of the entire family was increased.

Several parents were frustrated by the vagaries of nonspecific answers of physicians. They wanted concrete answers to such questions as: How long will she live? Will you know next week if we are going to get a remission? How long can we expect this remission to last? It was difficult for them to accept the physician's answer of "I don't know," or "I am unable to answer that."

All children had multiple absences from school, and this was a common concern to parents. However, most parents were surprised that it affected performance and grades as little as it did. When they realized this, their concern diminished considerably. Attempts to motivate the child or make the surroundings more compatible were helpful. One girl attended school much more readily after she was put in a class with a friend who had a seizure disorder. This appeared to facilitate a friendly relationship since both had a medical problem and allowed each to serve as moral support for the other.

The group proved to be a good means of information dissemination. The first part of each meeting was a "warming-up" period during which parents asked specific questions about the disease process, side effects of medication, clinic operation, interpretation of lab tests, and the value of a research protocol and its effect on medical care. This was a place where parents could relate to one physician and ask questions that had not been answered or understood when asked on the hospital wards and in clinics. Staff time was better employed when these questions were dealt with in a group rather than repeatedly with individual parents. Certain basic information was essential to all parents, some of which was communicated in an orientation letter given to them when their children entered the program. Parents reported that the group discussions were helpful in giving increased information about the disease and the "system." They helped parents and children feel more comfortable toward the clinic and staff.

Parents were helpful in identifying problems in the mechanics of our clinics. For instance, the rotation of house officers gave parents and children a feeling of insecurity due to lack of continuity of care. Clinic hours and difficulty in obtaining lab results were identified as problems. This input resulted in changes in some procedures which made the overall burden a little less.

Our institution is a teaching hospital, and daily rounds are usually a learning situation with discussion, questions, and answers often taking place at the bedside. Some parents objected to conducting bedside teaching rounds. They felt this caused alarm in the child and, in the case of leukemia, took some of the dignity away from him. The parents commented that they would not feel this way for a less grave situation. This occurred most often during the child's initial hospitalization when many parents protected him from the knowledge of the diagnosis and its seriousness.

Problems of the Siblings

Siblings of the leukemic children were also placed in stressful situations. On the one hand, they were fearful of loss of a brother or sister, and yet on the other hand, the sibling "got" to miss school and at times seemed to get special favors from relatives, friends, or others. This frequently caused jealousy, teasing, and other unpleasant interaction. The sibling often felt guilty after mistreating the sick child. It was important for the siblings to understand that leukemic children were not to have special favors, become spoiled, or "get by" with misbehavior. Parents who handled this best had frequent and open discussions with all children and allowed them to express their true feelings. Siblings modified their behavior considerably when they had a more complete understanding of leukemia and its management.

Most of the brothers and sisters of our patient children became aware at some point in the illness that it is frequently fatal. Parents felt this realization was most easily handled it if came from the parents rather than from a playmate or a television show. Most parents felt it was better to discuss the possibility of death early in the course of the disease. If handled openly, there were no instances of a sibling using this information to hurt the child with leukemia during arguments.

Problems with Friends and Acquaintances

Some of the most awkward and embarrassing problems to handle were caused by "others." They could be anyone from a close family friend to a chance acquaintance. Some of the problems developed because family members felt that they could not be as candid with friends as within the family.

Sometimes problems occurred whenever a friend or acquaintance learned of the diagnosis of leukemia in the presence of the affected child. Quite frequently there were inappropriate emotional responses of shock or pity. One mother had a traumatic experience which bothers her yet, months later. While waiting in line at the lab, a lady inquired what was wrong with her child. When told leukemia, the unthinking lady looked aghast and said, "My God, she's going to die!" When instances such as this occurred, most parents immediately became angry, and many reported that there were times when they wanted to physically assault such a person. Most felt their best approach was to quietly comment that this may no longer be the case and that they were certainly doing all they could to see that bad eventualities did not occur.

There was almost inevitably some problem with close friends of the parents. Most friends were well meaning but unable to talk with the parents about a dying child. It was difficult for them to know how to offer meaningful help in the most appropriate ways. Some made offers to help which were totally inappropriate and even inadventently hurt or antagonized the family. The most common happening, however, was that one by one friends started leaving them out of the usual activities until finally the parents felt isolated.

Some were fortunate enough to have a few close friends who were compassionate and understanding and at the same time supportive. These friends were of great value as the family circle of friends tended to diminish.

Problems of the Medical Team

The only "problem" from a staff standpoint was that the group meetings were emotionally fatiguing when deep personal feelings and problems were shared. Identification with these families was much more demanding for the staff than most of the routine hospital contacts.

The group was helpful in building trusting relationships and establishing open communication between parents and staff. All felt more comfortable in discussing medical and emotional problems without having the child present, which is often not possible in the clinic or hospital.

The group also provided a means by which staff could identify deficiencies in clinic procedures which were bothersome or inconvenient to patients and families. Several procedures were changed as a result of feedback from parents.

Comments by Parents

Throughout the first year that the group met, questions were raised by the staff and the parents about the usefulness of the group meetings. An attempt was made to find out how each parent felt about the experience or the reasons for nonparticipation. Several mothers made the comment: "I could say exactly what I felt in the group and I felt safe. Sometimes it's hard to talk about your feelings to your husband or to friends." Another comment was that "talking to other mothers eased the tension within me." Several mothers consistently attended while their own child was dying and felt that the group was the only place they could release much of the tension at that difficult time.

The staff wondered what the effects were on other parents upon hearing a very distressed mother talk about her dying child. One mother commented that "hearing about the child's relapse depressed me terribly and hit me harder than I expected, but it forced me to face reality about what could happen to my son, and I began to live day by day rather than living for the future." Another mother stated that "I feel terrible when I hear that another child is in relapse or dying. But somehow when I leave the group, I keep telling myself that my child is doing well now and I'm thankful for that."

Several mothers who attended group meetings expressed concern for others who did not. One mother said that the others "seem to be trying to kid themselves but sometime they will have to come face-to-face with the disease." Another mother told her husband, "I hate to go to the group this morning, but you know it's probably good to have to face reality each week."

The mothers who did not participate said, "The mothers in the group seem so pessimistic"; "the group made me feel more nervous for several days"; "I'm afraid I'll cry and not help anyone else, and I wonder if the group will make me worry more."

Some parents tried to put their child's disease and death out of their mind. The group experience only upset these parents. However, the vast majority were spending much time worrying about the child and his disease, and for them, the discussions were helpful.

CONCLUSIONS

The effects of parental group interaction on the families of leukemic children were assessed following a year of observation. During this period, 24 leukemic children, ranging in age from 2 to 16 years, were followed. Parents of these children attended some of the one- to two-hour weekly sessions during the children's course of treatment.

Observations resulting from these informal group meetings fell into several categories: factors affecting the patient; parents; siblings; family friends and acquaintances; and other members of the group, i.e., other parents and staff.

Many benefits accrued from the group sessions.

1. The cathartic effect gained from the informal sharing of information, problems, and experiences resulted in increased understanding between parents, staff, and families.

2. A need to lend extra emotional support during crises was recognized by parents and staff. Emotional support was particularly needed during periods of initial adjustment to diagnosis, intercurrent infection, relapse, when death became a probability, when treatment was discontinued, and both before and after death.

3. The staff members learned that didactic education of parents was best undertaken when stresses were minimal and that children were managed best when they consistently maintained a kind and supportive attitude.

4. Staff and parents learned to accept the child's need to express verbal and nonverbal anger toward treatments and those who administered them.

5. The problem of tactless comments about the child's condition was identified, and parents learned to more adequately cope with these situations.

6. The subjects of dying and death were aired, giving parents and staff an opportunity to understand their own feelings and helping to prepare them to discuss death with the sick child and other family members.

7. The difficulties of living with uncertainty were shared by the parents. Most of them reported that being able to ventilate and share their experiences with others relieved considerable tension.

8. Many problems related to disciplining the leukemic child, as well as siblings, were presented. Parents often had difficulty in dealing with their own feelings in this regard. They soon realized that discipline should be administered, insofar as possible, the same as in the preleukemic state.

9. Parents were of considerable help to one another in sharing solutions as to how they and their child could cope with problems related to therapy, e.g., pain, fear, bone marrow procedures, lumbar punctures, and loss of hair.

10. Perhaps the greatest benefit reported by parents was the opportunity to share and identify with one another at a level which was impossible for the professional staff.

Parents who shared together felt that they obtained a strength and an "at-peace" feeling which helped them endure the ordeal. The group became an important source of comfort, particularly during crises.

ACKNOWLEDGMENT

The authors gratefully acknowledge the advice and support of Jack Saiki, M.D., for his help in starting the group and consultation in preparing the manuscript.

REFERENCES

Ablin, A. R., Binger, C. M., Stein, R. C., Kushner, J. H., Zoger, S., & Mikkelsen, C. A conference with the family of a leukemic child. *American Journal of Diseases of Children,* 1971, *122,* 362.

Annual review of the group psychotherapy literature. *International Journal of Group Psychotherapy,* 1969, *19;* 1970, *20;* 1971, *21.*

Binger, C. M., Ablin, A. R., Feuerstein, R. C., Kushner, J. H., Zoger, S., & Mikkelsen, C. Childhood leukemia: Emotional impact on patient and family. *New England Journal of Medicine,* 1969, *280,* 414.

Bozeman, M. F., Orbach, C. E., & Sutherland, A. M. Psychological impact of cancer and its treatment. III. The adaptation of mothers to the threatened loss of their children through leukemia. I. II. *Cancer,* 1955, *8,* 1.

Friedman, S. B., Chodoff, P., Mason, J. W., & Hamburg, D. A. Behavioral observations on parents anticipating the death of a child. *Pediatrics,* 1963, *32,* 610.

Graham, J. R. *Certain aspects of group psychotherapy.* Unpublished material. Department of Psychiatry, University of New Mexico School of Medicine.

Kübler-Ross, E. *On death and dying* (6th ed.). New York: Macmillan Publishing Co., 1970.

Linder, R. Mothers of disabled children: The value of weekly group meetings. *Developmental Medicine and Child Neurology,* 1970, *12,* 202.

Natterson, J. M., & Knudson, A. G. Observations concerning fear of death in fatally ill children and their mothers. *Psychosomatic Medicine,* 1960, *22,* 456.

Siegel, A. A hospital program for young adults. *Archives of General Psychiatry,* 1970, *22,* 166.

Sorenson, E. T. Group therapy in a community hospital dialysis unit. *Journal of the American Medical Association,* 1972, *221,* 889.

Vernick, J., and Karon, M. Who's afraid of death on a leukemia ward? *American Journal of Diseases of Children,* 1965, *109,* 393.

GROUP TREATMENT OF FAMILIES OF BURN-INJURED PATIENTS

Marcia Abramson[1]

Probably no injury causes more physical and psychological trauma than a severe burn. Both the injury and the treatment that follows are frightening and painful, and the patient is often left with residual deformities that can radically alter his life. Varying degrees of fear, depression, grief, loss of hope, and psychotic reactions during the course of the treatment and during the long recovery period have been reported. In addition, the burn-injured person and his family are faced with the prospect of enormous medical costs and extensive hospitalizations that mean long separations from home and community. It is no wonder that a severe burn creates a severe crisis situation for patients and their families.

Interest in the psychological reactions of burn patients was first aroused at the time of the Cocoanut Grove fire in Boston in 1942. It was found that many of the persons burned at that time suffered from persistent and serious emotional problems (Adler, 1943; Cobb & Lindeman, 1943). Subsequent literature on the subject has supported these earlier findings (Hamburg, Hamburg, & DeGoze, 1953; Hamburg et al., 1953; Martin, Lawrie, & Wilkinson, 1968; Martin, 1970a, b; Andreasen et al., 1972). One of the significant outcomes of a study at the University of Iowa Hospitals and Clinics, previously reported in *Social Casework,* was that the relatives of burn patients undergo many of the same stresses as do the patients (Brodland & Andreasen, 1974).

During the early, acute stages of treatment, when the patient is faced with the initial physical and psychological shock to his system, the relative is often stunned and depressed. As the patient begins to cope with the active demands of the convalescence and the rehabilitation processes, the relative must also adjust to these changes. Because the focus of the medical staff must be on the patient, the relative often faces his anxieties about death and deformity and his boredom with a prolonged hospital stay without the active support of the professional staff. In addition, the families are faced with the trauma of watching a loved one suffer, often without being able to intervene in a meaningful way.

As a result of these findings, it was recommended that a group be organized at the burn unit of the University of Iowa Hospitals and Clinics

Reprinted from *Social Casework,* April, pp. 235–241, © 1975, Family Service Association of America, with permission.

[1]Associate Director, Department of Social Services, University of Iowa Hospitals and Clinics, Iowa City.

to help relatives cope with the stresses of being supportive to a seriously burned patient. It was apparent that relatives who remain for long periods of time with their burned family member form a natural group on the ward. They orient one another to procedure, offer each other support at times of stress, and develop an informal grapevine to disseminate information. It was anticipated that with the added leadership and participation of a social worker and a nurse to help focus the group's attitudes, feelings, and beliefs, the natural group could be utilized to achieve certain educational and counseling goals.

The original plan was to include only those persons who planned to remain with their relatives for the duration of the hospitalization and who would therefore be available to come to weekly meetings on a regular basis. It soon became apparent, however, that relatives who are not able to stay for the duration of the hospitalization are equally in need of support from the group and can contribute to the other members. It was also decided to include the relatives of patients who were returning for follow-up checks or reconstructive surgery. Recovery from a severe burn takes two years or more; the relatives can benefit from the continued support of the group and can help those persons whose relatives are still hospitalized to appreciate the problems that occur after discharge.

GROUP STRUCTURE

Initially, a sign was posted just outside the nurses' station announcing a weekly meeting and asking relatives to sign up if they were interested in attending. Subsequently, during the week following each patient's admission to the burn unit, the relatives were approached and asked whether they would like to attend the group.

The meetings were co-chaired by a social worker who was knowledgeable about the problems of families of seriously ill patients and a nurse who was familiar with the burn unit's medical and nursing procedures. The physical therapist and chaplain from the unit attended a few meetings in which the focus of group concern was on issues relevant to their services.

At the beginning of each group meeting, the purpose of the group was reiterated by the social worker: to help orient the relatives to the burn unit and give them the opportunity to share common concerns and questions with others undergoing similar stresses and to help the burn unit staff better understand these problems in order to be more helpful to them and to other families in the future. Although group members often already knew one another and were familiar with the patients, the social worker usually asked each member to introduce himself and describe the circumstances of the burn and the patient's current condition. Coffee was served, and group members were encouraged to talk with each other about their experiences in the hospital.

A notebook was kept on nursing care issues and made available to the rest of the unit nursing staff. Periodic meetings of nursing staff and the group leaders were held to share information and help the nursing staff understand and deal with the emotional reactions of family members. During a two-year period, meetings were held at weekly intervals, whenever there were two or more relatives present on the burn unit who wished to attend. In all, thirty-eight group meetings were held.

INITIAL REACTIONS

It was found that at meetings in which there was a preponderance of relatives of newly admitted patients, there were many specific questions about the medical and nursing care. Questions relating to shock, intravenous medications, diet, debridement, burn rounds, the use of silver nitrate, and the timing of procedures were raised, and relatives of patients who had been in the hospital longer were encouraged to share their relevant experiences. Only when the emotional implications of the procedures had been discussed did the nurse answer the specific question. If more experienced relatives were not present, the social worker would attempt to have the group members discuss the psychological implications of the various procedures before specific responses were given.

The need for specific information about procedures seemed to be closely related to the initial shock the relatives suffered during the early weeks of the hospitalization. At the same time that he had to begin to face the severity of the injury that had occurred to the patient, the family member had to get used to the sights, smells, sounds, and procedures of the unit. Explanations about the procedures often were not understood and had to be repeated; the relatives had to be helped to know what and whom to ask when they had questions. The group acted as a forum and catalyst for this procedure.

Mrs. L's husband was injured after suffering a seizure while burning trash. Mrs. L complained at the meeting that she never had an opportunity to talk with the doctor about her husband's condition. As she spoke to the group about her husband, it became clear that she had many misconceptions about his condition and his need for posthospital care. Underlying her inability to formulate questions for the medical staff was the fear they would tell her that he was in an even worse condition than she imagined. The group helped her to talk about her fear that her husband had suffered permanent mental deterioration from a recent seizure and would therefore require twenty-four-hour supervision upon discharge from the hospital. She responded well to the group's suggestion that she talk with the unit social worker about these fears and enlist her aid in formulating the questions to ask of the medical staff.

GROUP SUPPORT

More experienced members of the group have been able to share their experiences and solutions to problems with newer members in a way that can be highly supportive to the new members, as well as therapeutic to themselves.

At the first meeting he attended, Mr. P, whose children were burned in a house fire two weeks earlier, spoke of how other persons who had relatives on the burn unit had welcomed him to the unit, informed him about procedures, helped him to ask questions and understand what the doctors and nurses were telling him, and encouraged him to attend the group for further support and clarification. He discussed his children's different reactions to their burns. The group began to prepare him for the fact that his daughter, who was the more badly burned of the two but much more stoical than her brother, would probably begin to feel more pain and become increasingly depressed as treatment progressed. In later meetings, Mr. P spoke of how this discussion had helped him to understand his daughter's withdrawal and depression when it did occur and to deal with it as part of the normal reaction to a severe burn.

Among the problems discussed in the early stages of hospitalization were the primary relative's discomfort at being torn between the patient and the family at home, his need for support from other family and friends, and the visits from other family members, especially small children whose imagination about the burn was often much worse than the actual injury.

A phenomenon that occurred in the group was the mobilization of group effort to help a particular relative or patient. Sometimes it was a person like Mr. P, who needed information and support during the early stages of hospitalization. Other times it was someone who needed help in coping with the demands of a patient and could accept advice from the group more easily than from the staff.

Mrs. K, whose fifteen-year-old son was hospitalized with severe burns for several months, had promised her son at the time of his admission to the unit that she would remain with him throughout his hospitalization. After many weeks of constant attendance at his bedside, she was becoming emotionally and physically exhausted by the strain, and it was clear that she would end up a patient herself if she did not leave. All the encouragement, direction, and advice of the medical and nursing staff was to no avail until the other members of the group decided that it was time for her to take a few days of rest away from the hospital. They convinced her, and then her son, who later believed that it had been his idea to send his mother home.

Sometimes the group served as surrogate family for a patient who had no relatives available.

Carl, a fifteen-year-old who had been burned in a gasoline explosion, had no relationship with his family. As his sixteenth birthday approached, different members of the group expressed concern that the day not go uncelebrated. They spent part of two group sessions planning a party and delegated a group member to involve the staff and take up a collection. The party turned into a gala event for staff, patients, and relatives and clearly demonstrated the burn unit group's interest in one another.

Often relatives who were having difficulty coping with the patients, procedures, or staff were able to express some of their own feelings by focusing on the problems of others.

> Mrs. D, whose husband was burned in a farming accident while working as a migrant laborer, came a great distance to stay with him. She spoke little English, had few financial resources, and had much concern about her two small children who had been left at home with relatives. The usual problems experienced on the unit were compounded by her inability to communicate and her resulting isolation. The group spent several meetings giving her practical advice about financial resources and emotional support to cope with her husband's demands. The group also suggested ways to communicate better with the staff and activities that could help her become more involved with other people. Other patients who were having problems with finances and communication difficulties with staff and were also suffering from isolation were able to express their own needs indirectly while they were helping Mrs. D.

FROM ACUTE CARE TO REHABILITATION

One of the most stressful periods for burn patients and their relatives seems to occur when the focus changes from acute care to rehabilitation efforts. From being immobilized for days at a time, dependent, cared for by staff and relatives, and encouraged to express his feelings freely when in pain, the patient is suddenly faced with new instructions to be independent, take care of his own eating and toileting needs, do a prescribed number of exercises a day, and control his expression of negative feelings. The relative who has been so important in feeding, entertaining, and encouraging is often asked to leave if the patient continues to ask for assistance with tasks the patient is expected to do himself. For many patients, especially children, who have felt that the family member will stay only as long as he participates actively in the treatment process, and for their relatives, who suddenly seem to have no purpose, rehabilitation can be an anxious time. Patients complain about the nurses and physical therapists who are pushing them, or else they cooperate with staff instructions and take their frustrations out on the family member. Relatives find themselves caught between concern for the patient and fear of alienating the staff.

> Mrs. R, whose ten-year-old daughter, Marie, was burned when her dress caught on fire, found herself distressed by her daughter's expression of pain and the staff's expectations that Marie exercise control over her screaming. Believing that Marie's extreme fear increased her inability to cope with the pain of the exercises, Mrs. R became overwhelmed with the strain of being supportive while

trying to keep Marie and herself from alienating the staff by too much expression of concern. She expressed to the group her feelings that the staff wanted her to leave the burn unit.

The group was able to be helpful in a number of ways. It provided a place for Mrs. R to express her anger, not only toward the staff but also toward Marie for putting her in such an uncomfortable position. She continued to receive support and acceptance from the group despite her expression of angry feelings. She was able to express her anger directly to staff in the persons of the co-leaders without fear of retaliation. The co-leaders and group were able to help her examine and better understand her daughter's behavior and her own and the staff's reactions to it in a way that lent itself to the formulation of new solutions to the problems.

Relatives often use the group to express their pleasure in the fact that the burn crisis had made them appreciate strengths in themselves, the patient, and other family members that they did not know existed. A wife who had thought of herself as the dependent, helpless partner found she could assume the role of caring for the family farm and operating the machinery. She amazed the male members of the group when she described how she had changed the clutch on a tractor. One mother was delighted at the way her burn-injured adolescent boy, who previously had expressed a great deal of dissatisfaction with school and family life and had threatened to drop out of school, seemed to be able to redirect his energies toward finishing high school. Other mothers found that their teen-age children at home were willing and able to assume new responsibilities for themselves and younger children when a burned sibling kept the mother away from home for long periods of time. The expression of these strengths in the group and their positive reinforcement by other group members encouraged the participants to continue their efforts to cope effectively with the crisis.

PREPARATION FOR DISCHARGE

As the time for discharge from the hospital draws near, family members experience anxiety about how they will manage the patient at home. While the patient becomes increasingly concerned about returning to home, school, work, and other activities, the relatives begin to realize that at home they will be responsible, without the help of the physicians, nurses, and physical therapists, for exercises, wrappings, and dressing changes. The group experience permits the family member to express a natural ambivalence about taking on this responsibility alone. Returning relatives can share experiences and solutions to problems with those who are about to face them.

EVALUATION OF THE GROUP BY PARTICIPANTS

A few weeks after the patient's discharge from the hospital, every relative who attended two or more meetings was sent a questionnaire asking for his evaluation of the burn unit's relatives' group. Of the thirty-three letters sent out, twenty-three were returned. These relatives had participated in from two to twelve meetings of the group, with an average of four meetings per person.

When asked to indicate how helpful they found the group sessions, seventeen checked "very helpful," four "helpful," and two "not too helpful." When asked to comment on the ways in which they found the group helpful, many said the group meeting was a place to share problems with others who understood—both relatives and staff. One wife commented, "It was good to just be able to discuss some of my fears regarding my husband's condition with people who understood so well because they were going through the same ordeal." A mother added, "The nurse and social worker listened to everything I had to say. They were very reassuring when I needed it. I felt I could talk about any problem." Relatives indicated that they had come away with increased understanding of what patients go through physically and psychologically and had a better understanding of procedures and staff problems. The group meetings had helped them feel closer to one another and had relieved some of their tensions. Several commented that it was good for both the relative and patient for the family member to get away from the burn unit to talk. A husband commented, "I was able to release tension and ask questions about my wife's case without feeling like a nuisance."

When asked to comment on how the group failed to be helpful to them and what could be done to make it more valuable for relatives in the future, most replied that the group had fulfilled all their expectations, although there were some comments about the fact that a few relatives monopolized the conversation. Suggestions were made about timing, including making the meetings longer, scheduling them at a time when more relatives could attend, having more frequent meetings, and involving relatives as soon as the patient is admitted to the unit.

Relatives were also asked to comment on the problems that they and the patient faced on return home for which they had not been prepared. A number said that the most difficult adjustment was to the patient's moods and irritability. According to one mother, it was "mostly the change in personality which lasted—stubbornness." A wife said, "The only problem we had was getting adjusted to his moods, because mentally he was very unstable and at times he is very despondent." Another mother commented, "I didn't realize the full strain I was under. I did a lot of worrying and wondering if I was doing all of it right—the wrapping and such of my son."

OBSERVATIONS FROM THE WARD

In addition to what happened within the group and the reported benefits from group members after discharge, certain observations were made about the effect on the ward of the establishment of the relatives' groups. In the past, when many severely ill patients required much staff attention, relatives often reacted to the feeling that their patient was being neglected by expressing hostility toward one another or toward the staff. Cliques would form and one or two relatives or staff would become recipients of all the hostile feelings. With the advent of the group, the scapegoating of one another diminished. The relatives appear to have gained a greater understanding of why nursing and medical efforts need to be concentrated on certain sicker patients. The family members fill in with care and support for patients who do not need as much nursing attention, patients who would previously have felt neglected and uncared for. Furthermore, group meetings provided an opportunity for members to examine the emotional forces operating within the close-knit family of burn patients and their families. Some scapegoating of staff continued, but the group leaders were much better able to offer the relatives the opportunity to handle their anger and complaints in a manner conducive to productive change.

The group meetings also gave one member of the nursing staff the opportunity to share nursing concerns with the relatives, and other nurses were able to share their concerns with the nurse leader who brought them to the group. The group's reactions could then be conveyed to the rest of the nurses individually, by means of the group notebook and in staff meetings. The periodic meetings that the social worker and nurse co-leader held with the nursing staff permitted the sharing of information about patients' and relatives' psychosocial problems and needs and how these could best be met by nursing staff. As a result of these meetings, the nursing staff expressed a desire for more social work coverage so that they could have a better understanding of the patients and families as early as possible in the hospitalization.

The use of a nurse who was part of the burn unit staff and a social worker who had no direct responsibility on the ward seemed to be particularly effective. The nurse was knowledgeable about patients, procedures, and individual problems and in continuous communication with the rest of the staff. She demonstrated to the relatives the interest and concern that the staff must have for them, as shown by sending her. The social worker, on the other hand, because she was not identified as a member of the burn unit, could ask questions about issues that others took for granted and could focus primarily on the needs of the relatives, unlike other professional staff for whom the patient is the primary person. Thus, she brought a different point of view.

RECOMMENDATIONS

Although burn injuries are particularly stressful because of their suddenness, intensity, painfulness, and duration, there are many other medical problems that create significant stress for patients and families. Any illness that results in drastically altered life-styles or that causes temporary alteration in the patient's ability to cope can produce stress and crisis for the patient and his family. Cancer, chronic renal disease, cardiac illnesses, neurological problems, and birth defects are just a few of the medical problems that cause significant stress for patients and relatives. Relatives as well as patients need support from others who understand and who can provide some relief from the demands of the illness and treatment process. A group especially designed to provide such support for family members can ultimately help the patients and the medical and nursing staffs responsible for the care of such seriously ill patients.

REFERENCES

Adler, A. Neuropsychiatric complications in victims of Boston's Cocoanut Grove disaster. *Journal of the American Medical Association,* 1943, *123,* 1098–1101.

Andreasen, N. J. C., et al. Management of emotional problems in seriously burned adults. *New England Journal of Medicine,* 1972, *286,* 65–69.

Brodland, G. A., & Andreasen, N. J. C. Adjustment problems of the family of the burn patient. *Social Casework,* 1974, *55,* 13–18.

Cobb, S., & Lindeman, E. Neuropsychiatric observations. *Annals of Surgery,* 1943, *117,* 814–824.

Hamburg, D. A., Hamburg, B., & DeGoze, S. Adaptive problems and mechanisms in severely burned patients. *Psychiatry,* 1953, *16,* 1–20.

Hamburg, D. A., et al. Clinical importance of emotional problems in the care of patients with burns. *New England Journal of Medicine,* 1953, *248,* 355–359.

Martin, H. L. Antecedents of burns and scalds in children. *British Journal of Medical Psychology,* 1970, *43,* 39–47.

Martin, H. L. Parents' and children's reactions to burns and scalds in children. *British Journal of Medical Psychology,* 1970b, *43,* 183–191.

Martin, H. L., Lawrie, J. H., & Wilkinson, A. W. The family of the fatally burned child. *Lancet,* 1968, *295,* 628–629.

CHAPTER 12

COUNSELING SKILLS WITH THE BEREAVED FAMILY

Paul W. Power and Arthur E. Dell Orto

A severe loss may not only cause a crisis in family life, but may also cause a family to enter a state of bereavement that is intense and enduring. Family crises are usually temporary and are characterized by anxiety and a search ing for immediate solutions. With the family in bereavement the feelings of resentment, anger, and sadness can linger and cause a serious disruption to family functioning. If the loss is represented by the severe disability of a child or adult, continued grief could inhibit family efforts toward rehabilitation. In a family crisis experience the health professional usually assists the family to deal with the source of the crisis and helps family members to adapt. With family bereavement the emphasis is on the alleviation or the resolution of the grief. This intervention requires certain skills.

There is some overlap, however, with the skills outlined in Chapters 9 and 10. The abilities to listen, respond, provide support, impart information, and facilitate the family exchange of feeling are needed to help families deal with severe grief. To help families to cope with an irreparable loss also requires specific knowledge of the family, how its members handle grief, and a capability to apply this understanding at times when family emotions are intense. Often family members know how to adjust to the loss. Their difficulty resides in using their own courage to adjust and then find new satisfactions in living.

Although the topics of death and dying are usually associated with bereavement, there are events other than death that can cause intense family grief, such as the birth of a disabled child, the diagnosis of a chronic, severe illness, or the sudden unemployment of the family's breadwinner. When working with others, understanding the many forms of loss increases an individual's capacity to understand behaviors and emotions shown by others and to offer help appropriate to their needs (Schwab, 1979).

This chapter suggests a helping approach to assist families in bereavement. Three areas are emphasized: 1) general considerations to be aware of when helping a bereaved family, 2) contributions from family therapy that can serve as guidelines for intervention, and 3) an intervention approach.

GENERAL CONSIDERATIONS

Before beginning intervention with a bereaved family, the health professional should reflect upon certain ideas, an understanding of which will facilitate an effective helping approach:

Knowing yourself as a helper   During bereavement some family members may become extremely distraught. At these times the health professional may feel helpless, very anxious, fearful, and may become deeply emotionally involved. To experience anxiety and discomfort is normal, but they can hinder family helping. In assisting the bereaved family there is always going to be some agony, but if health professionals have an insight into their own defenses against grief and pain, then many feelings of discomfort can be controlled.

Understanding the stages of the grief process   Matz (1978) has identified different stages of mourning in response to a traumatic event. If a bereaved family is to reach an adaptive stage, family members will usually follow predictable steps. Matz has provided a conceptualization of behavioral reactions, although families may differ in how they react to the loss. The stages are: 1) *"If I deny it, it's not true."* The first response to a serious loss is usually denial, although Matz believes that the denial stage is "punctuated" by times of painful emotional awareness. The denial helps the family members to function and meet many of their daily responsibilities. 2) *"I have the power to undo it."* The denial gradually gives way to feelings of omnipotence. These feelings may be characterized by attempting to bring back the loss, by searching efforts, or may be expressed as anger at events or people the bereaved family regards as responsible for the loss. Unfortunately these efforts are doomed to fail, and gradually despair and helplessness occur. 3) *"I can't do anything about it."* Matz explains this is a time when the bereaved family members face the loss and begin to understand their feelings in order to reach an adaptive solution. The past may be reexamined, perhaps given up and partially replaced with hope. Depression also occurs, but hope may overcome it. 4) *"I am rebuilding and every now and then I remember."* The bereaved family members start to rebuild their lives. Social patterns are reestablished and new decisions are made to reach personal and family goals. According to Matz, painful memories will arise, but the family members appear to have more strength to deal with these emotions. With all of these steps, however, the phases themselves do not have clear-cut beginnings and endings. The move from phase to phase is gradual rather than sudden and dramatic.

Understanding intense grief reaction   Intervention approaches will differ between the family that has become almost completely dysfunctional because of the loss and the family that is still attempting to maintain its daily responsibilities. For example, when family members deny excessively the loss, are evasive in their communication, show an absence of basic self-caring, and have persistent anger, guilt, and depression, they are displaying very serious adjustment problems. The dysfunctional family is a closed system in which the level of nurturance is low. More extensive family therapy is usually needed for this family. In contrast, the family that is showing a reactive sadness has generally confronted the reality of the loss and still continues to meet its daily demands. Family communication styles are still intact. There may be some regression by the family members to more childish, aggressive behaviors, but this is temporary. Their sadness is actually a necessary part of the grieving process and the help provided to the family is often short-term. The assistance is mainly directed toward providing support for the alleviation of grief feelings.

Understanding the concepts of centrality, peripheral, preventable, and unpreventable   Dr. Bugen, whose article follows in this chapter, explains the meaning of these terms. They are important to understand because the health professional frequently assists the family to move from a belief in preventability to a belief in unpreventability. If the bereavement is central and the family members are convinced it was preventable, then, as Bugen states, the grief will be both intense and prolonged. Initial intervention with the family will entail an assessment of the relationship of the loss or trauma to the expectations, values, and beliefs of the family members.

Understanding the flexibility of goals for the bereaved family   Families who are experiencing loss will have different needs. Many family members are looking for some alleviation of the feelings of loneliness and depression, whereas others are searching for a way to integrate the loss into family life. A few health professionals believe that the family can be helped to accept the loss. The authors believe this is rarely so. Rather, they adapt to the loss and try to assimilate the chronic sorrow into their daily living. Other families, however, may need to have their family life reactivated. The loss has resulted in a temporary state of family confusion and disruption of customary roles. Activities have been suspended and family members are looking for a way to resume their customary patterns of living.

CONTRIBUTIONS FROM FAMILY THERAPY

Different ideas have evolved from the field of family therapy during the past 20 years. Chapter 8 identifies many of these concepts, but others can be emphasized that will facilitate intervention with the bereaved family. One of the most important overriding considerations, however, is that the family as a whole is viewed as the object of intervention, rather than its individual members. Any member of the family is both part of the problem and part of the solution and all family members must be involved in intervention. This is a corollary of the family systems approach (Bowen, 1976). Other beliefs from varied systems of family therapy that can be helpful are:

1. Family members have the capacity to recall the past, experience a present, and anticipate a future (Paul, 1967). When working with the bereaved family it is important to understand how people continue to reinforce and perpetuate the past in the present. Frequently this can prevent family adaptation to loss.

2. Over time formal and informal rules develop within the family structure that governs the actions of the individual family members (Jackson, 1965). For example, the family members may believe that all anger is destructive and therefore should not be expressed. There are further convictions about what is right or wrong, good or bad. Such beliefs may inhibit the working through of legitimate feelings stimulated by a loss.

3. Within a family there is usually "unfinished business." This may be shown by feelings of resentment, anger, or disappointment over an earlier event that has not yet been dealt with or expressed. Paul (1967) has often referred to this as the "family ghost." When the new loss occurs, old memories are revived as well as their accompanying guilt, hostilities, and sorrow.

4. A family changes when its conception of itself, or its way of thinking, changes (Ackerman, 1958). By family members learning to relate to each other in new ways the effects of a loss can be lessened. Upon impact of a severe loss the family members may feel a sense of failure, embarrassment, or inadequacy. They become vulnerable. Personal grieving over the traumatic event can provoke irritability and anger, which, in turn, negatively affect family communication patterns. Family members need to see the potential for support in each other, and this is often achieved when their way of thinking about the loss changes.

5. A constant adjustment to new roles is critical for both the patient and the family (Ackerman, 1958). The impact of a loss will generally create temporary role confusion, and if the family is to mobilize its resources for daily living demands, new family tasks may have to be assumed. Intervention efforts should consider the difficulty of this transition for

many family members, especially when there are younger children involved. Also, older siblings who are called upon to take over a parent's role are often placed in a stressful situation.

AN INTERVENTION APPROACH

Intervention should begin as soon as possible after the initial trauma, but this requires that workers be aware of family needs and are in a position to respond. Assuming this is so, an intervention approach is suggested that can be adapted to families experiencing varied forms of bereavement. The following ideas can serve as guidelines for intervention.

In assisting a bereaved family to adapt to a traumatic loss, it is important for the members to understand the source of their loss, then admit this loss and express their feelings about it. The intervention goal does not have to be family rebuilding, however; bereaved families have different needs. Some will only need a relief from initial anxiety or an opportunity to express their feelings, and others may simply have the need for more information related to the cause and circumstances of the loss.

The first meeting with the family, whether in the hospital, a clinic, an office, or the family home, is vitally important. It sets the tone for the remaining family contacts. For example, if the initial family encounter is characterized by the health professional's questions and an explanation of procedures, then the remaining family counseling will be a procedural explanation, almost an intellectual exercise, and not tap the emotions underlying the family's grief. On the other hand, if, during the first visit, the helper assumes the role of a listener, an assessor of family dynamics, and a facilitator for the expression of feelings, the remaining family counseling will help the family members to understand their grief and will assist in the alleviations of their feelings.

In the bereavement period good listening is shown by communicating a sense of caring and attending to the present family concerns. Active listening can help the family, because it communicates the helper's acceptance of the family and invites the troubled family members to share their worries and anxieties. It also implies that the helper suspends judgment and does not attempt to compare his experience with the family's experience. Active listening also promotes a trusting relationship with the family because it shows that the helper is vitally interested in the members and it encourages the members to continue speaking during the first interview.

In the beginning meetings with the family the helper should learn what the family understands about why the loss occurred, the effectiveness of the informal and formal supportive systems available to the family, and the family members' ability to cope effectively with stress. Matz (1978) has identified these goals as the determinants of successful grief resolution. The family must become aware of the basic source of the loss, because what may be perceived by the health professional as the cause of family grief may only be another symptom of a more serious problem. For example, the diagnosis of a terminal illness for a parent who has a long family history of alcoholism and being away from home for prolonged periods may renew feelings of resentment, especially if that person has undergone alcoholism rehabilitation before the diagnosis. Family members may still harbor deep emotions about the patient's earlier behavior. This represents "unfinished business," and the new diagnosis aggravates these feelings because it symbolizes another source of unpleasantness for the family.

Knowledge of support systems is also invaluable for the worker and family to assuage many feelings of grief. How individuals have previously dealt with stress can provide further ideas for the helper in assisting the family to adjust to their present difficulty. All of this information can be obtained by asking questions, but these should be carefully interspersed during the initial family meetings. Questions can frequently disrupt the family's flow of speaking or, if they are not timed properly, can indicate to the family members that a particular subject should not be discussed further.

One of the most valuable contributions of the helper during these beginning meetings is to assist the family members to express their feelings about the loss. The family should be given permission to grieve and realize that the experience of grief is a normal reaction. The family members can be encouraged to express the full extent of their feelings and thoughts resulting from the loss. Frequently the helper's response, "This is normal," is the most reassuring information for the family. The expression of family feelings is further encouraged when the helper reflects their emotions by such statements as "You are upset because... You must be disappointed because..." This reflection is not intended to operate at deep emotional levels but is a paraphrase of what has been said and a reflection of this to the family members (Anthony & Carkhuff, 1976).

It is important that the helper gently ask the family to look at old relationships that have been maintained and perhaps now have changed. It is not necessary to cheer the family up; family members with negative feelings should be helped to express them. The family members are relieved when they are able to acknowledge negative feelings and discharge them verbally. The bereaved are often prevented by family and friends from expressing the emotions that usually follow loss. Repetition, a frequent going over of the past, may be necessary for the family to verbalize its feelings and then to make sense out of the loss. The family must ask the unanswerable "whys" over and over again before adjustment to the loss can take place. Piece by piece the links with the past are reexamined, grieved over, given up, and partially replaced with the hope that what is lost may be compensated for or even replaced by another source of personal satisfaction.

Consequently, during these initial meetings the family is encouraged to talk, and the helper does not offer advice or give interpretations. Rather, facts and opinions are gathered. Moreover, this phase of family intervention depends upon the nature of the loss and how the family members initially responded to its impact.

When the helper has determined that the family members have a better understanding of the source of the loss, their reaction to it, and how adjustment could be achieved, and also believes that a trusting relationship has been established with the family members, he plans a course of action to meet the adjustment goals. The plans of action may take many forms, namely, providing support, reassurance, and information to help the family members move through the grief stages, and/or utilizing situational supports and resources. Grief resolution is encouraged by having a variety of well-integrated resources available to a family. Pastoral care, neighborhood crisis clinics, and friends can provide valuable assistance during the bereavement period.

The information imparted to a family should focus on more than the loss or its implications. Although the loss may become the most striking feature of family life temporarily, the remaining resources could be emphasized. These may not be obvious to the grieving family. These resources are often the established family strengths or environmental supports readily available to family members. Also, providing information may frequently mean reinforcing health care knowledge, suggesting new expectations for the family members, or reviving expectations for each other that might have been lost at the initial time of trauma. Through this information exchange process the health professional assists the family members to become aware of each other's needs, how to use the networks of support outside the home, and how to keep the family intact.

By support, the learning of new information, attending to each other's needs, and expressing their own feelings, the family starts to rebuild. If guilt feelings have dominated the family scene, renewed understanding can help the members move from beliefs in preventability to beliefs in unpreventability. Such a transition is usually difficult for the family members. Parents grieving for children tend especially to experience more difficulties than other bereaved persons in believing in preventability. Their convictions to change beliefs are facilitated by the trusting relationship with the helper. In conveying credibility and confidence the health professional assists the family to weigh the value of other choices and to perceive the problem of loss in another perspective.

During this time of intervention, the family assumes the responsibility for any needed change. Gradually the helper becomes less involved with the family as it tackles the adjustment problems or finds new interests, satisfactions, and creative activities. With the bereaved family there may be a terminating phase, but the members usually want the opportunity for periodic dialogue during the subsequent months. They may want someone they can turn to when the painful reality of the loss occasionally becomes over-whelming. Consequently, the helper stays in contact with the family, if only by an infrequent phone call, until it is perceived that the family is coping successfully and perhaps does not wish any further involvement with the helper. This is usually not true with the chronic conditions, but with death or a traumatic loss family members gradually cope and previous life pat-terns are reestablished, if only partly.

CONCLUSION

The occurrence of a family loss is usually a powerful, dynamic experience. In order for family members to cope effectively they often need skillful in-tervention. They need someone who can be there and listen, offer reassur-ance, and give validity to their feelings. For the family in bereavement in-tervention can take many forms, but it is always guided by the helper's conviction that underlying all approaches is the willingness to share an-other's loss. Such sharing is frequently the beginning of a resolution of the family loss.

The following articles in this chapter supplement the helping approach developed in the preceding pages. Kaplan, Smith, Grobstein, and Fischman discuss grief and mourning as part of the effects of serious illness on the family. They studied more than 50 families from the time of the diagnosis of leukemia until 2 months after the child died. In describing family responses, they learned that dealing with issues of mourning contributed to adaptive family coping. Bugen's article explains a model for prediction and intervention in human grief. He introduces important concepts for under-standing the grieving process which have a necessary implication for family intervention.

REFERENCES

Ackerman, N. *The psychodynamics of family life.* New York: Basic Books, 1958.
Anthony, W., & Carkhuff, R. *The art of health care.* Amherst, Mass.: Human Re-source Development Press, 1976.
Bowen, M. Theory in practice of psychotherapy. In P. Guerin (Ed.), *Family ther-apy: Theory and practice,* pp. 42–90. New York: Gardner Press, 1976.
Jackson, D. Family rules: Marital quid pro quo. *Archives of General Psychiatry,* 1965, *12,* 589–584.
Matz, M. Helping families cope with grief. In S. Eisenberg & L. Patterson (Eds.), *Helping clients with special concerns,* pp. 218–238. Chicago: Rand McNally Col-lege Publishing Co., 1978.
Paul, N. The role of mourning and empathy in conjoint marital therapy. In G. Zuk & I. Boszormenyi-Nagy (Eds.), *Family therapy and disturbed families,* pp. 186–205. Palo Alto, Cal.: Science and Behavior Books, 1967.
Schwab, R. Loss, pain, and growth. *Personnel and Guidance Journal,* 1979, April, 429–431.

FAMILY MEDIATION OF STRESS

David M. Kaplan, Aaron Smith,
Rose Grobstein, and Stanley E. Fischman[1]

Serious and prolonged illness such as childhood leukemia is a common source of stress that poses major problems of adjustment, not only for the patient but also for family members. It is important to emphasize family as well as individual reactions in coping with stress since the family has a unique responsibility for mediating the reactions of its members.

When individuals belong to families, they do not resolve their own problems of stress independently, nor are they immune to effects of stress that may be concentrated in another member of the family. Vincent (1967) states that the family is uniquely organized to carry out its stress-mediating responsibility and is in a strategic position to do so. No other social institution has demonstrated a comparable capability for mediation that affects as many people in the community.

Because the family has a commitment to protect its members under a wide range of stressful conditions and over long periods of time, physicians, social workers, and other professionals working with a severely ill child must extend their concern beyond the child, at least to members of the immediate family and perhaps to other close relatives. They must offer parents and other family members, as appropriate, help when they need it to handle and resolve specific problems of stress. If stress is great enough and sufficiently prolonged, the role of a family as a buffer for its members can be permanently impaired or even destroyed. To prevent this, more must be learned about effective individual and family coping—and more help given to improve this coping.

A better understanding of the process of coping with severe stress would have substantial clinical and preventive value. Adaptive coping by the family and its individual members—that is, mastery of the sociopsychological problems associated with stress—offers the greatest protection for family members confronted with stressful situations and the best assurance that the family will continue as a viable unit, able to meet the changing needs of its members after they have gotten over the stress.

Reprinted from *Social Work* *18*(4), pp. 60–69, © 1973, National Association of Social Workers, Inc., with permission.

The study on which this article is based was conducted, 1969–1972, at the Stanford University Medical Center with grant support from the American Cancer Society.

[1]Dr. Kaplan is Director of the Stanford University Medical Center, and Mr. Smith, Ms. Grobstein, and Dr. Fischman are staff members of the Departments of Pediatrics and of Community and Preventive Medicine, Division of Clinical Social Work, Stanford University School of Medicine, Stanford, CA.

This article describes the effect of serious illness on the family, delineates the family's critical role in resolving problems related to stress, and provides data needed for organizing preventive and clinical programs that will protect the family's stress-mediating function and mitigate the impact of stress on individual family members. The article is based on the authors' clinical review of more than fifty families with a child diagnosed and treated for leukemia at the Stanford University Department of Pediatrics. Each family was studied from the date the parents were informed of the diagnosis until two months after the child died.

IDENTIFYING EARLY REACTIONS

The aim of the study was to identify adaptive and maladaptive coping responses by the family as early as possible after diagnosis—within three weeks or four at most. It was hoped that developing a method of early case-finding would make intervention feasible during this crucial period and reduce the incidence of families who failed to cope adequately.

Early identification was attempted because studies of the concept of crisis suggest that both individual and family reactions to such threats as prolonged illness are fashioned from one to four weeks after the diagnosis is confirmed (see, for example, Caplan, 1964). Both adaptive and maladaptive coping responses become evident then. These responses tend to persist and to be reinforced throughout the course of the illness, which may run for years. Rapoport (1961) indicates that coping patterns are not as fixed and unyielding during these first weeks as they become in time. Therefore, the ideal time to discover that families are coping inadequately is during this early phase.

Families with a leukemic child constitute a high-risk group. The severe stress precipitated by the diagnosis of the illness generates many problems in addition to those involved in caring for the leukemic child. Both clinical and research observations indicate that a disturbingly large number of families who face this situation fail to cope successfully with the problems it poses (see, for example, Bozeman et al., 1955; Hamovitch, 1964). Binger et al. reported that following this diagnosis, at least one member in more than half the families in a 1969 study required psychiatric treatment (Binger et al., 1969). Bozeman et al. (1965) noted that in families with a leukemic child, school difficulties with the healthy children, divorce, and illness occurred frequently. In the study on which this article is based, 87 percent of the families in the sample failed to cope adequately with the consequences of childhood leukemia, and this failure created a variety of individual and interpersonal problems that were superimposed on the stresses posed by the illness itself. The success or failure of the family's coping behavior was assessed on the criterion that Friedman and his associates outlined:

Coping mechanisms observed in parents should be viewed in terms of how such behavior contributes or interferes with meeting the needs of the ill child and other family members (Friedman et al., 1971).

In addition to demonstrable risks associated with a fatal illness such as childhood leukemia, many critical problems of management that involve the family confront medical and social work personnel. Research has not yet provided data helpful for resolving these problems. The following are among the common unsolved questions of management:

1. What should the parents, the leukemic child, healthy siblings, and members of the extended family be told about leukemia—that is, about its course, treatment, and prognosis?
2. Who should give each family member the information deemed appropriate?
3. What advice should be given to parents who consider major family changes after they hear about the child's diagnosis—for example, having another child soon, separating from each other, remarrying, or moving to a new community?
4. What should be done to help parents who seriously disagree about the handling of fatal illness in the family?
5. What help can be offered to single-parent families faced with long-term illness?
6. During the period in which the parents are preoccupied with the leukemic child and tend to neglect the healthy siblings, how can the needs of these other children be protected?
7. What should be done to help parents who avoid visiting the leukemic child during hospitalization—and to help the child?
8. How can morbid preoccupation over the lost child be avoided?

COPING TASKS

The tasks of coping with stress occur in order and relate to the characteristics, sequential phases of the illness—that is, diagnosis, remission, exacerbation, and terminal state. These phase-related tasks must be resolved in proper sequence within the time limits set by the duration of the successive phases of the illness. Failure to resolve them in this manner is likely to jeopardize the total coping process of the entire family and the outcome of the stressful situation faced (Kaplan, 1968).

Successfully resolving any crisis depends largely on each individual's ability to experience with minimum delay the immediately painful consequences of a stress-producing event and to comprehend and anticipate, even though dimly, the later consequences—that is, the pain, sorrow, and sacrifice that the trauma will cause. Comprehension in this context means learning to accept one's new life circumstances, however painful, and then acting in accordance with the new conditions that follow the original crisis-precipitating event. The family, primarily through its adult members, can either facilitate or obstruct individual efforts to master a situation of stress.

The development of preventive or clinical programs that are capable of reversing maladaptive coping responses to any illness is contingent on having detailed knowledge of the process of adaptation specific to each illness, including relevant coping tasks and methods of task accomplishment. Because coping tasks vary significantly from one illness to another, it is first necessary to identify the problems posed by each illness.

The birth of a premature infant, for example, requires the family to anticipate the infant's possible loss. If it survives, the family must face the possibility of its being defective. Even when the prognosis is favorable, the parents must prepare themselves to care for an infant who has special early needs to yield in time to normal patterns. Many families with premature babies manage these tasks well, but a large minority do not. This minority continues to think of and treat the premature baby as though it were permanently damaged, even after its development follows normal patterns (Glasser & Glasser, 1969).

The family with a leukemic child is also suddenly confronted with major alterations in its circumstances that threaten cherished hopes and values for all its members and involve drastic alterations in their life-style. Each family member must comprehend these new circumstances and adapt to them by making suitable role changes, despite an understandable reluctance to face painful losses. While coping problems are unique for each illness, crises do fall into common groupings. Principles relevant for coping with leukemia apply with some modification to problems of family coping with other severe and fatal illnesses in children and adults.

FAMILY COPING

For any serious illness, coping demands and responses are not static, but change as the medical treatment of the illness changes. At any point in time, families confronted by childhood leukemia will have dissimilar experiences that reflect differences in the course of the illness as well as variations in medical treatment. Physicians and hospitals also have important differences in their philosophy of "managing" families who have a fatally ill member.

From the authors' observations, it is clear that certain methods of medical management facilitate family coping, while others hinder families struggling to master the consequences of leukemia in a child. For example, some physicians are vague and obscure when communicating with families concerning the diagnosis and prognosis. Others realistically describe the illness and its prognosis, but are eager to sustain hope by emphasizing possible breakthroughs in research. Still another group describes the illness realistically, but tries to focus the family's hopes on lengthy remissions during which the child may live comfortably and actively at home. The authors' experiences indicate that describing leukemia and its prognosis honestly and holding out hope of good remissions is the most helpful approach in dealing with patients and their families.

The marked differences in the medical management of families must be delineated before a demonstration program aimed at enhancing family coping with childhood leukemia can be established. However, it is possible and important at this point—without analyzing how this significant variable affects the coping process—to describe the essential factors in adaptive and maladaptive family coping with this fatal illness.

The typical experience with childhood leukemia today begins when a community physician who suspects a child of having leukemia refers that child to a medical center to confirm the diagnosis. The center usually makes this diagnostic evaluation with the child admitted as an inpatient. The family and the child (if old enough to understand the situation) await the news of the diagnosis with considerable apprehension; the parents may have received forewarning that serious illness is possible. However, the symptomatic behavior of the leukemic child prior to diagnosis rarely prepares the family adequately for the bad news to come, since the symptoms are rarely severe or frightening to the layman and may have been evident only for a short time.

ADAPTIVE COPING

Although what physicians tell parents about the diagnosis varies considerably, it is important for both parents to understand the essential nature of the illness as early as possible, preferably before the hospital that makes the initial diagnosis discharges the child.

According to the authors' observations, in families that achieve adaptive coping, parents understand that leukemia is a serious, ultimately fatal illness involving remissions and exacerbations but moving progressively toward a terminal state. These parents often reach this understanding within a few days after the diagnosis is confirmed. They do not spend an inordinate amount of time blaming themselves or others for the illness; instead, they accept the fact that the etiology of leukemia does not seem to be related to genetic characteristics or certain patterns of child care.

These parents do not arrive at this realistic understanding of the illness and what it holds for the future without considerable anguish. As a prelude to making the necessary changes in living that the child requires, they must accept the fact that they have a chronically and seriously ill child instead of a normal one. The realization that a child until recently considered healthy is seriously ill in itself provides reasons for family mourning. Furthermore, the recognition that there is neither a cure nor a good prospect of long-term survival (over five years) adds to the shock and grief these parents experience initially as they anticipate the eventual loss of their child.

Early comprehension of the consequences of a stress-producing event does not mean having detailed knowledge of what the future holds. The parents cannot know at the outset how long the child will live or what symptoms he will experience at each stage of the illness—but they should understand that since leukemia is a chronic and fatal disease, the diagnosis constitutes bad news and will involve painful losses and sacrifices for the family. The course of the illness varies with the type of leukemia; some forms have a rapid development and are short-lived, while other types continue for many years with proper treatment. The average life expectancy after diagnosis is from two to three years.

It is important for both parents to inform the family about the true nature of the illness. At the outset it is sufficient to tell all family members that the child suffers from a serious illness which will require regular and continuous medical care. Medical care is aimed at bringing the child home from the hospital.

Communicating the nature of the illness within the family leads to a period of grief that involves many if not all members. The diagnosis ushers in a phase of shared family mourning and mutual consolation that includes the leukemic child.

Those in the fields of health and social services have long known that mourning is a healthy, natural response to the news of impending loss. They realize what patients and family survivors must experience to accept fatal illness and death (see Lindemann, 1944). In the instance of childhood leukemia, each family member should have the opportunity to experience grief for current and anticipated losses. This should include the leukemic child, who gathers from his hospital experience and the behavior of staff and family that he is seriously ill.

The family as a group offers its members the potential of mutual support and access to its collective coping experience. When a healthy child becomes seriously ill, all members of the family need to find comfort and solace in each other in their grief. With such support they can face losses and make the sacrifices required by severe trauma.

Mourning may extend over a long period and be an intermittent process in which family members participate. Many losses are associated with a child's serious illness—such as goals that must be postponed indefinitely or relinquished forever. Some families are able to face the inevitable outcome realistically and talk about it frankly.

John D was the eldest of seven children, an active 12-year-old boy involved in many activities. The family was close, and Mr. D's job provided them with a reasonably good financial situation. The parents were understandably shocked when told that John had leukemia. Their initial reactions were typical of those of other parents, but they expressed their shock and grief openly and together. They understood that leukemia is a fatal illness for which there is no cure, respected and trusted the physicians, and made no attempt to seek corroborative or contradictory diagnoses from other physicians. The parents did not try to hide their feelings from each other but found strength and encouragement in grieving together.

From the start, Mr. and Mrs. D knew they must talk to their son about the diagnosis. They told him he had a serious illness that most children did not survive and encouraged him to trust the physicians, who would do everything within their power to keep him as well as possible as long as they could. John and his parents were able to cry together over the implications of the illness. Mr. and Mrs. D also talked with John's 10-year-old sister about the situation, since the two children were especially close.

The parents clearly wanted to be as honest as possible with John. The limited time remaining was doubly precious and was not to be wasted playing games or jeopardizing relationships. The pain of accepting their child's impending death would be even more unbearable if he turned away from them and no longer trusted them. They had never lied to him and were sure their frankness allowed them to trust, respect, and love each other.

At times the family had to express feelings of sadness by crying and mourning and no one tried to inhibit this. Mr. and Mrs. D allowed John time to himself but he was always free to go back to one or both of them with questions that were bothering him. He was a remarkable child whom everyone enjoyed. He was a bright, sensitive boy who wrote a science paper on leukemia for which he received an "A."

The D family's open discussion of survival with the child at an early stage attests to their unusual strength as a family. Not all families need to be as frank at the outset. Some may prefer merely to indicate to the child the seriousness of the diagnosis.

MALADAPTIVE COPING

Of the families studied, 87 percent failed to resolve successfully even the initial tasks of coping—that is, the tasks associated with confirmation of the diagnosis. Parents' reactions vary but fall into certain recognizable classes. Their most common reaction is to deny the reality of the diagnosis in as many ways as possible. Such parents avoid those who refer to the illness as leukemia. They themselves use euphemisms (for example, virus, anemia, blood disease) in speaking of the child's illness. They may even be fearful that the child will hear the news from someone outside the family.

> Mr. and Mrs. R refused to allow anyone to tell their 8-year-old daughter what her illness was or what implications it had. When the child asked her father what was wrong, he told her not to worry—there was nothing seriously wrong

—she had the gout, just as he did. One evening he called his neighbors for a meeting at which he asked them not to tell their own children that his daughter had leukemia for fear they would reveal the secret.

Reality-denying parents seek convincing reasons for their actions.

Mr. and Mrs. H said their 15-year-old son was not emotionally strong enough to be told about his diagnosis. When the child asked his parents what was wrong, they told him he had a long-term virus but would be O.K. After the child died several months later, his best friend informed the parents that their son knew he had leukemia but could not tell them he knew.

Parents who strongly reject facts cling to the possibility of a mistaken diagnosis and often seek other medical opinions to confirm their suspicions. Interestingly enough, parents who deny the existence of leukemia, who fight on many fronts to block out both thoughts and feelings associated with this illness, rarely deny their children the medical treatment offered for leukemia.

Mrs. T, 24 years old, was devastated when told her 4-month-old son had leukemia. Her mother encouraged her not to accept one physician's opinion but to see others, hoping that the diagnosis was wrong. As a result, the family was almost overwhelmed by financial problems, with bills from seven physicians and two university medical centers.

In some cases these parents deny the obvious symptoms of the illness and the effects of treatment.

The face of the once slender and attractive 4-year-old son of Mr. R became puffy and round soon after steroid treatment began. The physical change in the child was obvious to everyone except his father. When his wife reminded him of these changes, he became angry and refused to talk to her for several days.

Often these parents take elaborate precautions to keep the child unaware of the diagnosis.

Mr. and Mrs. B insisted that their 12-year-old son be protected from knowing the nature of his illness or how serious it was. They mounted a 24-hour watch over his hospital bed, never leaving the child alone. One parent or family member was always present. The child asked his parents to explain why they never left him as other parents did.

FEAR OF DISASTER

Such extreme precautions seem to stem from fear that the child's knowing about the illness will lead to disaster—for example, mental breakdown or suicide. Parents use this fear to justify concealing the diagnosis, but it often reflects their own inability to face the facts. One parent's open expression of fear or depression is perceived as confirming the other's worst fears and may lead to the other's repression of grief. One parent's emotion is frequently seen as "weakness," requiring the partner to inhibit expression of feeling because "someone has to be strong." The strong spouse who suppresses his own fears and grief is the one to be concerned about, not only for his sake but for the rest of the family, whose coping he jeopardizes.

> Mr. and Mrs. D, although quite close, seemed to have disparate ways of handling their grief. Mr. D was an open, sensitive person who cried whenever his son had a serious exacerbation of the illness. Mrs. D was secretive about her feelings, stating that both of them could not afford to break down because there were six other children to consider.

Some parents talk about postponing grief until the illness has reached advanced stages. These parents may have severe reactions in the later phases.

> Mrs. W, the mother of six children, resisted everyone's efforts to get her to express her feelings about the illness of her 4-year-old boy. Even when tears would have been appropriate, she refused to express any emotion. She rationalized the importance of remaining strong because she had to think of the other children. Because no one would promise her it would be better if she cried, Mrs. W insisted on waiting until later to cry and mourn. When her child's condition worsened, she was completely unprepared for the change. She became frantic and hysterical and required sedation. Even when her child called for her to be with him, she was so overwhelmed that she proved ineffective.

"Flights into activity" may accompany inability to grieve. Parents may try to escape from grief by becoming involved in new activities that keep them from thinking about the illness or the future—such as starting a new pregnancy, making other changes in family composition, or moving to a new home. Unfortunately, such activities increase the family's burdens and divert resources urgently needed to contend with the illness and its demands.

HOSTILE REACTIONS

Parents who refuse to accept the diagnosis occasionally display overt and massive hostility to members of the health center staff. If this lasts long, it usually evokes a counterhostility among the staff toward the family. The leukemic child is generally the chief victim of such family-staff warfare.

> Mr. and Mrs. A seldom left their child during his hospitalization. They refused to allow anyone to talk with them about his illness. Mrs. A would run away if anyone mentioned the word "leukemia." Both parents expressed great hostility toward everyone. Mr. A would curse the nurses; he refused to share pertinent information concerning his son's prior illnesses and infections with the physicians. As a result, the staff questioned his sanity.

Some families accept the diagnosis, but refuse to believe that leukemia is incurable or fatal even when the course of the illness confirms both facts. Shopping for a cure, resorting to faith healing, and placing the child on a special diet in the belief that food restriction will cure or arrest the illness are not uncommon practices among these families.

> Mr. H, a dairy farmer, refused to believe there was no cure for leukemia. He was sure the disease was transmitted to his 14-year-old son by the farm animals and therefore refused to allow the boy to eat milk products, restricting him to vegetables and grains. Mr. H also believed that iron-rich foods such as liver would enrich his son's blood. His theory involved overcoming his son's "bad blood" with "good blood."

In a few families the parents can accept the diagnosis and also can anticipate the additional care the illness will require of them. However, they fail to cope by refusing from the start to take on the actual care of the leukemic child because it is "too much for them to handle." These parents claim that they cannot help the child and should not be expected to care for him. This early abdication of parental responsibility is not to be confused with the later abdication that occurs in families only after the parents have taken care of the leukemic child for months or years.

> Mr. and Mrs. K could admit to themselves and others that their 3-year-old son had leukemia, but they could not cope with or adjust to the illness. They refused to visit the child when he was hospitalized, explaining that it was too hard on him when they left. Mrs. K claimed she was too ill to drive from their home to the hospital. Furthermore, since they couldn't take care of him when he was really sick, they didn't see why they should bother to visit him. They also refused to allow their 17-year-old son to visit the ill boy, stating that his school work would suffer and he would not be able to graduate with his class. The leukemic child was literally abandoned by his family, and no appeal from the staff changed their attitude. The child became withdrawn and frightened during each hospitalization.

DISCREPANT COPING

However capable one parent may be in facing and resolving the issues, the family's success in coping with childhood leukemia is in jeopardy if the parents take opposing positions at an early stage of the coping process. The family's ability to manage the illness depends on successful coping by both parents in the tasks that follow diagnosis. When the parents have different emotional reactions to leukemia and when they disagree on how to define the illness, whom to discuss it with, and what to tell others about it—then the essential ingredients for failure in individual and family coping are present.

> From the time the diagnosis was confirmed, Mr. and Mrs. D had difficulty communicating with each other. Mrs. D wanted to talk with her husband about their child's illness. He insisted that nothing could be accomplished by talking or crying over the situation. He offered no support to his wife, who constantly needed and expected him to comfort her. This gap in communication and

mutual support continued for over two years. Mrs. D's anger toward her husband finally became quite apparent. She was on one occasion able to receive comfort from her father, with whom she did not usually feel close, but never from her husband.

Discrepant parental reactions to the coping tasks that follow diagnosis may be responsible for 1) producing garbled and dishonest communication about the illness or preventing communication about it, 2) prohibiting and interrupting individual and collective grieving within the family, and 3) weakening family relationships precisely when they most need to be strengthened. Relationships between parents are undermined by dissatisfaction with the amount of support one gives to the other. Dishonest communication about the illness creates distrust and undermines relationships between parents and children. When parents fail to accomplish coping tasks that follow diagnosis, the net result is to compromise the family's ability to address itself to the next coping tasks, that is, preparing for and making the adaptations necessary in the siege phase of serious illness. Successful early resolution of the tasks following diagnosis is considered a most critical coping assignment because achieving further coping tasks depends on the effectiveness of this initial effort.

In the family system of reciprocal relationships, in which one function is to provide mutual assistance to members under stress, members expect others in the family to help them meet their needs—whether these needs are for emotional support or assistance with family functions and labors. When one family member fails to respond to what another considers legitimate expectations under stress, the inevitable resentment and dissatisfaction that follow decrease the effectiveness of the joint effort essential for successful family coping. The parents' failure to cope successfully with the initial tasks after diagnosis largely precludes sound coping by the rest of the family.

A family must have the closest possible cooperative relations to attain the discipline it requires for living through the siege imposed by a child's serious illness. Such close relations are based on trust, honesty, and mutual support and are virtually impossible to maintain if the family fails to handle the initial coping tasks adequately.

One purpose of the authors' study was to provide the groundwork for effectively assisting at an early stage those families who experienced difficulty in coping with severe illness—specifically, childhood leukemia. Preliminary attempts have been made to correct maladaptive family responses to the diagnosis of leukemia. The following case summary is an example of early efforts to develop appropriate techniques of intervention:

> The reaction of Mr. and Mrs. S to the diagnosis of leukemia was typical of many parents. The mother recognized the seriousness of the illness and felt frightened and depressed. When she cried and sought consolation from her

husband, he became angry. "What in hell are you crying about?" he asked. He refused to believe or accept the diagnosis. Mrs. S became angry with his failure to support her and they fought frequently.

Peter, their 13-year-old leukemic boy, resisted treatment procedures during his first hospitalization and an early rehospitalization, loudly proclaiming that the medication did not help and he knew he was "going to die." His parents had steadfastly refused to talk to Peter about the seriousness of his illness. When the project worker insisted, they finally consented to let the physician discuss Peter's illness with him because staff had continuing difficulty in managing him. The physician told the boy, while his mother was present, that he had a serious illness requiring continuous hospital and clinic care. Peter became upset and cried, but soon was less agitated. Just before his mother left the ward, he asked her to lean over so he could whisper to her. He threw his arms around her and they both sobbed bitterly. Then Peter said, "I'm all right now. You can go home." His mother, after a day or two, expressed pleasure that she and Peter were close once again. She was relieved that she no longer had to evade his questions or lie to him about his illness. He told her he now understood why she and his father were worried about him and why she cried. She had thought she had successfully concealed her worry and tears from him.

This case illustrates one method of reopening and clarifying communication in families whose members refuse to talk honestly with one another about leukemia. It is also clear that since coping is a family problem, coping tasks cannot be successfully resolved if key family figures are not included. In this instance, the reopening of family communication did not involve the father and an adolescent sister. After the boy died, the sister refused to go near his room. The family had to sell the house and move to a new home. These omissions limited the success of this interventive effort.

GUIDELINES

Certain guidelines for clinical management can be outlined at this point on the basis of the limited research data available. The following principles were derived from the author's study findings, plus consultation with a physician who had broad clinical experience.[2]

1. The successful management of the seriously ill child and his family is based on a trusting relationship with the physician treating the child. The psychiatrist is not a practical alternate for the physician, although he may serve as a consultant. Social workers, nurses, technicians, and other health and social service personnel who may be available can help deal with these problems, but they cannot take over for the physician.
2. Perhaps the most important function the physician or social worker can fulfill is to share the anguish, the grief, and the fears of these families

[2]The authors discussed clinical management of the leukemic child and his family with Dr. Dane Prugh, Professor, Department of Pediatrics, University of Colorado Medical Center.

without "turning them off." Listening without offering false hope is essential. Giving them long, intellectual descriptions of disease processes and chemotherapy alone is of small value.

3. The parents' denial of the significance of the illness is natural at the outset; however, persistent denial lasting for weeks and months should be probed gently but persistently. Sources of denial such as guilt may be mentioned to them as natural feelings. That the physician and the social worker can face the bad news with them offers the parents the hope that they can somehow survive the child's death.

4. Since families often must endure years of siege with a leukemic child, it is important to help them conserve their energies and resources for the long haul. Physicians and social workers should anticipate and discourage common family reactions that lead to such flights into activity as early pregnancy, divorce, remarriage, and changing jobs or residence. The most useful advice to families contemplating these activities is "Don't just do something, stand there." Each additional major change adds stress to an already overloaded circuit.

Appointments with the parents after the child's death are extremely valuable in assessing whether the family is managing adequately or needs additional help. All members of the family should be considered at that time since all are vulnerable as a result of the leukemic experience. Unresolved problems of grief are not uncommon long after the death of the child. The physician or social worker can help resolve problems of grief by indicating that such reactions are normal and that mourning often takes months to complete.

REFERENCES

Binger, C. M., et al. Childhood leukemia: Emotional impact on patient and family. *New England Journal of Medicine*, 1969, February 20, 414–417.

Bozeman, M. F., et al. Psychological impact of cancer and its treatment. III. The adaptation of mothers to the threatened loss of their children through leukemia, Part I. *Cancer*, 1955, *8*, 1–20.

Caplan, G. *Principles of preventive psychiatry*, pp. 39–54. New York: Basic Books, 1964.

Friedman, S. B., et al. Behavioral observations on parents anticipating the death of a child. In R. I. Noland (Ed.), *Counseling parents of the ill and the handicapped*, p. 453. Springfield, Ill.: Charles C Thomas Publisher, 1971.

Glasser, P., & Glasser, L. *Families in crisis*, pp. 273–290. New York: Harper & Row Publishers, 1969.

Hamovitch, M. B. *The parent and the fatally ill child*. Duarte, Cal.: City of Hope Medical Center, 1964.

Kaplan, D. M. Observations on crisis theory and practice. *Social Casework*, 1968, *49*, 151–155.

Lindemann, E. Symptomatology and management of acute grief. *American Journal of Psychiatry,* 1944, *101,* 1–11.
Rapoport, L. The concept of prevention in social work. *Social Work,* 1961, *6,* 3–12.
Vincent, C. E. Mental health and the family. *Journal of Marriage and the Family,* 1967, February, 22–28.

HUMAN GRIEF:
A Model for Prediction and Intervention

Larry A. Bugen[1]

This paper will present a model to facilitate both prediction and understanding of grief reactions. The model is presently intended only to apply to conventional grief in response to death, rather than "anticipatory grief" as formulated by Schoenberg et al. (1974). The generally accepted approach to conceptualizing grief reactions posits the existence of stages. Kavanaugh (1972) declared that seven phases can be identified in the grieving process: shock, disorganization, volatile emotions, guilt, loss and loneliness, relief, and reestablishment. Kubler-Ross (1969), emphasizing proaction, suggested five stages of "adjustment," including denial, anger, guilt, preparatory grief, and the "goodbye" stage. A separate set of stages was also proposed by Kubler-Ross to account for the grieving process of the dying themselves, in the mourning of their own incipient loss. The work of these pioneers in the study of dying and grief has led to an increasing social acceptance of the broad range of human grief response, and has encouraged mourners to express their sorrow without shame or guilt.

The "stage" concepts of grieving, however, contain a number of theoretical weaknesses and inconsistencies. First, both Kavanaugh and Kubler-Ross recognized that their stages are not separate entities, but subsume one another or blend dynamically. Second, the stages are not successive; any individual may experience anger, for instance, prior to denial, or perhaps disorganization before shock. Third, it is not necessary to experience every stage. Depression, or for that matter any volatile emotion, may never be a recognizable response to loss. Fourth, the intensity and duration of any one stage may vary idiosyncratically among those who grieve. For one mourner, sadness may be a short-lived experience, while anger is a more protracted stage; the duration of these two emotional stages might be reversed for someone else. Finally, little empirical evidence is offered by proponents to substantiate the theory of stages.

These flaws in the "stage" approach to understanding human grief suggest the need for a model that will 1) link pivotal determinants with consequent grief reactions in such a way as to allow for 2) predictive value, as well as 3) guidelines for constructive intervention. The model that will be outlined in this paper identifies two dimensions—centrality-peripherality

Reprinted from *American Journal of Orthopsychiatry* 47(2), pp. 196–206, © 1977, the American Orthopsychiatric Association, Inc., with permission.

[1]From the University of Texas at Austin.

Table 1.   Interaction of closeness of relationship and perception of preventability as predictors of grief

	Preventable	Unpreventable
Central relationship	Intense and prolonged	Intense and brief
Peripheral relationship	Mild and prolonged	Mild and brief

and preventability-nonpreventability—believed to contribute to both the intensity and the duration of the human grief response. Clinical illustrations of the model's formulations will be offered where possible, and the employment of the model as an aid in therapeutic interventions will be explored.

The thesis underlying the model to be presented holds that stages, in the strictest sense, do not exist in the grieving process. Instead, it will be proposed that the existence of *a variety of emotional states* is the essential point, and *not* the need to order them.

THE MODEL

The graphic illustration of the model (Table 1) is a 2×2 matrix, in which the vertical axis represents the closeness of the relationship between the mourner and the deceased, and the horizontal axis represents the extent to which the mourner believes the death might have been prevented. These two dimensions interact to create four reactive states reflecting both duration and intensity. As shown in Table 1, a mourner who considered the deceased a central person in his or her life and also believes that the death was preventable would be predicted to experience both an intense and prolonged grieving process. Perhaps the dynamic opposite is the mourner who had only a peripheral relationship with the deceased, and believes that the death could not have been prevented; here, the grieving process would be predicted to be both mild and brief. Dimensions of the model will be defined, and exampled presented, below.

CENTRALITY

The closeness of the relationship between the mourner and the deceased is directly related to the intensity of the grief reaction. If the relationship to the deceased is seen as central, the grief reaction will be intense. If the relationship is considered peripheral, the grief reaction will be mild. Any one, or some combination, of the following criteria may help define a central relationship.

1.   Centrality refers to a person whose presence and importance is so profound that, "I feel I have no life without him." This is perhaps the most powerful of all conditions, and the most likely to sustain a sense

of hopelessness. The mourner typically feels as though his or her life is meaningless or senseless without the loved one. Expressions such as "What am I going to do now?", "It's not worth going on," or "I wish I were dead, too" are very common. Age offers little protection from these feelings. The author recalls rather painfully a recent letter from a long-time friend of the family who was 76 years old. Two years had elapsed since the death of her husband, and little change could be found in her mood. Her despair and utter despondency were evidenced most vividly when she confided, "Well, another Christmas has passed. That means one less that I have to bear alone."

2. Centrality may refer, at a lesser intensity, to a person whose love is experienced as being a needed element in one's own life. For the dead to be considered central, it is not enough for the mourner merely to have loved the deceased. Mourners must see the nurturance and love of the dead as having been a vital source of daily support (a father's reassuring smile from the grandstand, for example, at the start of a teenage athlete's race), the loss of which is felt deeply and constantly.

3. Centrality may also refer to a person to whom the survivor had become behaviorally committed through daily activities. The most obvious example is the death of a child for whom a parent had daily set the alarm for school, made breakfast, washed dishes and clothes, gone out to meet after school, helped with homework, etc. But even an old cantankerous grandmother may be sorely missed when her close survivors realize in retrospect that delivering hot water bottles to a "storming old biddie" was one of the more vital moments in the day.

4. A person whose very existence serves as a reminder and symbol for our hope and beliefs may be a central figure. Thousands of individuals mourned President Kennedy's assassination with incredible intensity. It is striking that most of these mourners had never even met the President, yet experienced profound loss.

PERIPHERALITY

The other pole of this dimension is meant to describe distance and minimally important relationships. There may, in fact, be no relationship at all, as with neighbors who rarely speak to one another although living in close proximity. It is suggested that any grief reaction will be mild in the case of peripheral relationships.

1. Peripherality refers, at one extreme, to a person whose presence is both felt and respected, but whose loss is not viewed or experienced as irreplaceable. This may well fit the case of a coworker's death, in which the survivor had recognized the contributions of the deceased but had not extended the working relationship into the social arena. Peripherality

could also refer to a person whose presence is not recognized or necessarily respected. Such "strangers," in effect, elicit minimal grief reactions.

2. Pheripherality may also denote the behavioral view that our rewards and pleasures are not contingent upon the behavior or presence of the deceased. The obverse of this would also be true. In this case, the mourner recognizes that significant aspects of his or her life will not be affected by the death at hand—the loss will not affect the usual ways which the mourner obtains love, attention, etc. that give meaning to his or her life. Seligman (1975) described in some detail the situation just opposite to this, in which mourners believe that outcomes are independent of their responses; this will be discussed more fully below.

PREVENTABILITY

Establishing whether the mourner *believes* the cause of death was preventable or unpreventable is essential, since this dimension directly relates to the duration of a grief reaction. If the cause of death is believed to have been preventable, the grieving process will likely be prolonged. If the cause of death is considered to have been unpreventable, the grieving process will be relatively brief. To summarize:

1. Preventability refers to the *general belief* that the factors contributing to the death may have been sufficiently controlled so that the death might have been avoided. Whether or not the factors could actually have been controlled, it is the mourner's obsession that they *should* have been; the commitment, therefore, is to an idea rather than a fact. The use of "general" in the above definition is meant to connote all causative factors other than the mourner himself. Lambasting the hospital staff for their delay in using a respirator would be an example of this.

2. Preventability also refers to the specific "belief" of survivors that they themselves contributed to the death either directly or indirectly. A mother giving her daughter permission to attend a dance may "never forgive herself" if her daughter is killed in an automobile accident on the way home.

UNPREVENTABILITY

1. Unpreventability refers to the belief that nothing could have been done by any mortal to divert the forces contributing to the death.

2. Unpreventability refers to the belief that everything was done to divert the forces contributing to the death.

3. Unpreventability is demonstrated by attributions to, for example, God, fate, inevitability, luck, or misfortune.

In effect, the locus of control is believed to lie outside the realm of human influence. This belief absolves the mourner of both responsibility and guilt.

INTENSE GRIEF REACTION

An intense grief response may include the following physical symptoms: tightness in the throat, shortness of breath, sighing, loss of appetite, loss of sleep, and emotional waves lasting from twenty minutes to one hour (Lindemann, 1944). Psychologically, mourners may manifest general subjective distress, depression, uncontrolled crying, and debilitating anxiety leading to nightmares. The intensity of a mourner's grief may be so formidable that, Kavanaugh concluded, "few tasks in life cause more anxiety than consoling the bereaved!" (1972, p. 107). In relation to intensity, this author hypothesizes that:

1. A relationship exists between the intensity of our grief reaction and the extent to which we actually grieve for ourselves as compared to the deceased. With the death of a loved one, we certainly lose a part of ourselves. When we begin to recognize this lost part, this new void, we may begin to grieve for ourselves. As grief intensifies, an egocentric concern with oneself may be assumed on the part of the mourner. In fact, the psychoanalytic notions of narcissim will probably be associated with the most pathological cases of severe grief response. In most cases, then, what appears to be deep concern for the deceased is actually deep concern for the bereaved.

2. Experientially, the intensity of our grieving is directly related to a personal feeling of depression and a profound belief that our lives have been *hopelessly* altered. This conviction of helplessness and utter despair may be so severe that death of the mourner results. Examples are available in the realm of "voodoo" death (Cannon, 1942), spouse death at the loss of a loved one (Engel, 1971), and institutionalized helplessness (Ferrari, 1962; Schulz & Aderman, 1973). Seligman (1975) stated that when a

> ...person is placed in a situation where a particular outcome is—or *appears* to be—independent of his responses, he learns that his responses are ineffective. The affected individual may conclude that any responses he makes will be powerless to affect the outcome. The number of responses decreases; a "what's the use" syndrome develops; and helplessness becomes a self-fulfilling prophecy. If the outcome is a traumatic event—if it involves physical or emotional pain—the helpless subject may progress through successive stages of fear and anxiety to a deep depression, and, in some instances, death.

MILD GRIEF REACTION

Mild grief reactions may be characterized by an absence or mildness of physical symptoms. A loss is perceived by the mourner without significant physiological stress or acute psychological distress. Psychological symptoms such as sadness, loneliness, or irritability may well be experienced; severe despair and hopelessness, however, would not be present.

PROLONGED DURATION

Predicting the length of an appropriate grief reaction is an extremely difficult task. On the one hand, crisis theory suggests that most depressions will lift within a two-month period and an individual will find himself or herself beginning a process of reestablishment. Lindemann (1944) found, for instance, that with eight to ten interviews over a period of four to six weeks it was

> ...ordinarily possible to settle all uncomplicated and undistorted grief reactions. This was a case in all but one of the 13 Cocoanut Grove fire bereavement victims. (p. 144).

On the other hand, some clinicians maintain that the mourner must experience a full year of activities without the deceased in order to work through the grieving process. Christmas, New Year, and birthdays are seen as necessary transition periods in this case. For the purpose of this paper, prolonged grief will be defined as extending beyond a six-month period subsequent to the death. More specifically:

1. Prolonged grief exists when medical diseases such as ulcerative colitis, rheumatoid arthritis, or asthma are manifest in the mourner beyond the six-month interval following the death. Other symptoms, such as sleeplessness, oversleeping, or loss of appetite beyond the six-month interval may also connote prolonged grief.
2. Prolonged grief exists when the bereaved fail to extricate themselves from the deceased, while maintaining a relationship only with memorabilia symbolic of the death. A mother may lock a child's room, preserving it "as it was," and perhaps even sit in the room for hours each day. More common examples would include the need to retain the clothing of the dead, the need to frequently visit the graveside, or even to aspire toward the occupation of the deceased. It is interesting to note that most religions provide some ceremonial occasion for special interactions with the deceased. Such occasions represent opportunities to cherish sensitive and time-honored moments of recollection and would not be characteristic, by themselves, of a prolonged grief response.
3. Prolonged grief may be considered to exist in the special case of *helplessness proliferation*. Mourning is partly a belief in helplessness. The

bereaved is, in a sense, saying that, "I won't be able to go on without the deceased." The longer this "belief" is held on to, the longer the grieving process. This dynamism is very similar to what Seligman described as transfer of helplessness. Helplessness proliferation may be seen in the individual who first decides that he or she just can't make it to the Christmas party. This feeling soon proliferates to not needing friends, and eventually to being unable to maintain a job. By the end of the six-month period, this mourner may be ready for hospitalization or perhaps suicide.

4. Prolonged grief exists when the bereaved fail to find new, or reestablish old, patterns of rewarding interaction within their environment. In order to move beyond grieving, the bereaved must review their relationship to the deceased, accept their hurt in not having its pleasures any longer, and finally be willing to explore and establish new networks among the rich supply of resources still available to them.

BRIEF GRIEF REACTIONS

A brief grief reaction may exist when the anticipatory grief period was of sufficient duration to allow for a "working through process," so that a prolonged conventional grieving period is not necessary. In cases in which cancer has been the slow, deteriorating cause of death, most mourners have had opportunities to experience the full impact of their anticipated loss of a loved one prior to the death.

At one extreme, brief grief may reflect the intense process of painfully extricating oneself from the deceased and finding new patterns of rewarding interaction. This process may well occur within a two to six month period, and is usually facilitated by societal support groups or sanctions. The traditional Irish wake serves such a function by encouraging full grief expression on the part of the mourners.

At the other extreme, brief grief may reflect the *absence* of an emotional bond between bereaved and deceased. In such a case little remains to work through. Instead, the death may stimulate late pensivity regarding existential questions such as: "Is hard work worth the effort?", "What does exist after life?", and "How much in control of my life am I?"

EMPLOYING THE MODEL

As described above, four possible outcomes may be expected given the interaction of the two sets of determinants: 1) Given a central relationship between bereaved and deceased and the belief that the death was preventable, we would expect the grieving process to be both intense and prolonged. 2) Given a central relationship between bereaved and deceased and the belief that the death was unpreventable, we would expect the grieving process to be intense but brief. 3) Given a peripheral relationship between bereaved and deceased and the belief that the death was preventable, we would expect the grieving process to be mild but prolonged. 4) Given a peripheral relationship between bereaved and deceased and the belief that the death was unpreventable, we would expect the grieving process to be both mild and brief.

Four abbreviated case studies may help to further clarify each of the above grief reactions. The first two are from Lindemann (1944), the latter two from the author's own clinical experience.

Intense and Prolonged

"Some weeks after the Cocoanut Grove fire a young man aged 32, who had received only minor burns, left the hospital apparently well. . . . On the fifth day he had learned that his wife had died. He became restless, did not want to stay at home, had taken a trip to relatives trying to find rest, had not succeeded, and returned home in a state of marked agitation, appearing preoccupied, frightened, and unable to concentrate on any organized activity. His family returned him to the hospital. He was restless, could not sit still. . . and fell into repeated murmured utterances: 'Nobody can help me. When is it going to happen? I am doomed, am I not?' He complained about his feeling of extreme tension, inability to breathe and exhaustion. 'I'm destined to live in insanity or I must die. I know that it is God's will. I have this awful feeling of guilt.' Reviewing his morbid guilt feelings revealed the facts of the fire. When he tried to pull his wife out of the fire, he had fainted and was shoved out by the crowd. She was burned while he was saved. 'I should have saved her or I should have died too.' Eventually, after months of agonized grief this man jumped through a window to a violent death." (p. 146)

By definition, centrality refers to those whose presence and importance is so profound that, "I feel I have no life without them." The apparent meaninglessness of this man's life suggests the strong likelihood of a central relationship with his wife. The power and intensity of this condition is amplified many times over by the belief that he personally might have prevented her death. The interaction of these two determinants lends substance to a prediction that the grieving process would be both intense and prolonged. The intensity of this man's grief was certainly apparent. The severity of his despair and guilt also strongly suggest that his grief response would be quite prolonged. It was perhaps the hopelessness of assuaging such an incapacitating and prolonged grieving process which led to the suicide.

The *belief* that a death might have been prevented is the single most influential factor contributing to the prolongation of the human grief response. Preventability may be presumed to be a factor when any cause of death is unknown or when the mourner was present at the time of death. Another example of profound significance is crib death. Which parents have not shuddered at the approach of their child's third month of life and subsequently breathed a deep sigh of relief in welcoming the twelfth month. The combination of proximity and unknown etiology suggest both an intense and prolonged grief response for parents of any crib death.

Intense and Brief

"A woman, aged 40, lost her husband in the Cocoanut Grove fire. She had one child ten years old. When she heard about her husband's death she was extremely depressed, cried bitterly, did not want to live, and for three days showed a state of utter dejection. When seen by a psychiatrist she was glad to have assistance and described her painful preoccupation with memories of her husband. She had a vivid visual image of his presence, picturing him as going to work in the morning and herself as wondering whether he would return in the evening to play with the dog, his child.... It was only after ten days that she succeeded in accepting his loss and then only after having described in detail the remarkable qualities of her husband and his deep devotion to her. In subsequent interviews she explained with distress that she had become very much attached to the examiner and that she waited for his coming. She soon came to see these signs of her ability to fill the gap he had left in her life. She then showed a marked drive for activity, making plans for supporting herself, her little girl, resuming her old profession of secretary while making efforts to secure help from the occupational therapy department...." (p. 143)

This woman's vivid recollections of her husband's behavioral commitments each day (i.e., going to work, playing with dog and child) suggest a central relationship. Her belief that his love was a needed element in her daily routine contributed to her initial wish to die, and also outlined this man's importance to her. Nowhere in this case study is there any indication that she believed that his death might have been prevented. An intense but brief grief response would be predicted given such information. Her behavior bore this out, as she painfully wrestled with the agony of detaching herself from her dead husband, while also finding new patterns of rewarding interaction. The support of her psychiatrist certainly seemed to facilitate her coping with the process of reestablishment.

Mild and Prolonged

A relatively young doctor, aged 36, had just completed his residency and was working in a large metropolitan hospital. On a particular day he had to perform abdominal surgery on a 21-year-old female whose stomach had ulcerated to such an extent that immediate removal of half of the tissue appeared necessary. During the course of the operation, the patient began to hemorrhage and died within five minutes on the table. The final few minutes of agonized effort in this irreversible condition left the young doctor distraught. Believing that more expeditious use of clamps and diagnostic workups might have prevented the rapid deterioration of the patient's status, the doctor felt very much to blame and repeatedly muttered on his way out of the operating room, "Why did my first one have to be like this." During the next seven months irritability was an apparent beacon warning other hospital personnel that this doctor was about to operate on a "young woman." Supportive counseling by colleagues eventually helped this man work through the lingering doubts and preoccupation which accompanied him in these special circumstances.

Of the four reactions suggested in this paper, this condition is perhaps the most difficult to define. Most grief reactions which do linger are likely to be more intense than mild, or at least to begin as more intense states. As portrayed above, however, a personal belief that one is responsible for another's death may certainly trigger a prolonged reaction of this nature. The irritability mentioned in the narrative, though quite noticeable to hospital support staff, was not debilitating. The mildness of this doctor's response in part reflects the nature of his relationship to the deceased. Though her presence was both felt and respected, the doctor's usual daily rewards and pleasures were not contingent upon the behavior or presence of the deceased. Perhaps even more contributory to the mildness of this brief reaction is the notion that many doctors either deny or are reluctant to share their feelings. As Kasper (1965) strongly pointed out,

> While touched by pain and saddened by each patient's death, [doctors] often contrive to show their feelings in devious and distorted ways. (p. 268)

Mild and Brief

> While walking down a busy street in New York, an adolescent boy notices an elderly man staggering 30 feet ahead of him. Before he knows what happened the man collapsed and a crowd has formed around him. Stunned the boy rushes to the packed crowd quite aware this his own heart is pumping rapidly and his face is flushed. He is aware of being pushed by the crowd, someone screaming, "Get an ambulance," while someone utters, "It's too late." The lad is aware that the old man is dead, and that he has witnessed his first death. Slowly walking away, he takes time to stop in front of a store window a block away from the frightening scene he has just witnessed. Peering at himself with unknown intensity, he again becomes aware of his beating heart, his own flushed face, and sweating palms. Sensing the contrast between these sensations and their absence in the old man, the boy swallows hard and understands that for the first time he has feared his own dying. Then, as though a breeze propels him, he runs off very quickly. He knows that he has a baseball game to make and must concentrate on winning.

The adolescent boy in this vignette experienced both a mild and brief grief reaction, as would be expected on the basis of the known determinants. The relationship between the boy and old man is clearly peripheral, and the old man's loss is in no way seen as irreplaceable. In addition, there were no indications that the boy "believed" that the death was preventable. Given these factors, the boy's brief encounter with his own inevitable death is as predictable as is its quick denial. This scene, in fact, may capture the American way of life and death. We are forever being bombarded with images, scenes, and news of death through both electronic and paper media. The peripherality and anonymity of the countless victims allows us to escape from death and experience minimal pain.

THE INTERVENTION PROCESS

The grief model presented is a dynamic model. Not only can movement be monitored by the model, but actual interventions suggested. Positive movement essentially occurs in two ways: 1) an individual may move from a belief in preventability to a belief in unpreventability, or 2) an individual may shift a relationship with the deceased from centrality to peripherality.

The belief that a death was preventable suggests an intense grief reaction, according to the model. In order to mollify the intensity to a more mild and manageable state, a shift in belief towards unpreventability must occur. Traditional methods of grief work may succeed in encouraging a shift in belief or reduction of guilt. Such methods usually include empathic listening, unconditional positive regard, reassurance, physical presence and contact, and general acceptance. Attitude change research, however, suggests that stronger interventions must occur in order to change belief (Hovland, 1959). In addition to the above effective techniques, the clinician must recognize the cognitive structure supporting the belief of preventability. Every conceivable strategy that can contradict this belief should be used to dissuade the mourner, particularly when he or she feels personally responsible for the death.

The first case study presented the situation of a young man who was overwhelmed with guilt regarding the death of his wife. Recognizing that the alleviation of his intense grieving was dependent upon an attitude change toward unpreventability, every credible source should have been consulted. These might have included: 1) a doctor who would stress the physical incapability of the mourner to save his wife due to smoke inhalation and subsequent fainting; 2) a priest who might argue against the patient's belief that it was God's will that he die; 3) an engineer who might enumerate various elements of the physical structure at the scene of the fire which made the survivor a victim of that particular environment; and 4) other widows and widowers who might have experienced guilt feelings of their own and were willing to track their own movement toward unpreventability.

Where a mourner does not know the cause of death, a belief that the death was preventable is most likely. Every effort should be made to establish the cause of death, particularly in situations where the death occurred suddenly in the presence of the mourner. For instance, by seeking a consultation from a number of pathologists, a sufficient understanding of an autopsy report may reveal biological causes and dispel the notion that prompter action by the mourner may have saved the victim's life.

The belief that a death might have been prevented is such a powerful dynamic that some doctors take every conceivable precaution to ensure that such a belief never establishes itself. One rather controversial strategy is never to let relatives make life and death decisions regarding surgical techniques. This should be the doctor's domain, particularly in cases of potential child mortality. Should the patient die, the family is thus spared the guilt of having made a "wrong" decision. Though such strategies have merit according to the model, the trend of the times is to increase the decision-making prerogative of the public in cases of euthanasia, abortion, and living wills. This increases control but decreases the sense of preventability. Controversy surely lies ahead.

The second major shift in any grief reaction is a change in relationship from centrality to peripherality. In order to curtail a prolonged grieving process, this shift must occur. Individuals who believe that they now have no life of their own or who cling to symbolic vestiges of the deceased will perceive their world only through grief-colored glasses. An active helping process with such individuals can work toward two goals: 1) facilitating the needed detachment of the mourner from the deceased, and 2) facilitating the mourner's process of reconstructing new patterns of living. The first detachment step is a sensitive stage requiring the skills and patience of an understanding person. Talking through the hurt and pain, encouraging the mourner to review his or her life with the loved one, and learning to say good-bye are difficult processes that can be influenced by others. The essential key to this process requires working through the common idea that the dead, one's family, friends, society, and God will somehow disapprove if we even think of having a new life on our own. Understanding this hesitancy and guilt, it behooves family, friends, ministers, and perhaps psychologists to sanction this needed "letting go" process, while encouraging in addition the required reconstruction process.

The middle-aged woman in the second case study represents a good example of this working-through process. An unnecessarily prolonged grieving process was curtailed through the help of the "examiner," most likely a psychiatrist. The woman needed to review her relationship with her dead husband and accept his loss as a first step. Secondly, she needed assurance from someone—in this case, the examiner—that she was still respectable and lovable. She did not need to feel guilty for being attracted to the examiner. Only then was she ready to "fill the gap" and make new plans not only for herself, but also for her children.

In conclusion, it must be stressed that this model is not being presented as a panacea for either understanding or working through human grief. It is offered, however, as having potential value as a resource in working with the bereaved. Understanding that a belief in preventability will most likely lead to an intense grief reaction, for instance, may provide a pathway through the thicket of congested feelings and swirling thoughts. It is hoped that the torturous grief of the mourner may be in some measure assuaged by the application of the model.

REFERENCES

Cannon, W. "Voodoo" death. *American Anthropology*, 1942, *44*, 169-181.

Engel, G. Sudden and rapid death during psychological stress: Folklore or folkwisdom? *Annals of Internal Medicine*, 1971, *74*, 771-782.

Ferrari, N. *Institutionalization and attitude change in an aged population: A field study and dissidence theory.* Doctoral dissertation, Western Reserve University, 1962.

Hovland, C. Reconciling conflicting results derived from experimental and survey studies of attitude change. *American Psychology*, 1959, *14*, 8-17.

Kasper, A. 1965. The doctor and death. In H. Feifer (Ed.), *The meaning of death.* New York: McGraw-Hill Book Co., 1965.

Kavanaugh, R. *Facing death.* Baltimore: Penguin Books, 1972.

Kubler-Ross, E. *On death and dying.* New York: Macmillan Publishing Co., 1969.

Lindemann, E. Symptomatology and management of acute grief. *American Journal of Psychiatry*, 1944, *101*, 141-148.

Schoenberg, B., et al. Anticipatory grief. New York: Columbia University Press, 1974.

Schulz, R., & Aderman, D. 1973. Effect of residential change on the temporal distance to death of terminal cancer patients. *Omega*, 1973, *2*, 147-162.

Seligman, M. *Helplessness: On depression, development, and death.* San Francisco: W. H. Freeman & Co., 1975.

PERSONAL STATEMENT ......
Ted

Changing from a fully functioning, young, athletic college student to a comatose, nonverbal invalid can take place in a matter of seconds. To recover may require years; some may never recover. For me, being alive today is a miracle. Following the motorcycle accident which resulted in a brainstem contusion, my family was informed that it was unlikely that I would live. The following presentation is my perspective on my personal struggle to beat the odds. Not only was I able to win, but I was also able to rise above the physical and emotional strain placed on my life.

PERSONAL STATEMENT

As a college student I was at the point in my life of having everything going for me. I was happy as a student at the University of Maine, had a girlfriend, and was actively involved as a member of the track team. My preoccupations at that time centered around my independence, my future, and the variety of other joys and pleasures which were part of my life and that of my friends.

The summer prior to my senior year in 1975 I was employed as a construction worker. To reduce the amount of time I would have to spend traveling to my home, I was living in a tent. It was a taste of the pioneer life, living in the outdoors, working and basically enjoying my sense of independence from my family. This need for independence and self-sufficiency had been an issue in the relationship with my parents and had caused some conflict between us. At this time I had no idea that I would soon become the most helpless, dependent person imaginable.

On August 23, 1975, I was riding my motorcycle, enjoying the beauty of the Maine summer's evening. My last recollection was that I
was out of control. The next thing I remembered was that it was November and I was in a
hospital. Having no speech and being partially
paralyzed, my life at that time was one of confusion, desperation, and challenge. I had a hard
time putting the pieces together, but I somehow
realized that I was hurting. I knew that I
needed people to maintain my life supports
since I could not do anything on my own. My
decision at this time was if I am going to survive, I must draw people to me. I could not act
up because I may drive them away.

What made a difference to me at this time
was the support given to me by my family and
friends, who were always there. Their presence
and encouragement made me want to make an
effort to do as much for myself as others had
hoped for me.

Being unable to speak since I came out of
my coma, I was in a position of having to deal
internally with the many issues that I was terrified and uncertain of, such as will I ever be
able to speak, walk, or even approximate a
semi-normal life. This is where the encouragement and input from the medical staff really
made a difference for me. They conveyed a feeling of confidence and support that made me
want to try even though I did not know how far
I would be able to go. At this point in time the
personal relationships I had were just as important to me emotionally as the life supports were
to me physically.

There was a critical turning point in my
attitude when I began to attain some degree of
independence. I became angry. I could not verbalize this anger, but it was there. It began to
consume me. I went through the range of emotions, such as bitterness, hatred, disappointment, and fear. Here I was, 21 years old, a
practical vegetable. How can I go on. I had a
choice again: either rise above it or die emotion-

ally, physically, or both. I chose to live, to fi-
guratively reach out and grasp whatever bit of
life I could. I attribute this choice primarily to
my experience as a member of the track team—
having to be independent and reach inside
myself to tap resources I did not think were
there: To go the extra Mile.

However, having made the choice, I had to
still have the external motivation to go on. My
nurses provided that. They were realistic, non-
patronizing, attentive to me, and made me work
hard. I saw them in the same light as a coach
who was there primarily to help me win. At the
same time they gave me constant input, again
being unable to verbalize, I was in need of the
monitoring from the outside world. It is terrifying to think what would have happened to me if
I was ignored.

I often wonder how many severely injured
or ill people are life in isolation and become
stagnant because they are nonresponsive like I
was. This is the thought I carry with me to this
day: "How lucky I was that people did care."
During my hospitalization, my brothers from
the fraternity maintained a constant vigil. Their
presence was an additional support to the family and medical personnel, especially during the
difficult times when I was faced with major
choices, such as "Why try or why struggle."

As time passed, my attitudes of
hopelessness, hatred, anger, and self-pity began
to give way to hope and optimism. In retrospect
I believe this can be attributed to the small
gains that I was able to make. I could feel,
begin to speak, and regained a variety of body
controls. While great gains were not made, there
was significant progress to have me appreciate
the fact that I was moving, no matter how
slowly.

A traumatizing thought for me was how
would I have coped if I had to remain a semi-
conscious vegetable for the rest of my life. When
I considered the potential realities of what could

have happened I suddenly become most appreciative.

As I reflect upon where I have been and where I am today: able to walk, talk with a slight impediment, and remember most things, I find myself aspiring to qualitative improvements in my life. I wish that my speech could continue to improve and that I could walk better, although if I had my choice, I would choose speaking clearer over walking better.

Interpersonally I have many friends, but I am missing one important dimension and that is a girlfriend. Prior to the accident I had a girlfriend; after it, I did not.

At this time my major stumbling block is myself. I cannot see what any girl would see in me. Deep inside I guess I am hoping that I will make more gains prior to seeking out a relationship. My rationale is that the more improved I am, the better chance I have of not being rejected. However, I am aware enough to realize that the gains I make may not be tremendous and that I have to accept myself the way I am before another person could accept me. What I have going for me is my ability to place myself in situations where I can learn and experience new things. This is part of my personal rehabilitation effort to maximize my chances for success. I do not know how far I can go but I know that I will try.

MOTHER

Ted has asked me to record some of my reactions to his accident, illness, hospitalization, and handicap. I look back over the past 2½ years and I find my memory is fragmentary, surrealistic, and shrouded in fog. Therefore, I will present these thoughts as chronologically as I can but in a more or less stream-of-consciousness style; that is the way I remember them.

The call from the accident room of the Eastern Maine Medical Center came at 6:40 pm

on Tuesday, August 23, 1975. The doctor
reported that Ted's condition was "grave" and
that he had stopped breathing several times. I
felt very calm as I reminded the doctor that he
had been an associate of my late father (a physician and member of the staff at EMMC for many
years), and that I wished everything to be done
for my son. Ted's father and I rushed to the
hospital prayerfully fearful.

Ted was in the Critical Care Section, con-
vulsing and surrounded by aides, doctors,
nurses, tubes, machines, wires—and he was dirty. Ted's father was sure he would live; I was
sure that he would die.

The rest of the night was unreal—we
learned as much as we could about the accident—we called our daughter, relatives, and
physicians—signed papers—listened to
reports—a 5% chance to live.

Most terrible of all was that there was
nothing I could do but wait helplessly. For a
month of coma, I waited. Through several infections, operations, x-rays, I waited. I asked,
"Why?" There was no answer. I was terrified,
and still there was so very little I could actively do.

School began, and I returned to work. This
was a very great help to me—my mind was
taken up and I was active. We all experienced a
sort of "yo-yo" condition—way up with hope
one day, down with despair on the next.

Friends, students, acquaintances, and
relatives were extremely supportive. Finally,
Ted came to. His eyes opened, he moved—not
much but a little. He would blink twice for
"no" and once for "yes." I really think I had
hoped it would be like a soap opera—he would
open his eyes, say, "Where am I?" and get up
out of bed and come home. If I had ever known
how very long it would be! He was moved from
CCU to the neurological section of the hospital.
This was somewhat traumatic for us all because
the care was not so careful or so intensive.

About this point I really came to grips with the problem. I had stopped my why's and self-pity, swallowed **some** of my overweening pride, and accepted the fact that whatever happened, God's will, not mine, would prevail. At last I could cope.

Daily visits were the rule. Ted still could not speak, but we discovered that he could read. Physical therapy was started; he could sit up with help. He looked awful—retarded—painfully thin like a survivor of Bergen-Belsen. Our physicians were optimistic and had stopped repeating: "The condition is stable; he's holding his own; his vital signs are good." How I hate those words! Tubes were removed one at a time—food, real food, was given. I was amused; Ted ate everything. He'd always been an exceedingly fussy eater, and I used to threaten, "Someday you'll be so hungry, you'll eat that!" Vindication #1!

On Thanksgiving Day he came home to dinner. He still could not speak, had to be tied into the wheelchair so he'd not fall out, had a suprapubic cateheter, and had to be fed. But he could smile; he could communicate (sort of); and oh, how he could eat! More. chicken soup?

From that point on he came home each Sunday and by Christmas he could talk—not always intelligibly, but talk. Astonishing to us all was Ted's personality change. He was cheerful, cooperative, and happy (this was very different from the sometimes surly, self-conscious, and somewhat withdrawn person we were used to). Somewhere along the line he'd learned to laugh at himself and to know he had to accept our help. Vindication #2; I'd told him **that,** too!

In February Ted was allowed to come home for a week. I was very apprehensive about this. He was pretty helpless—catheter still, not very mobile, had to be dressed. The one thing I'd **never** wanted to be was a nurse. I resent sick people, and mechanically (with tubes and such), I'm a klutz. However, I buoyed my sagging con-

fidence by figuring I was as smart as some of
the aides who'd been caring for him at the hospital (pride again). We both survived the experience. Ministering to a 6-foot 2-inch baby is different.

It was very difficult to return him to the
hospital. But in another month he was home for
good. We tried to keep everything as normal as
possible. The only physical changes in the
house were removing thresholds and one rug,
and rearranging furniture for easier passage of
the wheelchair.

Again fortune smiled and sent us a young
man who stayed with Ted 2 days of our working
week, a girl 1 day, and our housekeeper the
other 2. These individuals were all involved in
the rehab process and were inventive therapists.
I worried and tried to stave off any pitfalls. (I
am still too protective.) Hospital therapy was
continued on an outpatient basis, and Ted
worked very hard to recover. We all did.

A word here about the hospital—Ted was at
EMMC for 7 months. He received excellent care,
and we were supported by the interest and the
involvement of the entire staff. Everyone from
the lady who pushed the dinner cart to the
senior physicians were exceedingly cooperative.
I liked especially the honesty, humor, and realistic approach which everyone seemed to have.
Questions were always answered; my only problem was in knowing what questions to ask.
Ted's sister, Debbie, took over at this point. She
was preparing for two degrees, one in psychology and one in nursing. She knew what to question. Her sense of the ridiculous also smoothed
some rough seas. When Ted started to talk
(croak?), she spent the afternoon telling him
jokes about people with speech impediments. He
loved it! Whenever there was a new problem,
Debbie found the book where we could study
and learn.

Ted's physical progress was coming. I
hoped to keep his mind active and pushed him

to plan and to return to school. I shuddered
when he could not do things which seem so
easy to us who have no physical handicaps, but
I tried to be less fearful for him. We, his family,
took him to restaurants, to stores, to sports
events so that he'd be used to society. He moved
from the wheelchair to crutches and, oh joy, in
August he participated as an attendant in a
friend's wedding. Everyone was ecstatic.

He returned to college, commuting for the
first semester and living at his fraternity the
second. He graduated. Out of 1600 black-clad
seniors, he was the one with **one** crutch.

Now he walked, talked understandably, had
a part-time job, and was accepted to graduate
school. It was difficult for me to let him start
off to the unfamiliar "big city" with so many
problems. But I felt that he had to be independent and live his own life. He does.

How do I feel now? I have intense pride in
his achievements and his hard work. I am
greatly indebted to so many people for their interest and support. Most of all I'm grateful that
he has been able to recover and that we as a
family—my husband, my daughter, and I—have
had the resources to help him. I hurt when he
falls, but I try to accept it. We all try to be as
realistic as possible about the future and to face
it all with gratitude, with faith, and with
humor. When people ask me, and they do, how
does one survive a period such as this, I quote
Pearl Buck, who had one of her suffering characters reply: "I really cannot face it, but I
must."

FATHER

I was working in the garden when Charlotte
came running out saying, "Teddy's had a
motorcycle accident and it's bad." I went cold
and thought, "Oh, my God, he's dead. Can Charlotte stand it?"

From then on I did what had to be done,
driving cautiously to the emergency room, going

to critical care, seeing Teddy mechanized and
with blood on his face but not really marked. I
don't remember my thoughts. I do recall thinking, "He's not dead yet." I called people. Without being reminded, I'm not sure who beyond
my sister-in-law. Billy Deighan was sitting in
the waiting room (Billy was with Teddy when
the accident happened). I don't remember what
he or I said. Debbie (Teddy's sister) and her
friends arrived. We sat in the CCU waiting room
waiting with others who were waiting as we
were. It was a close community; we became
close.

There were the crises. I prayed he would die
rather than become a vegetable. I don't remember the point at which I knew he would live. It
wasn't many days after the accident. At that
time I came back to earth and realized what was
and what might be. I cried.

From then on it was a treadmill on which I
thought about the outcome as little as I could
force myself to do. The details of the first 6
months or so are blurred. I probably prefer it
that way.

As Teddy improved my biggest concern was,
"How much are his intellectual and reasoning
faculties damaged? And if they're not what
dents will being crippled put in his psyche?"

My background as an engineer puts a lot of
trust in absolutes. If this is done, that will
result. Although I know what statistics are, the
2-year limit on improvement weighed heavily.
Would he improve to the point where he would
see the future as promising?

At the present stage in his recovery I'm
sure he has answered the questions I had, and
if no further physical improvement is made,
he'll still be able to make his way. The fact that
I see continuing improvement is added frosting
on a cake that is already much larger than I
dared hope.

RECOMMENDED READINGS
FOR SECTION III

Aguilera, D., & Messick, J. *Crisis intervention—Theory and methodology.* St. Louis: C. V. Mosby Co., 1974.

Anthony, W., & Carkhuff, R. The art of health care. Amherst, Mass.: Human Resource Development Press, 1976.

Becker, M., & Green, L. A family approach to compliance with medical treatment. *International Journal of Health Education,* 1975, *18*(3), 3–13.

Bocian, M., & Kaback, M. Crisis counseling: The newborn infant with a chromosomal anomaly. *Pediatric Clinics of North America,* 1978, *25,* 643–650.

Breu, C., & Dracup, K. Helping the spouses of critically ill patients. *American Journal of Nursing,* 1978, January, 51–53.

Buscaglia, L. *The disabled and their parents: A counseling challenge.* Thorofare, N.J.: Charles B. Slack, 1975.

Croog, S., Lipson, A., & Levine, S. Help patterns in severe illness: The roles of kin network, non-family resources, and institutions. *Journal of Marriage and the Family,* 1972, February, 32–41.

Dixon, S. *Working with people in crisis—Theory and practice.* St. Louis: C. V. Mosby Co., 1979.

Eichel, E. Assessment with a family focus. *JPN and Mental Health Services,* 1978, January, 11–14.

Foley, V. *An introduction to family therapy.* New York: Grune & Stratton, 1974.

Glasser, P., & Glasser, L. (Eds.). *Families in crisis.* New York: Harper & Row Publishers, 1970.

Haley, J. *Problem-solving therapy.* New York: Harper & Row Publishers, 1976.

Hall, J., & Weaver, B. *Nursing of families in crisis.* Philadelphia: J. B. Lippincott, 1974.

Jones, W. Grief and involuntary career change: Its implications for counseling. *The Vocational Guidance Quarterly,* 1979, March, 196–201.

Kaplan, B., & Cassel, J. (Eds.). Family and health: An epidemiological approach. Chapel Hill: Institute for Research in Social Science, University of North Carolina, 1975.

Kaplan, D., & Mearig, J. A community support system for a family coping with chronic illness. *Rehabilitation Literature,* *38*(3), 79–82.

Kevner, J., et al. The impact of grief: A retrospective study of family function following loss of a child with cystic fibrosis. *Journal of Chronic Diseases,* 1979, *32,* 221–225.

Mooney, T. O., et al. *Sexual options for paraplegics and quadraplegics.* Boston: Little, Brown & Co., 1975.

Noland, R. (Ed.). *Counseling parents of the ill and the handicapped.* Springfield, Ill.: Charles C Thomas Publisher, 1971.

Panieczko, S., Cornelius, D., & Frank, W. *Sex and disability—An annotated bibliography, '75-'77.* Washington, D.C.: Regional Rehabilitation Research Institute, George Washington University.

Quigley, J. Understanding depression—Helping with grief. *Rehabilitation Gazette,* 1976, *19,* 2-6.

Schwab, L. Rehabilitation of physically disabled women in a family-oriented program. *Rehabilitation Literature,* 1975, *36,* 34-43.

Schwab, R. Loss, pain, and growth. *Personnel and Guidance Journal,* 1979, April, 429-431.

Sex education, counseling, and therapy for the physically handicapped. Washington, D.C.: American Association of Sex Education and Counselors (AASEC), 1979.

Simos, B. Grief therapy to facilitate healthy restitution. *Social Casework,* 1977, June, 337-342.

Stewart, S., & Johansen, R. A family systems approach to home dialysis. *Psychotherapy and Psychosomatics,* 1976/77, *27,* 86-92.

Within reach—Providing planning services to physically disabled women. Everett, Wash.: Planned Parenthood of Snohomish County, 1977.

Younghusband, E. (Ed.). *Case-work with families and children.* Chicago: University of Chicago Press, 1965.

Zuk, G., & Boszormenyi-Nagy, I. (Eds.). *Family therapy and disturbed families.* Palo Alto, Cal.: Science and Behavior Books, 1967.

CONCLUSION

In discussing the many excuses offered by rehabilitation counselors for reducing the expectations others have regarding the professional's behavior, Sink (1979) cites a prevalent one: "The family doesn't cooperate. They are over protective, don't approve of the vocational objective, or they won't let the client go to work" (p. 3). The goal of this book has been to bring the family into sharper focus as a vital force in the rehabilitation process. It indicates that within the family many influences exist that can aid or deter rehabilitation. Although many health professionals believe that the family is to blame for its lowered patient expectations, just the realization that one patient's psychosocial environment is being attended to is a step toward the possibility of greater rehabilitation productivity.

Physical disability or chronic illness affects the entire family, and the chapters of this book have been organized to illustrate how disability affects family members, and, in turn, how family members influence the patient. Some of the possible negative or constructive family influences that can reinforce the client's rehabilitative behavior include: the emotional reaction of the patient and the family members from the trauma of a disabling condition, the varied cultural and societal influences on the modern family, communication patterns within the family, and the kind of information the family members understand about the disability or illness and their level of expectations for the patient. Margolin (1971) reports unpublished data that indicates that the quality of interpersonal relationships within the family is more important than the disability itself (Treischmann, 1978). It is the conviction of the authors that these influences must be understood before a rehabilitation plan is developed. In becoming aware of these influences the health professional can then show the family's effectiveness in assisting a client's rehabilitation.

The chapters in this book also explain the different skills for helping the family to play an instrumental role in rehabilitation. An explanation of how these skills can be applied to varied family circumstances makes it more of a reality for the health professional to provide services to family members as part of a client's rehabilitation. The rehabilitation act of 1973, as amended, authorizes provision of services to members of a handicapped person's family when such services are necessary to the adjustment or rehabilitation of the handicapped individual. This book shows how to give such services to help the family adjust to the disability and to aid in the rehabilitation of a family member.

It is imperative that the family not disintegrate because of stress of dealing with the disability. Research shows that most family members are able to adjust to the increased stresses resulting from disability (Abrams, 1978). To facilitate this adjustment appropriate and timely intervention is needed. Through such intervention with key family members, or by securing counseling services for them, the health professional may be able to influence the family's reaction to the client's condition in a way that leads to acceptance and support, rather than rejection.

There are many other roles for helpers when working with the client's family. They may establish supportive services, such as support groups for spouses, that may be of particular help to two groups of spouses. Spouses of clients with a sudden-onset disability, such as a heart attack, continue to experience particular stress for as long as a year. Spouses of clients with progressive, deteriorative disabilities may experience increasing stress as the client's condition worsens. With the cooperation and guidance of the patient's physician, the helper can encourage the client's family to provide many types of home treatment assistance that will augment the client's rehabilitation progress. The health professional can also teach the family ways to reinforce rehabilitation gains of the client (Abrams, 1978).

The themes that have been developed in this book are well illustrated by the personal statement of Lois and the two following articles. Lois's story contains much of this volume's material in microcosm. She explains the emotional impact that the diagnosis and progression of diabetes had on her, and identifies how she coped with the not-too-apparent implications of the illness. As her vision gradually grew worse, and the disease itself became a troublesome factor for her, she had to deal with depression and dwindling hope. It is a battle that she fought at times alone and at times with family support; the family support was a strong resource, particularly in her earlier years. Lois's account is a testimony of what one person can do to handle the progressive experiences associated with a disease. It shows the almost hidden influence of the family on a person's confidence for the future.

The article by Shellhase and Shellhase highlights the importance of the patient maintaining "an active membership in his family" (p. 545). They discuss the family reaction to trauma and present an important assumption that the patient's orientation to the family can be influenced both positively and negatively by the individual's relationships within the rehabilitation setting. In discussing the varied professional supports to the family, these authors emphasize the continuing attention to the family as a unit during the rehabilitation experience. Ruth Lindenberg's article is a review of the literature of practitioners and educators who have studied family influences on the attitudes and behavior of disabled persons. In reporting the family influences on rehabilitation outcome, the rehabilitation programs, which include families, and rehabilitation personnel attitudes, she concludes that working with families has been a missing component of rehabilitation practice. Her article suggests how the rehabilitation process can be greatly enhanced by including family strategies, and identifies some of the obstacles preventing this involvement. Both articles are valuable complements to the material developed in the book. They provide further evidence that a more effective model in rehabilitation is one that recognizes and utilizes psychological and family factors in the patient's environment.

Assisting patients and families to cope with severe disability and traumatic illness is usually a long-term process. It involves the efforts of health professionals who are attuned to the needs of the patient and who are alert for cues suggesting how the family can be supportive. Families can offer tremendous support to the disabled. Yet however significant family members can be in meeting the needs of the disabled, "their own needs and those of the rest of the family must also be recognized and dealt with" (Connors, 1978, p. 38). Family members themselves need support. To provide such support implies that the health professional is aware that the process of the family adjusting to physical disabilities is never an easy task, nor is it one that is accomplished with finality and then put aside. Assisting the family to adjust is also helping the family to become a more influential force in the patient's rehabilitation. Throughout all these endeavors the health professional is continually working with families so that they are in a position, as Malone (1977) states it, "to avoid those situations which can be avoided, to change those situations which can be changed, and to accept those which cannot be altered" (p. 97).

REFERENCES

Abrams, K. The role of the family in rehabilitation. *Rehabilitation Brief,* 1978, *1,* 1-2.

Connors, K. *Families and disabled adults.* A monograph prepared for educational use at Howard Community College, Columbia, Md., 1978.

Malone, R. L. Expressed attitudes of families of aphasics. In J. Stubbins (Ed.), *Social and Psychological Aspects of Disability,* pp. 97-102. Baltimore: University Park Press, 1977.

Margolin, R. Motivational problems and resolutions in the rehabilitation of paraplegics and quadraplegics. *American Achives of Rehabilitation Therapy,* 1971, *20,* 94-103.

Sink, J. When you care enough to offer the best excuse. *Journal of Rehabilitation,* 1979, January/February/March, 3.

Treischmann, R. The psychological, social, and vocational adjustment to spinal cord injury: A strategy for future research. *Final Report,* Easter Seal Society of Los Angeles County, 1978, April.

WORK WITH FAMILIES IN REHABILITATION

Ruth Ellen Lindenberg[1]

Studies show that family influences have direct bearing on the attitudes and behavior of disabled persons and suggest that these influences may be importantly related to the outcome of rehabilitation. Articles and pronouncements of some practitioners and educators suggest the need to view the disabled persons within the larger systems that surround them. Certain rehabilitation programs do include work with families, although these manifestations are rare. This article will: a) review findings that relate to family influences on the disabled; b) offer suggestions that may stimulate the inclusion of the family in rehabilitation practice; c) explore programs that include work with families which might serve as models; and d) examine the extent to which the family is perceived by rehabilitation counselors and educators as a component of the rehabilitation process.

FAMILY INFLUENCES ON REHABILITATION OUTCOME

Limited studies are available that include family influences among variables studied. In studying 62 hemiplegics who had received extensive counseling at the Institute for Rehabilitation Medicine in New York, Weisbroth, Esibill, and Zuger (1971) examined physical status, demographic data, cognition, and vocational program, but included no variables related to family influences. Scholl, Baumann, and Crissey (1969) deplored that earlier follow-up studies left the relationship of multiple variables largely unexplored, but proceeded to mount a study of the vocational success of the visually handicapped that included only one variable related to family influence, i.e., socioeconomic status of the rehabilitant's family of origin. This factor was found, incidentally, to be of no significance.

A few studies show that persons living in a family unit, whether that of origin or procreation, fare better in vocational success than unattached persons. Neff (1959) found success in employment associated with positive family attitudes toward the client and active family support when he studied the employment status of 217 former clients of the Jewish Vocational Service in Chicago one year after they completed their program. Age, intelli-

Reprinted from *Rehabilitation Counseling Bulletin* 20(1), pp. 67–76, © 1977, American Personnel and Guidance Association, with permission.

[1]Professor, Department of Social Services, Cleveland State University.

gence, disability, and even previous employment experiences were unrelated. Clients who were rated high on likelihood of employability at the time program was completed and who were known to have high family support, were employed in greater numbers a year later. Also, those clients with lower predicted employability, but with high family interest, did better in gaining employment than those without family support. McPhee and Magleby (1960) in a study involving 288 clients of the Montana Bureau of Vocational Rehabilitation four to nine years after termination of program found significant differences between the substantially employed, the unsubstantially employed, and the minimally employed in the areas of education, motivation, age, stable marriage, and family relationships. Differences were observed among each of the groups in nine specific areas. For example, more of the substantially employed than the unsubstantially employed and the minimally employed were married, had children, lived with and supported their families, participated in social activities with family members, had greater feelings of accomplishment related to family, attended church, and reported no family problems associated with their rehabilitation. Similar findings linking marital status and support of dependents with success in employment were evident in the follow-up study of 163 discharged tuberculosis patients treated at Cook County Suburban Hospital in Chicago (Weiner, 1964). Olshansky and Beach (1975) examined the characteristics of a group of physically disabled persons who could not secure employment subsequent to training at the Community Workshop in Boston. These investigators found a heavy incidence of separated, divorced, and widowed persons. Wardlow (1974) and Sandovsky (1974) in studies of program "discontinuers" found discontinuance related to such factors as homesickness, family problems and emotional difficulties. Similar findings have been reported for clients with psychiatric problems (Freeman & Simmons, 1963; Neuhaus, 1968). Jarvik, Salzberger, and Falck (1974) found similar characteristics with deaf clients.

Galloway and Goldstein (1971) offered group therapy to families of 40 clients in rehabilitation programs and studied its impact on clients as contrasted with a control group. Although the experiment had problems because of some parents discontinuing and because three therapists of differing orientations led the therapy groups, ratings of clients on factors such as work organization, perseverance, productivity, work adjustment, and vocational objectives were significantly higher for the experimental group in their first four months in program. At the end of the first year, more experimental group clients were participating in advanced school and training programs, achieving better grades and reporting greater satisfactions. These clients reported increased understanding by their parents and greater satisfactions at home. Those clients on the job experienced fewer job changes, while more control-group clients were on the job with higher ratings by employers on work traits and vocational objectives. This fact was attributed by the researchers to good counseling, i.e., clients with better potential were encouraged to seek further schooling or training rather than early placement.

On the other hand, some studies report adverse outcomes of some types of family involvement. In closely studying a small group of families with a disabled member, Klausner (1969) noted that the rehabilitation was sometimes retarded because caring for a disabled person had high value for families who had built their lives around this function. In such cases, the family tended to view the prospect of independence for a disabled member less enthusiastically. Klausner concluded that it is not the individual who is disabled but the family, and that consequently the family becomes the logical unit of rehabilitation interventions. Rosenstock and Kutner (1967) point to the entry of a family member into rehabilitation as a family crisis affecting role complementarity. If previously set family roles do not shift with the new role of the person entering into rehabilitation, there will be conflict and lack of support for his or her more independent behavior. Fordyce (1971) discussed reinforcers in the home that sustain nonwork behavior and the necessity to work with the family to shift contingencies that reward behavior not conducive to change. For example, consider the inherent conflict between the reinforcements of the parents who resist their retarded son's learning to use public transportation and those of the travel trainer working to encourage travel self-sufficiency.

Studying the effect of parental attitudes on congenitally blind children, Lairy and Harrison-Covello (1973) noted the slow overall development of children whose mothers were unable to overcome their depression and to alter their overprotectiveness. Citing a matched study of blind adults at the New England Rehabilitation for Work Center, Krause (1962) reported the greater vocational success of clients who did not live at home during the period of their training and attributed this to the fact that independent living in a new milieu discouraged dependent relationships. Freeman and Simmons (1963) demonstrated that the predictions and expectations of family members of discharged mental patients influence the behavior that subsequently occurs. If successful behavior is predicted, it is more likely to occur. If regressed behavior is anticipated, the patient tends to live out this script. Beppler and Kroll (1974) in a follow-up of 34 disabled homemakers trained at the Harmarville Rehabilitation Center learned that the development of organizational and managerial skill, although critical for homemaker's progress, had to be reinforced by family participation for success.

REHABILITATION PROGRAMS WHICH INCLUDE FAMILIES

Rusalem (1969) recognized that successful rehabilitation cannot occur without family participation and cited the need to bring the family into critical phases of the process. Although it is his opinion that agencies are increasingly providing family counseling and other family oriented services, there is little evidence that this practice has impacted the rehabilitation field as a whole.

A look at some of the programs which might serve as models for agencies wishing to include families is in order. Rehabilitation programs dealing with children have the best record. In Peoria, Project Self-Help, which serves a group of multiply handicapped children (ages three to eight) in the public school program, includes family counseling as an integral part of the program (Highfill & Anderson, 1975). Beck (1973) established guidelines for programs of short-term group treatment of parents of handicapped children. Philage and Kuna (1975) reported that seeing parents and children with learning disabilities in separate and conjoint therapy groups achieved results not obtained by previous methods. Rehabilitation programs for the visually handicapped child were early comers in work with parents. The programs of the Boston Center for the Blind (Hall, 1974) and the Birth Defects Clinic of the Colorado Medical Center (Froyd, 1973) document this approach. Connor and Muldoon (1973) are convinced that family counseling needs to be built into the rehabilitation of the blind of all ages. The record for work with parents of agencies serving deaf children has also been commendable. Examples are the Children's Diagnostic Center in Vancouver, British Columbia (Freeman, Malkin, & Hastings, 1975) and the Langley Porter Project in San Francisco (Regional Rehabilitation Research Institute, 1974). Parents work side-by-side with children and teachers in the Bill Wilkerson Speech and Hearing Center in Nashville (Wildman, 1968). Aggressive work with families of the young adult deaf (Hurwitz, 1971) in a comprehensive rehabilitation program at the St. Louis Employment and Vocational Center was found to be essential to help them gain perspective on the rehabilitant and to define the role that they would need to play in the rehabilitation process. Bennington (1972) in an unusual program utilizing Satir-Gestalt techniques helped families with a deaf member learn and practice communication as a group by nonverbal methods; this helped to improve tenuous family relationships (Satir, 1972).

Experiments in work with families of other disability groups are reported in the literature. Nau's work (1972) with disadvantaged families in the Arizona Job College Family Rehabilitation Project is well known for its combination of helping strategies, such as counseling, education for living skills, and vocational skills development. Similar models according to Nau have been employed in Danish folk schools and in work with disadvantaged families, including American Indian families. Erba (1972) writes of sessions with the family as an adjunct to psychotherapy with renal disease patients who are undergoing dialysis. In addition, family work has been conducted as an adjunct to treatment with other specific disability groups, e.g., orientation groups for parents of adolescents who are mentally retarded and in a workshop setting (Scott, Debellis, & Price, 1969), self-help groups for parents of cleft-palate children (Irwin & McWilliams, 1973), and family groups in burn treatment centers (Abramson, 1975). Stroke victims' families seen in admission conferences at a Veterans Hospital pointed to the value of these sessions in helping them voice concerns, gain necessary information, and begin early planning for family members (Oradei & Waite, 1975).

REHABILITATION PERSONNEL ATTITUDES

Extensive search of the leading journals and periodicals of the rehabilitation field as well as reports of demonstration and research projects over more than a 10-year period was undertaken in an attempt to locate programs describing rehabilitation practice with families (H.E.W., Rehab. R&D Projects, 1955–1970; Vocational Rehabilitation Index, 1974). Foregoing sections of this article report the only programs described in the literature suggesting that such practice is indeed limited.

Muthard and Salomone (1969) studied a sample of 378 rehabilitation counselors employed in state rehabilitation programs and rehabilitation facilities as well as educators and representative leaders in the field to ascertain their perception of functions and roles. Counselors saw their primary functions as affective counseling, vocational counseling, case supervision, and placement. Leaders in the field, not in direct practice, wanted more emphasis on work adjustment counseling as compared to affective counseling. Rehabilitation counselor educators saw need for more emphasis on more affective and interpersonal counseling, but nothing in the findings of the study indicated that this should include family counseling.

Review of a sample of the curricula of rehabilitation counseling programs, as well as conferences and task force reports on training rehabilitation personnel, give little evidence that preparing students for work with families rates a high priority (H.E.W., SRS 73-25038, 1972; H.E.W., Region IX Task Force 1973; H.E.W., 4th Inst. Rehab Serv; Trela, 1972). Several university programs, however, do offer courses emphasizing counseling with families.

Although it appears that rehabilitation practice does not generally encompass work with families, a number of writers seek to change this. Christopherson (1962) points to the fact that rehabilitation reverses the law of the survival of the fittest and poses a new and higher moral law. In doing so, rehabilitation must be aware that restoration of function and work capacity in a disabled person is but one part of its responsibility; total success depends on concern for interpersonal and family competence. Scott (1965) deplores the fact that rehabilitation relationships are conceptualized in individualistic and psychological terms:

The focus of rehabilitation is on the individual. The problem of disability is thought to be like a trait, something that is inherent in an individual. The process is not usually thought of as part of a complex social system involving family, friends, and community. When rehabilitation fails, explanations are ordinarily psychological, such as the disabled person not being ready for service or resisting or failing to accept his handicap...Rehabilitation is a sociological process and of a type involving the whole individual (p. 136).

New directions in training suggested by Sussman, Haug, and Joynes (1970) would require a many-faceted counselor role in which the counselor would bring discrete systems together in linking and creating new subsystems. McCoy (1975), in the area of rehabilitation of the deaf, concludes that parental involvement has been a revolutionary breakthrough in the field and a primary factor in improving the chances of the deaf. Trela and O'Toole (1974) implore the counselor to get out of the office and meet clients in their natural settings. Olshansky (1972) articulates the dilemma of the counselor:

The counselor finds it difficult to understand that he(she) is involved in many conflicting and interconnected systems which may hinder the counselor and client from functioning effectively. Unless attention and thought are given to the idea of systems and ways of coping with various systems at different points in time, the counselor will continue to experience frustration (p. 231).

Usdane and Ayers (1972) recognized that the field has been deeply committed to rehabilitation as an individual process, but indicate that the time has come for new approaches.

Traditional counseling models have placed heavy emphasis on individual counseling, which are psychologically or vocationally oriented within the context of a super-ordinate, subordinate relationship. A newer model makes the counselor a broker or a merchandiser of services. The time is ripe for a model based on an ecological perspective that views the individual within the context of family relationships and broader interactional networks. In such a model, the family would become the target of intervention. The model would also suggest a more egalitarian relationship with responsibility for decision-making and control of the rehabilitation process shared among clients, families, and rehabilitation workers. What then are the roadblocks to change? Infatuation with traditional individual modes of treatment, bureaucratic pressures, resistance to "role blurring" may be factors contributing to lack of change. Productive strategies for change need development.

CONCLUSIONS AND RECOMMENDATIONS

The foregoing review of the issue regarding family work in rehabilitation points to several conclusions. First, the rehabilitation field in general reported little outcome research examining whether, as a result of rehabilitation services, persons in fact possessed better work capacity, more finely honed living skills, greater personal satisfaction, and enhanced opportunity for actualization of human potential. More attention needs to be paid to identifying and studying variables related to outcome, family influences among them. Second, although there is already evidence that work with families influences outcome, it has for the most part been a missing component of rehabilitation practice. The individual is still perceived as a free-standing entity rather than a member of a larger interacting system. Practice remains the captive of a model, which by emphasizing individual counseling, puts the family out of bounds. Third, practitioners, especially in the public vocational rehabilitation programs, seem reasonably content with the status quo. Rehabilitation counselor educators do not appear to be deeply disquieted with things as they are. Fourth, models for interventions with families exist in selected settings. These can be utilized in other settings once there is greater consciousness of the value of bringing families into the picture.

What appears to be most indicated is consciousness raising, calling attention to the need to consider the family a component in the intervention network. A number of strategies already exist that could be employed to do this. These strategies include contact with family members of new clients at the onset of program for joint goal setting and program determination; orientation groups for families of new clients; progress reviews that include client and family; and ongoing family therapy when role adjustments of family members impede the progress of the disabled persons struggling to assert themselves. Families themselves can be utilized to help other families, and closer relationships can be established with community service agencies to facilitate collaborative work. There is no dearth of approaches and techniques once there is conviction that they are critical for improved practice. Since funding sources increasingly demand accountability, and consumers' involvement is beginning to shape service planning and delivery, the present time is ripe for a change in perspective. This perspective confirms that the rehabilitation client is part of a "social network," "communication system," or "nuclear family" that shapes and affects the client's behavior and treatment.

REFERENCES

Abramson, M. Group treatment of families of burn injured patients. *Social Casework,* 1975, *56*(4), 235–241.
Beck, H. *Group treatment for parents of handicapped children* (Report). Washington, D.C.: Public Health Service, Department of Health, Education and Welfare, 1973.

Bennington, K. Counseling the family of the deafened adult. *Journal of Applied Rehabilitation Counseling,* 1972, *3*(3), 178-187.

Beppler, M. C., & Kroll, M. M. The disabled homemaker: Organizational activities, family participation and rehabilitation success. *Rehabilitation Literature,* 1974, *35,* 200-206.

Christopherson, V. A. The patient and the family. *Rehabilitation Literature,* 1962, *23*(2), 34-41.

Connor, G., & Muldoon, J. A statement of the needs of blind and visually handicapped individuals. *New Outlook for the Blind,* 1973, *67*(10), 352-362.

Erba, G. Rehabilitation counseling considerations in end stage renal disease. *Journal of Applied Rehabilitation Counseling,* 1972, *3*(2), 25-36.

Fordyce, W. Behavioral methods in rehabilitation. In W. Neff (Ed.), *Rehabilitation psychology,* pp. 74-108. Washington, D.C.: American Psychological Association, 1971.

Freeman, H. E., & Simmons, O. G. *The mental patient comes home.* New York: John Wiley & Sons, 1963.

Freeman, R., Malkin, S., & Hastings, J. O. Psychosocial problems of deaf children and their families: A comparative study. *American Annals of the Deaf,* 1975, *120*(4), 391-405.

Froyd, H. E. Counseling families of severely visually handicapped children. *New Outlook for the Blind,* 1973, *67*(6), 251-257.

Galloway, J. P., & Goldstein, H. K. *A follow-up study of the influences of group therapy with relatives on the rehabilitation potential of rehabilitation clients* (Final Report). New Orleans: Delgado Community College, 1971.

Hall, G. C. *Parent's role* (Report). Boston, Mass.: Boston Center for Blind Children, 1974.

Highfill, T. J., & Anderson, R. The social work function in the early help program for preschool handicapped children. *Child Welfare,* 1975, *54*(1), 47-52.

Hurwitz, S. N. *Habilitation of deaf young adults* (Final Report). Vocational Rehabilitation Program for the Deaf in a Comprehension Vocational Facility. St. Louis: Jewish Vocational and Employment Service, 1971.

Irwin, E. C., & McWilliams, B. J. Parents working with parents: The cleft palate program. *Cleft Palate Journal,* 1973, *10*(10), 360-366.

Jarvik, L. S., Salzberger, R. M., & Falck, A. Deaf persons of outstanding achievement. In A. B. Cobb (Ed.), *Special problems in rehabilitation,* Chapter 8. Springfield, Ill.: Charles C Thomas Publisher, 1974.

Klausner, S. J. *Disabled families: A study of the link between the social contributions of the disabled and the retardation of their rehabilitation in the family context.* Philadelphia: Philadelphia Center for Research on the Act of Man, 1969.

Krause, E. Dependency for the blind: Family vs. therapeutic work setting. *New Outlook for the Blind,* 1962, *56,* 353-357.

Lairy, E. C., & Harrison-Covello, A. The blind child and his parents: Congenital visual defect and repercussions of family attitudes on the early development of the child. *American Foundation for the Blind Research Bulletin,* 1973, January.

McCoy, V. Major current trends: Rehabilitation and education of the deaf and hard of hearing. *Rehabilitation Literature,* 1975, *36*(4), 102-107.

McPhee, W. M., & Magleby, F. L. Success and failure in vocational rehabilitation. *Personnel and Guidance Journal,* 1969, *38*(2), 497-499.

Muthard, J. E., & Salomone, P. R. *The roles and functions of the rehabilitation counselor.* Washington, D.C.: American Rehabilitation Counseling Association, 1969.

Nau, L. Why not family rehabilitation? *Journal of Rehabilitation,* 1973, *39*(3), 14–17.

Neff, W. R. *Success of a rehabilitation program: a follow-up study of the vocational adjustment center.* Monograph 3. Chicago, Ill.: Jewish Vocational Service, 1959.

Neuhaus, E. C. *Behavioral characteristics of rehabilitated mental patients.* Unpublished report. Mineola, N.Y.: The Rehabilitation Institute, 1968.

Olshansky, S. Eleven myths in vocational rehabilitation. *Journal of Applied Rehabilitation Counseling,* 1972, *32*(3), 229–236.

Olshansky, S., & Beach, D. Special report. *Rehabilitation Literature,* 1975, *36*(8), 251–253.

Oradei, D., & Waite, N. Admission conferences for families of stroke patients. *Social Casework,* 1975, *56*(1), 21–26.

Philage, M. L., & Kuna, D. A new family approach to therapy for the learning disabled child. *Journal of Learning Disabilities,* 1975, *8*(10), 22–31.

Regional Rehabilitation Research Institute, University of Florida. *Research applied to policy and practice.* Gainesville, Fl.: *Series A (1),* 1974.

Rosenstock, F., & Kutner, B. Alienations and family crisis. *Sociological Quarterly,* 1967, 395–405.

Rusalem, H. *Delivering rehabilitation services* (Report). National Citizen's Conference on Rehabilitation of the Disabled and Disadvantaged. Washington, D.C.: Department of Health, Education and Welfare, Social and Rehabilitation Services, 1969.

Sandovsky, R. Correlates of motivational indices in rehabilitation settings. In A. B. Cobb (Ed.), *Special problems in rehabilitation.* pp. 348–350, 365. Springfield, Ill.: Charles C Thomas Publisher, 1974.

Satir, V. M. *People making.* Palo Alto, Cal.: Science and Behavior Books, 1972.

Scholl, G. T., Baumann, M. K., & Crissey, M. S. *A study of the vocational success of groups of the visually handicapped* (Final report). Ann Arbor, Mich.: University of Michigan, School of Education, 1969.

Scott, E., Debellis, E., & Price, R. Formation of a hard core project. *Journal of Rehabilitation,* 1969, *35*(3), 30–32.

Scott, R. Comments about the interpersonal processes of rehabilitation. In M. Sussman (Ed.), *Sociology and rehabilitation,* pp. 132–138. Washington, D.C.: American Sociological Association, 1965.

Sussman, M., Haug, M. R., & Joynes, V. A. Modern models of rehabilitation counselor roles. *Journal of Applied Rehabilitation Counseling,* 1970, *1*(3), 6–15.

Trela, J. E. *Role of facilities in training rehabilitation personnel.* Cleveland, Oh.: Vocational Guidance and Rehabilitation Services, 1972.

Trela, J., & O'Toole, R. *Social rehabilitation and poverty: Cleveland inner city project.* Cleveland, Oh.: Vocational Guidance and Rehabilitation Center, 1974.

U.S. Department of Health, Education & Welfare, Social and Rehabilitation Service, *Rehabilitation Research and Demonstration Projects, 1955–1970,* Final Reports and Resultant Publications of Projects.

U.S. Department of Health, Education & Welfare, Rehabilitation Services Administration (SRS 73-25038), *New dimensions in training rehabilitation facilities personnel,* Special Report 1972-1.

U.S. Department of Health, Education & Welfare, Rehabilitation Services Administration. *Region IX task force on graduate preparation in rehabilitation counseling,* 1973.

U.S. Department of Health, Education & Welfare, Vocational Rehabilitation Service, Series #67-50. *Training methods in vocational rehabilitation: Fourth institute on rehabilitation services.*

Usdane, W., & Ayers, G. *New dimensions in training rehabilitation facilities personnel.* Conference paper, Third Annual Conference, International Association of Rehabilitation Facilities, Chicago, Ill., 1972.

Wardlow, D. A nine month's drop-out study. Hot Springs Rehabilitation Service. In A. B. Cobb (Ed.), *Special problems in rehabilitation,* pp. 348, 366. Springfield, Ill.: Charles C Thomas Publisher, 1974.

Weiner, H. Characteristics associated with rehabilitation success. *Personnel & Guidance Journal,* 1964, *17*(3), 687–694.

Weisbroth, S., Esibill, N., & Zuger, R. Factors in the vocational success of hemiplegic patients. *Archives of Physical Medicine and Rehabilitation,* 1971, *52,* 441–446.

Wildman, E. S. A program for parents of deaf infants. *Journal of the Tennessee Medical Association,* 1968, *61*(4), 391–394.

ROLE OF THE
FAMILY IN REHABILITATION

Leslie J. Shellhase[1] *and Fern E. Shellhase*[2]

The wisdom of man's needed link to his kin has asserted itself repeatedly throughout the history of the human experience. Within the helping professions, much attention has been directed toward the identification and utilization of the resources of the family for the alleviation of a wide range of problems that may threaten family and individual functioning (Hill, 1965). The experience of the family is the earliest and the most basic of primary group experiences that man can have. Experiences within that group have much to do with the developing capability of its younger members. The adult members of a family turn to that group for reassurance of identity, self-worth, and even purpose of life. Many of the corrective experiences that humans undergo to extend their capabilities now occur as the family is named as the basic unit to be treated.

In this article the role of the family is considered in relation to one of its members in response to the tragedy of physical disability. In earlier times, the family was seldom assigned a significant role in the treatment of the physically disabled because of the high mortality rate that resulted from many disabling traumatic events (Mechanic, 1965). Because of recent medical advancements, the longevity of the disabled has been extended. This change means that a great number of the physically disabled survive and return to their families after spending a period of time in a specialized rehabilitation center. This higher recovery rate creates the realistic requirement that a life for the disabled patient must be planned for in an environment removed geographically and by purpose from the treatment facility. In most instances the home to which the patient goes is where he was a member prior to his injury. This likelihood creates both the opportunity and the necessity for initiating work with the patient and his family almost at the instant of admission of the patient to the rehabilitation center.

This work with the family is essential if the family is to retain a close engagement to the disabled member. There are many aspects of the process

Reprinted from *Social Casework*, November, pp. 544–550, © 1972, Family Service Association of America, with permission.

This article is based on a paper presented at the Annual Forum of the National Conference on Social Welfare, Dallas, TX, May 17, 1971.

[1]Professor, School of Social Work, University of Alabama, Tuscaloosa.

[2]Statistician, Partlow State School and Hospital, Alabama Department of Mental Health/ Division of Mental Retardation, Tuscaloosa.

of accommodation to disability that must be carried out by the individual patient. He must adjust his self-concept and his personal goals to include the realistic limits imposed by his disability. He must develop new capabilities which depend upon the personal resources that he still possesses following the disabling event.

The patient does not carry out his adaptive process in solitude. Within the treatment setting he acquires a number of working colleagues, including both staff and fellow patients. In addition to working with others in the treatment setting, it is essential that the patient continue to maintain an active membership in his family. He must have the engaged commitments of his family in his own rehabilitative career if the gains he makes through this process are to have real and lasting meaning.

NO PREPARATION FOR CATASTROPHE

The family member who becomes the patient in the rehabilitation process comes to that position with minimal role preparation. Even the customary notions of life as a continuum of health interspersed with episodes of illness do not fit the circumstances of the rehabilitation patient. The route to disability is one for which there are few omens. Disability is most frequently the result of traumatic experience which assuredly had not been sought and for which there had usually been little forewarning. The traumatic event constitutes a break in the experiential thread of the patient's life. The ability of the individual to order and reorder his life and, to a considerable extent, his social environment becomes greatly limited.

At the onset of disability, the changed life circumstances of the rehabilitation patient may approximate, in their demands and constrictions, those of a wider range of illnesses that are more time-limited and transitory in their demands upon the individual. The sick role has been well described for some time (Parsons, 1964; Mechanic, 1965). The idea that the ill person will accept a dependent position within the social structure of the treatment situation has depended upon the promise to the patient that he would thereby be delivered back to health and from the continuing necessity of maintaining himself in the sick role. For the patient with a disability, there are the changed circumstances that do not promise any such payoff. Restoration of former functioning is seldom a realistic goal. Indeed, much of the initial exchange between the patient and those treating him consists of study and determination of what should be realistic expectations regarding the future experience and capabilities of the patient.

It is understandable that at the outset of this venture the patient occupies a position at some distance from that of his therapists. The patient, recently beset by catastrophic disability, relies primarily on his earlier orientation to health and illness. He sees only the healthy state as equilibrium and

anticipates its return through the workings of the natural process (Zborowski, 1969). In contrast, those treating him are oriented to the reality that the
disabling condition represents a pivotal event in the patient's life and that
his potentials are now recast in light of his present condition. This situation
between the patient and his therapists contains many elements of conflict.
The resistance of the patient to this new reality is often so strong that
lengthy time and endeavor are required by those treating him to bring about
a reorientation in the patient. It is at least this early in treatment that the
wisdom of treating the family unit asserts itself. Disability has fate-altering
potentials for families as much as for individuals.

ACCEPTANCE OF REALITY

Anyone who survives a disabling experience can scarcely regard its effects as
other than humbling. Disability, by its nature, takes away from the abilities
of an individual (Meyers, 1965). In a therapeutic sense, however, it is cen-
trally diminishing in its effects. The accommodation to disability is an
essential early part of the rehabilitation process. Within that frame, acceptance of disability is not a defeating experience; rather, it leads to a new
realization and assessment of oneself from which the rest of one's life is
planned. The fact that this positive construction is held by the treatment
staff does not ease the experience of personal accommodation by each
patient.

Reality in this situation is indeed harsh, and its comprehension does
not necessarily bring acceptance by the individual that his life now exists
with greatly redefined parameters. The process by which the disabled person accepts this new definition is analogous in some ways to a process of
religious conversion. However, in contrast to the religious experience in
which the individual voluntarily renounces his old self in favor of a newly
defined self, in the disabling experience the individual is stripped of his
former potentials without any deliberate efforts on his own part. Unlike the
religious conversion in which the individual is drawn to the promise and
uplift of the new self that is offered him, the disabled person has not sought
this new role. He is, rather, disabled from the maintenance of his former
role and functions without having acquired any new capabilities. Viewed in
this light, the newly disabled individual is in a life circumstance more nearly
analogous to that of the newly incarcerated convict or the newly institutionalized mental patient (Goffman, 1957).

In common with the convict and mental patient, the disabled patient
finds himself abruptly in an environment that has little relation to the one
within which he had been before. In each of these circumstances, the individual is characterized by the relative powerlessness that he possesses. The
circumstances that brought him to the new situation—sentencing for the

convict, commitment for the mental patient, and usually traumatic injury for the disabled patient—have tended to strip the individual of identity and capability.

The process of mortification that occurs upon entry to a total institution is less severe than the redefinition of self and function that occurs following traumatic catastrophe (Kriegel, 1969). The imprisoned convict retains a potential for influencing his environment which is recognized by his "keepers." The potential of the mental patient in the past has been dealt with for its demonic and disruptive qualities and, more recently, has been managed for its therapeutic contribution (Shellhase, 1961). By comparison, the disabled patient has a greatly limited potential for influencing his environment. Often, the patient arrives at the rehabilitation center so quickly following the traumatic event that he does not yet fully accept the reality of his loss. He is still oriented to the life situation which has been ended by his disability. Seldom will he have comprehended the enormous changes that are being forced upon him. Both the patient and his family are often still numbed from the disabling event and have not yet begun to take stock of the full meaning to them of the disability (Duff & Hollingshead, 1968).

ROLE OF REHABILITATION STAFF

Within the rehabilitation setting there are various people who initiate the reorienting process within the patient and his family. Most important are the staff who have a specialized knowledge of disability and are trained to understand and respond to it. Their authority within the rehabilitation situation is derived from their status as staff of the rehabilitation treatment center. Their staff status, in turn, is derived from their identity as professionals and paraprofessionals within the relevant helping disciplines in the setting. These people carry the value system of rehabilitation. It is the staff who define the environment of the rehabilitation setting, provide continuity within the setting, and transmit the culture of rehabilitation (Duff & Hollingshead, 1968). The complex of relationships and transactions among the treatment staff which is necessary for the development and maintenance of this culture will not be elaborated upon in this article, although the authors recognize that these endeavors affect the experience of the individual patient in rehabilitation.

There is a cumulative culture in every rehabilitation setting, and it does contribute to the social environment of the patient. Evidence of this culture is to be found within the treatment plans for each patient. These plans respond to the perceived need of the patient and are constructed from the rehabilitative resources and intentions of the treatment setting. To a considerable extent the patient's experiences with the treatment staff provide him with a mirrored portrayal of his new identity. In the absence of accustomed physical function, he looks to the staff to define and predict the realistic alternatives.

ROLE OF FELLOW PATIENTS

If the treatment staff provides a mirror by which the patient can view himself, a second set of people—the patients—provides a lens through which he looks at his current surroundings. They share with the newly arrived patient the distinction of being the reason for the work endeavors of the staff. If it is the staff who carry the continuity of the rehabilitation environment, it is the patients who assume the task of interpreting the environment and its demands to the newly disabled patient. The attitudes and values of his fellow patients are usually not so different from those of the new patient himself (Glaser, 1963). The long days of hospital living provide much opportunity for the sharing of knowledge and impressions with fellow patients. If there is a treatment culture, there is also a patient culture which is created from the recurrence of common experience and reaction to the therapeutic endeavors. It is by access to this body of knowledge that the patient learns from more than his own experiences. He draws from it his own determination of how he will enter into the treatment transaction.

The only reasonable role objective of the patient is that of becoming a patient with whatever benefits that may eventually provide him. Clearly, the objective of the disabled patient is to progress out of the treatment setting and get back to the life which had provided him with a system of satisfactions. There are no conclusive studies on this matter; however, there is recurring evidence to suggest that an element in successful rehabilitation is the maintenance by the individual of a central identity which is located outside the rehabilitation setting and which does not become untenable because of the limiting demands of the disabling condition. It is, perhaps, such an individual who can best adjust within the rehabilitation experience and gain the most from it. It is the patient who can view the rehabilitation experience as a time-limited one linking his past life to the promise of a future life who can best assess the relatedness of this experience to his own personal goals. The contribution made to this experience by the continuing relationship that the patient has with his family is obvious. His dependence upon his family assumes new and more extensive proportions as they constitute his major link to a world larger than the treatment setting.

It is the premise of this article that such an orientation of patient to family does not exist solely by chance and that it can be influenced both positively and negatively by the individual's career within the rehabilitation setting. If such a relationship exists, there is a necessity for the management of the rehabilitation experience and the social environment of the patient within both the treatment setting and his broader experiences, especially in his relationships with the other members of his family. To accomplish this goal, the rehabilitation staff and, by extension, the patient himself must attend to what goes on within the total life of the patient; this care must be taken in regard to his progress through the physical aspects of rehabilitation as well as in regard to the social, emotional, and fate-determining elements of his current and future life experiences.

This act requires an early and continuing engagement by the family in the rehabilitation experience. The break in the continuing thread of the patient's experience brought on by the traumatic and disabling event occurs not only to the patient but also to his family. For the patient, accommodation to this change is forced upon him by the unrelenting reality of his disability. It may mark its insistence through reduction or absence of physical function. It may manifest itself through persistent pain and discomfort. The helplessness of the patient to move beyond or to ignore this set of circumstances provides him no option but acceptance. This acceptance in itself is a difficult and pain-filled task. An even greater task confronting the patient is his acceptance of the reality of the uncertain potential of rehabilitation (Bloom, 1965).

The progress of the patient can be assessed with some accuracy in regard to his acceptance of disability and his engagement in the rehabilitation process. The experience of each individual patient is unique, but there are sufficient common elements and occurrences for the observant helping person to perceive and place in some order. If there is a means of systematizing the experience of the disabled patient, this process provides for the organizing of knowledge which is generated from such experience and the utilization of that knowledge in the preparation of additional helpers in the rehabilitation process. It is suggested by the authors that the effect of disability upon the total family and the effect and contribution of the family to the rehabilitation process can also be systematized and transmitted.

FAMILY REACTION TO TRAUMA

Just as the traumatic event is usually instantaneous and unheralded for the individual patient, the family also is ill-prepared for the traumatic event and its consequences. Many of the same defensive measures made by the patient himself are made by the family. Just as the patient goes through a process of denial in which he tries to wish away the reality of his disability, so his family also goes through a period of emotional turbulence.

A family may regard the tragic disabling event as of divine ordination and seek to determine and act upon its portent for the family members. For example, parents may regard the traumatic injury of a child as the consequence of some shortcomings on their part. Because parents do participate extensively in determining the child's environment and experience, there may be some realistic base to this concern. If the child was injured on a motorcycle that the parent provided or if the child was injured by a firearm negligently left loaded, the burden of guilt felt by the parent may be extremely heavy. It is highly unproductive to the family's needs for one of its members to be so immobilized by guilt that the necessary functioning of the family is impaired or threatened.

One helpful response by the treatment staff is to provide the opportunity for parents to share with other parents their concerns and the resolutions that they have made to their own reaction to the disabling tragedy. There is a demonstrable gain to the parent who can provide support to another during the stressful time that both are coming to a workable acceptance of their children's disability.

The impact upon family shows itself in several fashions. The disruptive effect of the event is usually manifold. The economic impact involves heavy demand upon the family's financial resources. The high costs of medical care can be aggravated through the loss of earning power, if the patient had been the breadwinner; the priority of family objectives, which had appeared reasonable and attainable prior to the accident, may need to be altered. The reorganizing of family objectives often results in considerable change in role and function of a number of family members. If a housewife must assume the role of breadwinner and manager of the family household, these new duties may place her and all family members in situations of adaptive stress. The objectives of the family may have to be revised substantially.

The change in role and function among family members is not limited to the income-producing activities of the members of the family, even though such activities are both important and highly visible. In addition, the full range of activities and transactions which contribute to the maintenance of the family as a group undergoes extensive change. Established patterns of decision-making activities are no longer workable if they had depended upon the able-bodied presence and participation of the now-disabled member. In addition to the earlier purposes of the family—the nurture and rearing of children, the providing of an emotional and psychic base for all members, and the maintenance of ego-supporting and satisfying activities—the family is now required to devise and implement an accommodation to the reality of the disability within the family group.

The authors suggest that most families are able to carry out such adaptive endeavors with a minimum of external intervention. Instances of total and unremitting denial and rejection by the family of the disabled member and his needs, while not rare, are infrequent. The methods of response by the professional to situations of pathological disengagement by the family are becoming increasingly refined. At the same time, the accuracy of prognostic evaluation of such endeavors is also probably on the increase. In most instances of working with the family of disabled patients, the central task is not the identification and eradication of pathological processes within the family. The task involves more assisting the family toward an understanding and acceptance of the realities of the patient's disability. The work of the family is to accommodate itself to the permanence of the disabling condition and to reallocate both the sentiment and substance of family resources to maintain the family intact through such experience; at the same time, it must participate in and support all rehabilitative endeavors to maximize the gains that the patient makes toward the highest possible level of functioning as a member of the family and as participant in the larger world.

Although it is essential that the family continue to maintain a sense of membership for the disabled person, it is imperative that the family regroup itself, its resources, and its functions in such a way as to continue their existence as a unit. Survival of the family is crucial. The threat to the family of the presence of a severely disabled member, especially if he had been a stalwart in the family, may be strong enough to lead to the disintegration of the family unit. This breakdown may occur by the somewhat orderly process of dispatching children to the homes of relatives, purportedly for a time-limited period, or it may occur as a rout with family members abandoning all commitment to the family.

VARIED PROFESSIONAL SUPPORT TO FAMILY

There is no single approach that can always be sufficient to the needs of the disabled person and his family. A comprehensive practice can be developed which provides for the assessment of family strengths and needs in relation to accommodation to the reality of continuing disability in one of the members. Such an assessment is, most likely, a service procedure in existence in most rehabilitation centers. Most frequently, the focus of such an assessment is upon the needs of the patient in the rehabilitative process and upon the availability of resources from the family to meet these needs. Usually there is some endeavor to interpret to the family the nature of ongoing needs of the patient which must be met by the family once the patient has come home. For example, the family may be informed of the kinds of preventive measures they should carry out in order to prevent pressure sores from developing. If the patient is on medication, the family may be instructed in the signs that would indicate untoward response by the patient.

The professional who is concerned about the survival of a patient and his family must concern himself also with the ongoing function of the family. He must move to a ready assessment of the relative strengths and weaknesses of the family. He must look to the family's optimum use of its existing strengths, with attention to the maintenance of an adequate level of both material and personal resources. He must shore up the resolve and capability of the family to continue to handle its own affairs in the face of uncertainty and adversity resulting from the traumatic incident, which may have led to turbulence within the family's personal counsels.

Just as the patient himself must be given support in order that he may endure and, perhaps later, accept the reality of his disability, so also must the family members be provided with a range of supportive services, so that they can move beyond the first awesome response to the traumatic accident to an adaptation to adequate functioning which utilizes modes of support that are new to them. In these endeavors the professional takes as a central orientation the overall functioning of the family as a unit. At the same time he must keep in balance his concern about the patient. If a family's comprehension of the condition and needs of the patient is shown by their placement of the patient in a back bedroom with minimal attention from the family, there is obvious need for further attention to this family. At another extreme of response, if the needs of the patient become expressed by him as demands and the family subordinates its own needs in slavish attention to the patient, there is equally compelling need for external intervention to achieve a better balance within the family. It is of utmost importance that the professional allow time for acceptance by the family members, who at the outset of agency contact may be almost as immobilized by the threat of the disability to the future family as is the victim himself.

These endeavors with the family of the disabled patient should be initiated early in the rehabilitative process. The concerns with keeping the family current should go far beyond the professional's familiarity with the patient's course of treatment. A process of helping the family to accommodate to the reality and complex demands of the disability upon the family as a unit should be undertaken early.

Among the techniques to be used in the helping process are those which move a family toward more sensitive and insightful use of the relationships that exist within every family. The stress that disability places upon the family does not always call forth the highest and most effective level of functioning. The family may need help in assessing its effectiveness and in examining its goals in order to determine whose needs are being met and whose are neglected. The techniques of family therapy, developed largely in response to behavioral problems, have applicability to work with the families of disabled patients.

Throughout the endeavors to create a positive and working engagement by family members in the future of the severely disabled member, one must remember that the sick member is not in a static condition. He is engaged in a complex process of rehabilitative services. The goal of these services is to return the patient to his family prepared for the maximum resumption of his role within the family.

In summary, it is through the early and continuing attention to the family as a unit during the rehabilitation experience that the patient is never far removed from them, affectively and interactionally. In this way the trip home is never a long one.

REFERENCES

Bloom, S. W. Rehabilitation as an interpersonal process. In M. B. Sussman (Ed.), *Sociology and rehabilitation,* pp. 114-131. Washington, D.C.: American Sociological Association, 1965.

Duff, R. S., & Hollingshead, A. B. Sickness and society, pp. 89-103. New York: Harper & Row Publishers, 1968.

Glaser, W. A. American and foreign hospitals: Some sociological comparisons. In E. Freidson (Ed.), *The hospital in modern society,* pp. 63-66. New York: The Free Press, 1963.

Goffman, E. Characteristics of total institutions. In *Symposium on preventive and social psychiatry,* pp. 43-84. Washington, D.C.: Walter Reed Army Institute of Research, 1957.

Hill, R. The American family today. In A. H. Katz & J. S. Felton (Eds.), *Health and the community,* pp. 127-140. New York: The Free Press, 1965.

Kriegel, L. Uncle Tom and Tiny Tim: Some reflections on the cripple as Negro. *The American Scholar,* 1969, *38,* 412-430.

Mechanic, D. *Medical sociology,* pp. 61-63. New York: The Free Press, 1965.

Meyers, J. K. Consequences and prognoses of disability. In M. B. Sussman (Ed.), *Sociology and rehabilitation,* pp. 35-51. Washington, D.C.: American Sociological Association, 1965.

Parsons, T. *The social system,* pp. 436-447. New York: The Free Press, 1964.

Shellhase, L. J. The group life of the schizophrenic patient, pp. 1-11, 144-155. Washington, D.C.: Catholic University Press, 1961.

Zborowski, M. *People in pain,* pp. 67-72, 110-121, 168-170, 201-213. San Francisco: Jossey-Bass, 1969.

PERSONAL STATEMENT . . . . . .
Lois

T'was the eve of the new year I came on the
scene
My father was ecstatic, my mother serene.

Was a healthy happy baby, my family I adored
When a so-called catastrophy struck when I was
four.

We went to Dr. Harrington who sent us to the
city
Mom's suspicions then were verified as they
said with pity:

"Cut out all the sweet things, start a routine
quite athletic.
Though she's just a little girl she must be
energetic."

From dancing school and skating, then hikes
and jumping rope
We soon hit on a schedule full of promise and
good hope.

Blessed with wonderful parents and big
brothers too
And growing up in a neighborhood with many
friends so true.

My school years have really been fine with
nary a hitch
Instead of a so-called catastrophy, I'm a happy
diabetic.

> (Lois, written in eighth grade)

Diabetes in its basic form—a lack of sufficient
production of insulin by the body, requiring
control by diet, exercise, and the addition of artificial insulin—has been a minor disease with
which to be afflicted since childhood. As my
autobiographic poem implies, I enjoyed what I
considered a normal, happy childhood, with
plenty of exercise and only minor frustrations
due to diet and daily insulin shots. My parents

treated me as normal and equal to my brothers
and friends, allowing me to accept my disease
as but a small individuality in my life. Mother
was, by nature, a mom who enjoyed playing
with her children and all the entourage of
neighborhood children, so her watchful eye on
my needs was essentially undetected. Because of
good parent interaction in a neighborhood of 5
to 10 girlfriends, my diet needs were known to
my friends' moms, and when I came to visit, or
overnight, diet remained intact. My thanks goes
to all involved in continuing my sense of normalcy.

As the years went on, I learned the limits
and exchanges of my diet and what tolerances
good exercise allowed me. Dancing was an almost daily endeavor of 2 to 4 hours, while other
sports were added in season. Yet, above the
exercise, there was music—piano, voice, violin,
and every school singing group I could join.
School grades remained high, in upper level
classes, which I worked to maintain, but enjoyed too.

I was accepted at the college of my choice in
the fall of my senior year. I had selected a small
girl's college in northern New England which
promised a good opportunity to live away from
home and pursue my teaching/psychology degree. Having spent three summers at a "regular" camp with no difficulties in diet, I was
unprepared for the dietary and lack of exercise
problems that surfaced in college during the
first semester. After completing the semester
and winding up in the hospital with a carbun-
cle, the doctor suggested I not remain in a dorm
setting with cafeteria food because of the inability of the school to provide me a proper diet.
Happily, I was able to shift to an equally good
college closer to home, where I could commute
to school. Here I remained for the completion of
my 4-year degree.

In retrospect I wish I had felt more prepared to cook my own food and had been able to

room with another one or two persons in an
apartment or room with kitchen privileges. In
that way I could have perhaps continued the living away from home during my college years. I
also needed to find more sources of exercise,
which I believe could have been found with
more time up there. With the dayhop commuting to the college nearer home, valuable time for
exercise was spent in travel.

With the completion of my psych/ed degree,
I started elementary teaching about an hour's
ride from home. I lived away from home in a
room with kitchen privileges as did two other
girls. Diabetically I did very well on my own
diet, but still missed the formal exercise I had
enjoyed in youth.

In 1967 I was married and moved to another state where my husband was completing
his Ph.D. There I taught for 2 more years, and
maintained moderately good exercise and diet
control.

We then returned to our home state, took
up residence about an hour from home, where I
again taught. During the second year, January
1971, I began to have eye hemorrhages in rapid
succession, which threatened to destroy all my
sight. It was diagnosed as diabetic retinopathy.
Thanks to intensive laser beam therapy, and
many changes in life-style, I maintained usable
sight of my right eye. It was necessary to stop
driving a car, limit my exercise to walking (with
a companion), and avoid lifting anything in excess of 5 pounds or bend or strain muscles (particularly abdominal). Pregnancy or small
adopted children were ruled out, if I wished to
try to save my remaining sight.

Within 6 months, at the end of the school
year which I taught, the hemorrhaging stopped
and my sight became somewhat stable. At my
husband's insistence, we moved into my
parent's home, because he felt that I could not
do all the housework required in our apartment. Within the next year my husband left.

After a few months, I registered myself with the State Rehabilitation Commission which helped me find a job as a receptionist in a nearby town. Four months after beginning work, it was found I had developed a rapidly grown cataract, compounded with glaucoma, and was operated upon. My supervisor asked me not to return after the forecast of 6 weeks recovery period.

Later that spring, I began volunteering at a halfway house where I taught guitar—a skill I had developed since losing my sight in 1971. I also bought a Siberian husky pup, which was trained by me in obedience classes, to be my constant companion in case my sight should become worse, and for greater mobility (guiding me in walking). She remains my special dog. Although her basic obedience does not qualify her as a guide dog, she is my companion dog.

The summer of 1973 was a very depressed period for me. I felt I was a leech on my parents, as I had no job and required driving to so many places. My diabetes was more erratic due to lack of sufficient exercise, diet, and (a factor I had no realization was a diabetic complicator) emotional turmoil.

I struggled and finally turned the corner by deciding to begin again. I filed for divorce after the 14 months of separation, and began considering returning to school. My sight remained stable with only one usable eye (since the cataract surgery). The diabetes continued to be ruled by emotions and still too little diet adjustment for my limited exercise (walking about 1 mile a day).

Late that summer an old school friend stopped by to see my parents, found me walking with the dog, and an old flame bloomed. He was only home for a week to take part in a relative's wedding, but he was my inspiration as he encouraged me back to my old happy self. We continued to write during the following year as I trained my dog and went to college for master's

level courses, and when we again met the test of
time seemed to be pulling us closer and closer
despite all my reservations.

During the spring of 1974 I asked for mobility training from the State Commission for
the Blind, after I had experienced a scare while
walking with my dog at heel from a sidewalk
curbing into the street, to hear a screech of
wheels at my blind side. Although I had stopped
and looked and listened, I had not distinguished
this car, and my dog merely obeyed my com-
mand to "heel." With the commission's help, I
was acquainted with the white cane and its use.
I also acquired financial aid from them so that I
was able to register in the fall of 1975 as a full-
time student. Through this training I grew tremendously, regaining lost confidences and
more, in a new field to which I could clearly
relate. Being driven to and from the school required my parents' help and my boyfriend's until, in December, my dad went into the hospital
for lung cancer surgery and, in February, my
boyfriend's business required him to leave the
area. I was able to continue school with my
mother's driving until dad was again able to
help out. I remained in close touch with my
boyfriend and, in fact, one week after graduat-
ing from the university, we were married and
moved to his place of business.

There I gained employment and we began to
raise huskies. Diabetically, my eyes remained
stable and diet and exercise were moderately
balanced. Emotional upsets continued to trigger
blood sugar jumps but I became more aware of
these as causes and addressed them more
directly.

It was during this period that diabetic
amyotrophy became evident. Away from diabetic specialists its diagnosis was not determined for almost a year, during which time exercise became more restricted due to pain and
weakness of the thighs and pelvic region. This
condition is presently scheduled for full exami-

nation of the extent of the involvement of the problem and I shall be pushing for a physical rehabilitation program which would be safe to pursue. Regrettably, this is an area of diabetic complication in which not much research has been done as yet.

Diabetes in and of its basic form—insufficient insulin production, requiring regulation of diet, exercise, and insulin injections—has not been more than a minor problem for me. It was not until exercise was limited that diet and insulin control became troublesome. Even then it was not until I had a close encounter with frostbite (in part due to diabetic neuropathy) and then battled diabetic retinopathy (which is tenuously holding in a legally blind status) that diabetes became a real worry. Now with diabetic amyotrophy becoming unmasked, the frustrations of divergent diabetic side effects are high. As of yet, no kidney or heart problems have become evident, but one fears that it is only a matter of degenerative time.

So, despite recent strides in the understanding and hopeful curing of diabetes, I regret to say that I remain glum as I have no sense of reprieve from these complications. Feeling that I have maintained moderately good control of my diabetes within stable diabetic tolerances, I am depressed to see myself developing various diabetic complications while a brittle diabetic friend who is 7 years longer a diabetic has had no complications to date.

I don't know what the future holds for me. My sight is holding steady and has been for almost 5 years. The amyotrophy is said to be time limited to 18 to 24 months, but residual loss is not discussed. I do not feel that I need to find a diabetic specialist who will talk openly and listen carefully to me during these tenuous years. I feel I have that relation with my ophthalmologist and hope to do the same diabetically. With the same support and care professionally as I have from my husband and parents, I will be more able to maintain a positive outlook in the future. There are still many things I can do and enjoy such as our dogs, my job, and our friends—that make the losses—sight, mobility, and children—easier to handle. After all, maybe the amyotrophy will recede to a manageable level and the sight will remain as it is, or be improved with the help of research. Then I will be able to live out a practically normal life (as I see it).

Index

use of creative play, 377-378
psychological aspects of chronic illness, 128-147, 208-210
psychological management of, 139-143, 190-191
psychosomatic illness, 74
rejection by parents, 137, 176-177
restricted mobility, 131, 142
school and peer relationships, 141
secondary gains, 236, 335-336
sensory impairment, 131
separation fears, 120-121, 130-131
of short stature, 185
sibling relationships, 135, 138-139
special facilities and programs, 126-127
threat of death, 132
treatment procedures, 182-183
Chronic disabling illness, 14-20
behavioral and emotional responses, 16-17
comprehensive care for, 18-19
coping mechanisms, 15-16
dependency, 17-18
effects on family, 133-139, 152-160
emotional impact in children, 117-127
environment, 15, 18
giving in-giving up complex, 17
goal-oriented approach, 19
holistic view, 14-20
medical model, 18-19
mourning process, 15
personal statement (Joe), 21-23
physician's reactions to, 139
psychological aspects, 128-144
effect of illness, 133
family reactions, 133-139
nature of illness and management, 130-132
premorbid personality and needs, 129-130
specific emotional reactions, 136-139
psychosocial development and, 16, 133
readaptation, 16, 18
responses to, 16-17
sick role, 16
treatment plan, 16

Classification of families, 46, 48-69
literature review, 46, 48-69
systems of, 48-63
developmental family stage, 51-52
family theme or dimension, 55-59
initial problem or diagnosis of identified patient, 52-55
style of adaptation, 49-51
types of marital relationships, 59-63
types of families, 63-66
chaotic, 66
childlike, 66
constricted, 55, 63, 74
impulsive, 65-66
internalized, 64-65
object-focused, 65
Cleft palate, 119, 180
Colitis, ulcerative, 74, 185
Communication skills, 162
family patterns, 70, 327
Community resources, 42, 138, 175
Compensating for disability, 114
Comprehensive care, 18-19, 339-341
Compromise stage, 252-253
Congenital malformations
adaptation of parents to birth of infant, 195-207
attachment to child, 200-201
period of reorganization, 201
personal statement (Karen), 220-223
personal statement (Maria), 27-34
Convulsive disorders, 183-184
Coping mechanisms, 79-80, 94-105
aids to survival, 15-17
by children, 96, 186-188
chronic disabling illness, 15, 158-159
cognitive styles, 97-100, 103
minimization, 97-98
vigilant focusing, 97, 99-100
defensive adaptive maneuvers, 103
denial of implications for future, 15, 187
by families, 146-147, 174-175
role changes, 158-159
by family with leukemic child, 475-488
adaptive coping, 479-481
coping tasks, 477-478
discrepant coping, 484-485
family coping, 478-479

Psychosomatic illness, 72, 74
family therapy and, 331–332
Psychotic families, 54–55
Punishment, illness viewed as, 76

Reactive patterns in families, 161–164
acceptance stage, 163, 528–529
anxiety stage, 162
assimilation stage, 163, 253
Readaptation, 16, 18
Reality, acceptance of, 528–529
Reconciliation, families in crisis, 408
Reconstruction phase of assimiliation, 253
Reestablishment following family crisis, 417–418
"Reflux" stage, 353–354
rehabilitation, 247, 254–255
Rehabilitation
accommodation, 247, 252–253
anxiety stage, 162, 247–251
assessment of family strengths, 533–535
assimilation stage, 163, 247, 253
comprehensive, 163–164
counseling skills needed, 513–515
group model, 425–427
role of counselors, 520–521
disabled patients, 527–528, 531
acceptance of reality, 163, 528–529
personality of, 93
effect of family dynamics, 343–351, 513
phenomenology of disability, 344–350
family approach, 242–256
family assessment, 244–245
patient adaptation, 247
stages, 246–255
family influences on, 321–351, 513–520
family reaction to trauma, 531–533
changes in role and function, 532–533
government programs, 513–514
impact of family involvement, 161, 164, 513–515
intervention goals, 44, 321–323
communication, 322
competencies, 322

flexibility, 322
normalization of family relations, 322–323
involvement of professionals, 348–350, 520–521, 529–530
programs that include families, 518–520
reflux stage, 247, 254–255
role of family, 331–342, 518–520, 526–535
role of fellow patients, 530–531
role of staff, 520–521, 529–530
spinal cord injured, 242–256
support groups, 514–517, 533–535
Religious beliefs, 162, 175
effect on reaction to disability, 45, 87
Renal disease, 184–185
effects on family, 157
Research needs, 82, 215–217
Resignation, 252
Resistance, techniques of, 15
Resource persons, 359–360
Responsibility and power
families with disabled child, 387–390
marital relationships, 60–62
Rheumatoid arthritis, effects on family, 154
Roles
chronic illness and changes in structure, 38, 152–158
complementarity of, 38
definition, 37
of family members, 37, 327
flexibility and marital adjustment, 166–167
for helping professionals, 359–360
of husband and wife, 45, 166–167
importance of role intactness, 77
sick role expectations, 238–239

Sadness, 199–200
adaptation of parents, 199–200
Scapegoating, 54–55, 338–339
Schooling for sick children, 132
Search for meaning, 15–16
family crisis, 414
Secondary gain from illness, 16, 236, 335–336
Self-control, 103